T0175615

Essentials of Global Health

Essentials of Global Health

Edited by
BABULAL SETHIA BSc, MB BS, FRCP, FRCS
Consultant Cardiac Surgeon, Royal Brompton and Harefield NHS Trust
Past-President and Global Health Lead of the Royal Society of Medicine, London, UK

PARVEEN KUMAR DBE, BSc, MD, DM, DEd,
FRCP (L&E), FRCPath, FIAP
Professor of Medicine and Education, Barts and The London School of Medicine and Dentistry, Queen Mary University of London, and Honorary Consultant Physician and Gastroenterologist, Barts Health NHS Trust and Homerton University Hospital NHS Foundation Trust, London UK

Associate Editors
FELICITY KNIGHTS MA (CANTAB), MBBS, MPH
Former Academic Foundation Doctor, Newcastle upon Tyne Hospitals NHS Foundation Trust / Northern Academic Foundation Programme, Newcastle upon Tyne, UK

DANIEL KNIGHTS MA (CANTAB), MBBCHIR, MPH
Former Academic Foundation Doctor, Newcastle upon Tyne Hospitals NHS Foundation Trust / Northern Academic Foundation Programme, Newcastle upon Tyne, UK

Foreword Writers
SALLY C DAVIES DBE, FRS, FMedSci
Chief Medical Officer for England, UK.

MICHAEL MARMOT MBBS, MPH, PhD, FRCP, FFPHM, FMedSci
Director of the International Institute for Society and Health. MRC Research Professor of Epidemiology and Public Health, University College, London, UK

ELSEVIER

ELSEVIER

Notices

Knowledge and best practice in this field are constantly changing. As new research and experience broaden our understanding, changes in research methods, professional practices, or medical treatment may become necessary.

Practitioners and researchers must always rely on their own experience and knowledge in evaluating and using any information, methods, compounds, or experiments described herein. In using such information or methods they should be mindful of their own safety and the safety of others, including parties for whom they have a professional responsibility.

With respect to any drug or pharmaceutical products identified, readers are advised to check the most current information provided (i) on procedures featured or (ii) by the manufacturer of each product to be administered, to verify the recommended dose or formula, the method and duration of administration, and contraindications. It is the responsibility of practitioners, relying on their own experience and knowledge of their patients, to make diagnoses, to determine dosages and the best treatment for each individual patient, and to take all appropriate safety precautions.

To the fullest extent of the law, neither the Publisher nor the authors, contributors, or editors, assume any liability for any injury and/or damage to persons or property as a matter of products liability, negligence or otherwise, or from any use or operation of any methods, products, instructions, or ideas contained in the material herein.

Every effort has been made to contact everyone across the world who was involved in helping create this book. If you note any omissions please inform the publisher so that we can rectify those at reprint.

ISBN: 978-0-7020-6607-8

Printed in Poland

Last digit is the print number: 9   8   7   6   5   4   3   2   1

Content Strategist: Pauline Graham
Content Development Specialists: Ailsa Laing, Louise Cook
Content Coordinator: Susan Jansons
Project Manager: Anne Collett
Design: Miles Hitchen
Illustration Manager: Karen Giacomucci
Marketing Manager: Deborah Watkins

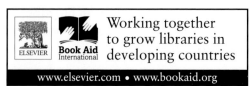

CONTENTS

FOREWORD BY PROFESSOR DAME SALLY C DAVIES

Essentials of Global Health is a unique book resulting from the collaboration of more than 127 medical students and recently qualified doctors from around the world. The varied viewpoints of its authors give the book a unique perspective on the current global health agenda.

This is reflected in the diversity of topic areas that the book examines. They include health economics, health systems and policy, climate change, and many other challenges not often included within undergraduate medical school curricula.

Most of the case scenarios in the book are based upon personal student experiences and give practical insights into health challenges faced by local communities.

Global health has always, and will always, be complex given the multiple interlocking factors which impact upon all our lives. This is recognised in the United Nations Sustainable Development Goals (SDGs), the set of targets running to 2030 covering a huge range of social and economic policy. The SDGs recognise that those who want to solve one of the world's problems must be aware of the rest, and as a global community we must pull together to create sustainable change.

It is therefore imperative that all who engage in the provision of healthcare understand the variety of interconnected challenges within the global health agenda.

Essentials of Global Health offers a timely insight into the issues facing the current, as well as future, generations. I recommend it highly.

There are three reasons why people devoted to global health should be concerned with industry. First, industry produces things that can improve or damage health: food, pharmaceutical products, tobacco, alcohol, as well as housing, infrastructure and motor vehicles. Second, industry employs people. The nature of employment and working conditions can be good for health or bad. Third, industry has environmental and social impact which, in turn, can be health-damaging or health-enhancing. Then, of course, there is trade, which can be a force for good or evil, depending on the set of trading arrangements. All of that is in this book on global health.

Surveys in the US and Europe show that people's perceptions of the major threats to the world are inequality and climate change. Most things that are of such importance in society are likely to affect health and the distribution of health. And, if they affect health, they will have an impact on global health. All of that is in this book on global health.

When, as chair of the WHO Commission on Social Determinants of Health, I called for global action, I said we needed a social movement. Others pointed out that taking an explicit human-rights' approach is a way to advance the cause of health equity. Still others talked of using the law. Some focused, less theoretically, on international institutions and other mechanisms to achieve progress on health equity. Discussions of all of these are in this book on global health.

I emphasise social determinants of health – the conditions in which people are born, grow, live, work and age; and inequities in power, money and resources (Monnat, 2017). Others from the health sector look to universal health coverage and disease control. All of these are in this book.

In addition to the content of the book, which will be illuminating to anyone – student or practitioner – concerned with global health, there is something else that shines through. This work of deep and comprehensive scholarship and advice was put together by students and young doctors (with the brilliant guidance of two experienced senior editors).

One of the most exciting professional moments of my life was when the International Federation of Medical Student Associations (IFMSA) invited me to address their meeting in Copenhagen. The level of enthusiasm in the room was palpable. At the end of our encounter I said, and have repeated to student groups many times, that this gathering gives me hope, optimism, faith. If the future of global health depends on the enthusiasm, commitment, knowledge and belief in social justice of these young people then we are in good hands indeed. That spirit is captured in this book.

Monnat SM: *Deaths of despair and support for Trump in the 2016 presidential election*, Pennsylvania, 2017, PennState.

PREFACE

The concept of this book arose during discussions at the Royal Society of Medicine in London between the editors and members of the Students for Global Health (was Medsin UK). In recent years, there has been a surge in the appreciation of global health challenges amongst young people. The realisation that these challenges are relevant across the world has promoted a demand for information about factors that influence the health and well-being of individuals and populations.

The discussion of global health challenges is often limited in undergraduate curricula. This is not entirely surprising as the concept of global health as an entity is not universally recognised. However, a large body of students appreciate the global interplay of health and illness as well as the need to learn about the factors which impact on effective well-being.

In 1948 The Constitution of the World Health Organisation enshrined '…the highest attainable standard of health as a fundamental right of every human being'. Sadly, achievement of this aspiration has been compromised by political inertia as well as deficiencies in local governance. Current international health care structures have so far failed to effectively address the major inequalities in health although the Sustainable Development Goals hope to achieve significant progress by 2030. It is essential for all who work in the health care environment, including medical students, doctors and allied health care professionals, to recognise and address these problems.

Essentials of Global Health offers an introduction to the major concepts and challenges in health care. This book seeks to be informative and easily digestible. It illustrates the overlapping roles of Society, Politicians, Global Organisations and Health Professionals; the appreciation of these relationships is essential for the delivery of effective health care.

Although it is not a textbook, it is unique in that it brings together contributions from students and young doctors from over 30 countries. The authors of this book present a multicultural vision of global health. After reading their work, we hope that readers will be stimulated to explore and, hopefully, to contribute to the global health agenda in pursuit of health equity for all.

BS
PJK

If you are reading this book, then the chances are you are something like us. You probably read the news and hear about growing crises in our national health systems, and the way we care for our world. You probably own products from several continents, and are not surprised to come into contact with individuals from other countries - as colleagues or friends. You have probably watched the growth of brands like Coca Cola and McDonald's and wondered how they have managed to spread like wildfire across the face of our world.

Growing up in our generation, we recognise the impacts of globalisation, commercialisation, and increasing movement of people and disease. We also know that we will be the ones who will suffer the ill-health consequences of climate change, antibiotic overuse and broken health governance systems. But we are optimistic about our future, believing that we can also be a part of the solution. Young people are already engaging across the spectrum of global health, from advocating at high level summits on sustainable development and climate change, to immersing themselves in resource-poor health systems on student electives. This book contains many of these examples, and we hope they will inspire you as they inspire us. We are no different from you: we had a spark of interest, seized an opportunity and learned as we went along. However, if you are like us, then you will also see that simply learning is not enough. We hope you will join us in stepping beyond learning to taking action, like the young people in these case studies. Whether by setting up or volunteering for a community project, speaking to your council or health service, signing a petition, or collaborating with students in other countries, there is no time like the present.

This is the first book of its kind, written by students and junior professionals for their peers. Our team of contributors numbers 127, from over 30 countries. We believe this has led to a richness and diversity of personal narratives that few books can claim. As we're sure you can imagine, working across cultures in such large numbers has not been easy, requiring careful communication, team-work and patience. However, our team has persevered, and so, our mutual goal, this book, has been realised. If this is a metaphor for the future of global health at large, then we believe there is still hope.

FK and DK (on behalf of the contributors)

Most contributions to this book originally came from medical students across the world who, at the time of writing, had not yet graduated. In the interim, many have graduated and become doctors. Every effort has been made to contact all of you, but if we have missed anyone please let us know.

Salma M. Abdalla, MBBS, MPH
Research Fellow, Boston University, School of Public Health, Boston, USA

Eirliani Abdul Rahman, BA (Hons), MSc
Cofounder and Executive Director YAKIN (Youth, Adult Survivors and Kin in Need) - a not-for-profit, Singapore, Singapore

Ellen Adams, MBChB, BSc
Foundation Year 1 Doctor, Glasgow, UK

Christine Andreasen, MD
Resident, University of Copenhagen, Copenhagen, Denmark

Guendalina Anzolin, MSc
MSc Student/Freelance Journalist, Department of Global Economic Governance and Policy, SOAS, University of London, London, UK

Rev Canon Aston Baker Bagarukayo
Development Studies Centre, Mbarara, Uganda

Hope Bagarukayo
Development Studies Centre, Mbarara, Uganda

Paula Baraitser
Senior Lecturer, King's College London, UK

Laura Bertani, MD
Resident Physician, Ventura County Medical Center, Department of Family Medicine, Ventura, CA, USA

John Jefferson Besa, MD
General Practitioner, College of Medicine, University of the Philippines Manila; Philippine General Hospital, Manila, Philippines

Anand Bhopal, MBChB, BSc (Hons), MA (Dist)
Foundation Year 2 Doctor, Wishaw General Hospital, NHS Lanarkshire, Glasgow, UK

Nicolas Blondel, MBBS, iBSc
Global Public Health, Foundation Doctor, Colchester General Hospital, Colchester, UK

Ragna Boerma, MD, PhD
Junior Doctor, GGZ Ingeest, Department of Psychiatry, Amsterdam, The Netherlands

Isobel Braithwaite, MBBS, BSc, MSc
Junior Doctor, University College London NHS Trust, London, UK

Helena Chapman, MD, PhD, MPH
Research Scientist, University of Florida, Department of Environmental and Global Health, Gainesville, FL, USA

Joseph Cherabie, MD, MSc
Medical Resident, University of Kansas School of Medicine Wichita, Internal Medicine, Wichita, KS, USA

Omar Cherkaoui
IFMSA President 2016/17

Alice Clarke, MA (Cantab), MA (KCL)
Medical Student, University of Bristol, Bristol, UK

Alice Cozens, MBChB, BSc, DRCOG
GP Registrar, Cambridge University Hospital Trust, Cambridge, UK

Amanda Craig, MSc, BA
Auditor, UK

Josephine de Costa, BA/LLB (Hons I), Grad. Dip. Arts (Env. Sci)
Medical Student, School of Medicine, The University of Sydney, Sydney, NSW, Australia

Jessica Dean, MBBS(Hons), BMedSci(Hons), LLB HMO (Hospital Medical Officer)
Faculty of Law and Faculty of Medicine, Nursing and Health Sciences, Monash University Melbourne, VIC, Australia

Marieke Dekker, MD, PhD
Consultant Neurologist, Department of Internal Medicine, Department of Pediatrics and Child Health, Kilimanjaro Christian Medical Centre; Department of Neurology, Radboudumc Nijmegen, Moshi, Kilimanjaro, Tanzania

Roopa Dhatt, MD, MPA, BSc
Dirext, Women in Global Health, Washington DC, USA

Stijntje Dijk, BSc (Medicine)
Medical Student, Erasmus Medical Center, Rotterdam, The Netherlands

Naheed Dosani, MD, CCFP(PC), BSc
Palliative Care Physician, Lecturer, Department of Family and Community Medicine, Division of Palliative Care, University of Toronto; Assistant Clinical Professor, Department of Family Medicine, Division of Palliative Care, McMaster University, Toronto, ON, Canada

Robbert Duvivier, MD, PhD
Senior Lecturer in Medical Education, University of Newcastle, Newcastle, NSW, Australia

Benjamin Ebeling, MD
Doctor Resident, Copenhagen, Denmark

Mennat-Allah Elbeheiry, MBBCh, PMHE
Health Economist, Cairo, Egypt

Ismail El-Kharbotly, MBBCh
Resident of Surgical Oncology, Department of Surgical Oncology, The National Cancer Institute, Cairo University, Cairo, Egypt

Rose Ekitwi
Functional Adult Literary Coordinator, Baptist Union of Uganda, Kampala, Uganda

Germán Ángel Emanuel Escobar
Undergraduate Biology Student, International Student in the Federal University of Minas Gerais (UFMG), "National University of the Northeast, Biology and Life Sciences; National University of the Northeast (Castilian: Universidad Nacional del Nordeste, UNNE) Biology and Life Sciences", Corrientes, Argentina

Maria Espanol, MD
Pediatric Resident Physician, Nassau University Medical Center, New York, NY, USA

Sebastian Fonseca, MD, MA, PhD Candidate
PhD Candidate Global Health and Social Medicine, Department of Global Health and Social Medicine, King's College London, London, UK

Christopher Fourie, MBBCh
Engineering Sciences Student, University of the Witwatersrand (MBBCh), University of Salzburg (current), Johannesburg, South Africa

Molly Fyfe, MPH, PhD
Senior Research Manager, King's Centre for Global Health; Cambridge Assessment Admissions Testing, Cambridge, UK

Pravesh Gadjradj, BSc, MD/PhD Candidate
Department of Neurosurgery, Erasmus MC: University Medical Center, Rotterdam, Leiden University Medical Center, Rotterdam, Netherlands

Sam Gnanapragasam, MBBS
Foundation Year Doctor, GKT School of Medicine, King's College London, London, UK

Anya Gopfert, MBBS, BSc
Senior House Officer, University of Bristol, Bristol, UK

Angeli Guadalupe, MD, MSc
Resident Physician, Department of Pediatrics,
Davao Regional Medical Center, Tagum
City, Philippines

Renzo Guinto, MD
Doctor of Public Health student, Harvard
T.H. Chan School of Public Health,
Boston, MA, USA/Manila, Philippines

Manuel Hache-Marliere, MD
Critical Care Research Fellow, Critical Care
Medicine, CEDIMAT, Santo Domingo,
Dominican Republic

Fadi Halabi, MD
Resident Physician, Washington University in
St Louis, St Louis, MO, USA

Fiona Headley, MBBS, BSc
Foundation Year 1 Doctor, Barts and the
London School of Medicine and Dentistry,
London, UK

Thomas Hindmarch, MA (cantab), MBBS
General Practice Academic Clinical Fellow,
University of East Anglia and Norwich GP
School, Norwich, UK

Charlotte Holm-Hansen, MD
Pediatric Resident, Department of Pediatrics,
Sealand University Hospital, Soro,
Denmark

Johanne Iversen, MD
Resident Anaesthesiology, Sykehuset
Innlandet, avd GjÃ¸vik, Brumunddal,
Norway

Xiaoxiao Jiang
China

Ishita T. Johal, BDS
Dentist, Birmingham, AL, USA

Mubashir Jusabani, MD
Intern, Department of Internal Medicine,
Kilimanjaro Christian Medical Centre,
Moshi, Kilimanjaro, Tanzania

Mike Kalmus Eliasz, MBBS, AKC
Independent Global Health Consultant and
Foundation Year 2 Doctor, Independent
/ Barking, Havering and Redbridge
University Hospitals NHS Trust,
London, UK

Mustapha Kamara, MBBS
Research Assistant, Department of
Epidemiology, University of Florida,
Gainesville, FL, USA

Rockie Kang, MSc MD Candidate
Bart's and the London School of Medicine
and Dentistry, University of London,
London, UK

Maxwell Kaplan, PhD
Dean John A. Knauss Marine Policy Fellow,
Biology Department, Woods Hole
Oceanographic Institution, Woods Hole,
MA, USA

**Elizabeth Kay, BBDS, MPH, PhD, FDSRCPS,
FDSRCS, FFGDP**
Foundation Dean and Faculty Associate
Dean, Peninsula Dental School, University
of Plymouth, Plymouth, UK

Jelte Kelchtermans, MD
Pediatric Resident, Department of Pediatrics,
Jackson Memorial Hospital, Miami,
FL, USA

Wajiha Jurdi Kheir, MD
Resident in Ophthalmology, American
University of Beirut Medical Center,
Department of Ophthalmology, Beirut,
Lebanon

Jesper Kjær, MD
Codirector, Psychiatric Research Academy,
Department of Affective Disorders, Aarhus
University Hospital, Aarhus, Denmark

Felicity Knights, MA(Cantab), MBBS, MPH
Former Academic Foundation Doctor,
Newcastle University, Newcastle upon
Tyne Hospitals NHS Foundation Trust,
Newcastle upon Tyne, UK

Daniel Knights, MA (Cantab), MBBChir, MPH
Former Academic Foundation Doctor,
Newcastle upon Tyne Hospitals NHS
Foundation Trust / Northern Academic
Foundation Programme, Newcastle-Upon-
Tyne, UK

Anne Kobusingye
Persons with Disabilities Development
Organisation Coordinator, Kabale, Uganda

Christian Kraef, MD
Hamburg, Germany

Freya Langham, MBBS, BMedSci(Hons), DTMH
Medical Registrar, Alfred Health, Melbourne,
  Australia

Jae Hyoung Lee, MD
Medic, Republic of Korea Air Force, Seosan,
  Korea

Alexandre Lefebvre, MD
Anesthesiology Resident, Department
  of Anesthesiology, Pharmacology and
  Therapeutics, University of British
  Columbia, Vancouver, BC, Canada

Ana Beatriz Lobato, MD
Family Medicine Resident, Federal District
  Health Department, Brasilia, Brazil

Ljiliana Lukic
Croatia

Ivan Lumu, MBChB, MPH
Senior Medical Officer, Infectious Diseases
  Institute, Makerere College of Health
  Sciences, Kampala, Uganda

Gerald Makuka, MD
General Practitioner, Nyangoto Health
  Centre, Tarime District Council, Nyangoto,
  Tarime, Tanzania

Akansha Mimi Malhotra, MBBS
Foundation Year Doctor, GKT School of
  Medicine, King's College London, London,
  UK

Nazia Malik, MBBS, BSc
Senior House Officer, Centre for Primary
  Care and Public Health, Blizzard Institute,
  Barts and The London School of Medicine
  and Dentistry, London, UK

Altagracia Mares, MD
Department Salud Publica, Universidad
  Autónoma de Nuevo León, Monterrey,
  Mexico

Farhan Mari Isa, MD
Junior Doctor, Department of Medicine,
  Syiah Kuala University, Banda Aceh,
  Indonesia

Timothy Martin, MBBS (Hon), BMedSc (Hon), MPH, DCH
Paediatric Resident, Royal Children's
  Hospital, Melbourne, Australia

Amelia Martin, MB ChB
Foundation Year Doctor, GKT School of
  Medicine, King's College London, London,
  UK

Martha Martin, MBBS
Foundation Year Doctor, GKT School of
  Medicine, King's College, London, UK

Jonathan Meldrum, MBBS, MA (Oxon)
Resident Physician, Department of
  Emergency Medicine, Yale New Haven
  Hospital, New Haven, CT, USA

Arthur Mello, MD
Family Medicine Resident, Federal District
  Health Department, Brasilia, Brazil

Basem Mohamed, MD, MBBCH, MSc
Consultant at the World Health
  Organization, Health Workforce
  Department, Geneva, Switzerland

Baher Mohamed, MBBCH
Doctor, General Practitioner and Masters
  Student, Global Health Institute of
  Geneva, Geneva, Switzerland

Yazan Mousa, MD
Junior Medical Doctor, Nottingham
  University Hospitals NHS Trust,
  Nottingham, UK

Latif Murji, MD
Resident Physician, Department of Family
  and Community Medicine, University of
  Toronto, Toronto, Canada

Meggie Mwoka, MBChB
Doctor (Medical Officer), University of
  Nairobi, Nairobi, Kenya

Jake Newcomb, MD
Resident Physician, NewYork-Presbyterian
  Hospital, New York, NY, USA

Dat Nguyen-Dinh, MD
Resident, University of Montreal, Montreal,
  QC, Canada

Kingsley Njoku, MBBS, MPH (pending)
Doctor of Medicine, Institute of Applied
  Health Research, University of
  Birmingham, Birmingham, UK

Chra Noori-Abdulla, MBChB
Medical Intern, Sydney, Australia

Samuel Ognenis, MBBS
Resident Medical Officer, Fiona Stanley
  Hospital, Perth, WA, Australia

Miriam Orcutt, MBBS, MSc
Medical Doctor and Research Associate,
  Institute for Global Health, University
  College London, London, UK

Martha Paisi, MSc, MMedSci
Post-Doctoral Research Fellow in Public
  Health Dentistry, Peninsula Dental School,
  Plymouth University, Plymouth, UK

Storm Parker, MBBS, BSC Hons
Senior House Officer, Barts and the London
  School of Medicine and Dentistry,
  London, UK

Samantha Pegoraro, MD
Medical Doctor and Freelance Journalist,
  Rome, Italy; Climate Change and
  Health Coordinator, Italian Climate
  Network

Alexandra Peterson, MBBS (Hons)
Foundation Year 1 Doctor, NHS Lothian,
  Edinburgh, UK

Anika Rahim, MBBS, BSc (Hons)
Foundation Year 1 Doctor, Oxford Deanery,
  Oxford, UK

Sakina Rashid
Medical Student, Kilimanjaro Christian
  Medical University College, Moshi,
  Tanzania

Anna Rasmussen, MD, MSc
Health Policy MD, University of
  Copenhagen, Copenhagen, Denmark

Sadie Regmi, MBChB, BSc (Hons)
Registrar and Academic Clinical Fellow,
  Imperial College London, London, UK

Kevouy Reid, MBBS
Medical Intern, The University of the West
  Indies, Mona Campus Faculty of Medical
  Sciences, Kingston, Jamaica

Isaac Rukundo, BSc Educ
Graduate Teacher of Mathematics and
  Physics, Ministry of Education, Science,
  Technology and Sports, Department of
  Education, Kampala, Uganda

Aliye Runyan, MD
Obstetrics and Gynecology Resident, Wayne
  State University, Detroit, MI, USA

Abilash Sathyanarayanan
India

Iza Sanchez-Siller, PhD
Researcher, School of Education, Humanities
  and Social Sciences, Tecnológico de
  Monterrey, Monterrey, Mexico

Sebastian Schmidt, MD
Resident in Psychosomatic Medicine,
  Psychosomatic Medicine and
  Psychotherapy, Schön Klinik Hamburg
  Eilbek, Hamburg, Germany

Vita Sinclair, MBBS, BSc ACCS
Anaesthetic Trainee, South London School of
  Anaesthesia, London, UK

Anjum Sultana, HBSc, MPH
Graduate Student, University of Toronto,
  Toronto, ON, Canada

Shela Putri Sundawa, MD
Pediatric Resident, University of Indonesia/
  Cipto Mangunkusumo Hospital, Jakarta,
  Indonesia

Anna Szczegielniak, MD, MSc
Junior Doctor–Psychiatry Resident and PhD
  Candidate, Department and Clinic of
  Psychiatry and Psychotherapy, Medical
  University of Silesia in Katowice, Poland,
  Katowice, Poland

Avin Taher, MD, MBChB
Kurdistan Region of Iraq, Erbil, Kurdistan,
  Iraq

Yassen Tcholakov, MD MIH
Public Health and Preventive Medicine,
   Faculty of Medicine, Department
   of Epidemiology, Biostatistics and
   Occupational Health, McGill University,
   Montreal, Canada

Kim Patrick Tejano, BSPH, MD
Post-Graduate Intern, College of Medicine,
   University of the City of Manila, Manila,
   Philippines

Charlotte Thomassen-Kinsey, BA (Hons), MSc
Durham University (BA), Leeds Beckett
   (MSc), Leeds, UK

Kelly Thompson, MBBS, MLitt, MPhil, BA
Programming Specialist Women in Global
   Health, Manasquan, NJ, USA

Daniel Tobón-García, MD, MPH(c)
Masters in Public Health Candidate,
   Universidad de los Andes, Bogota D.C.,
   Colombia

Elizabeth Tomlinson
UK

Gabriel Tse
Canada

Eleanor Turner-Moss, BSc (Hons), MBBS, Mphil
Academic Clinical Fellow in Public Health,
   University of Cambridge, Cambridge, UK

Jack Turyahikayo, MBChB, Mmed
Physician, Makerere Palliative Care
   Unit(MPCU), Internal Medicine, Palliative
   Care, Kampala, Uganda

Maria van Hove, MD
Foundation Year 1 Doctor, Worthing
   Hospital, Worthing, UK

Michael Van Niekerk, MBChB
Medical Officer, Khayelitsha District
   Hospital, Cape Town, South Africa

Aaminah Verity, BSc, MBBS, MSc, DTMH
Doctor NHS, London Deanery, London, UK

Waruguru Wanjau, BSc, MBChB
Medical Officer Department of Medicine,
   Samburu, Kenya

Emily Ward, MBBS, BSc
Clinical Leadership Fellow, NHS Education
   for Scotland, Dundee, UK

Alistair Wardrope, MBChB, MPhysPhil
Academic Foundation Doctor, University of
   Sheffield/Sheffield Teaching Hospitals
   NHS Foundation Trust, Sheffield, UK

Nick Watts, MBBS, MA, BSc
Executive Director, Lancet Countdown on
   Health and Climate Change, London, UK

Margot Weggemans, MD
PhD candidate, University Medical Center
   Utrecht, Utrecht, Netherlands

Elizabeth Wiley, MD, JD, MPH
Preventive Medicine Resident, Johns Hopkins
   Bloomberg School of Public Health,
   Baltimore, MD, USA

Kimberly Williams, MD, MSc, BSc
Resident Physician, University of Calgary,
   Calgary, AB, Canada

Felicia Yeung, MBBS
Foundation Year Doctor, GKT School of
   Medicine, King's College London, London,
   UK

Chérine Zaim, MD candidate
Medical Student, Faculty of Medicine,
   University of Montreal, Montreal,
   QC, Canada

ACKNOWLEDGEMENTS

We would like to thank our many colleagues and friends who have helped in the preparation of this book. Our co-editors, Felicity and Dan Knights, were instrumental in coordinating the contributions from all of the section and chapter authors. Their commitment and enthusiasm for this project was outstanding. We were constantly impressed by the quality of the authors' manuscripts, often written by individuals for whom English was not their first language.

We would like to acknowledge and thank the following people for their input during the early stages of the manuscript: Rizkia Chairani Asri, Maria Jose Cisneros Cacares, Ahegl Emanuel, Rael Garcia, Regina Ivanovna, Bethany Jones, Benjamin Skov Kaas-Hansen, Vishal Kumar, Rizki Meizikri, Jules Nkurunzi, Webby Phiri, Trudie E Roberts and Sankhya Saroj.

We would also like to thank the Royal Society of Medicine and the International Federation of Medical Students Association for supporting this project. All funds generated through sales of this book will be used by these two organisations for global health projects.

Pauline Graham, Ailsa Laing, Louise Cook and Anne Collett from Elsevier have guided the project through from start to finish. We are indebted to them for their commitment to this book. We would also like to thank Zoë Mullan (Editor-in-Chief of the open-access journal Lancet Global Health) for her help and insights. It has been a pleasure working with them all.

ABOUT THE EDITORS

Mr B. Sethia
Babulal Sethia studied medicine at St Thomas' Hospital in London, and is currently a Consultant Congenital Heart Surgeon at the Royal Brompton Hospital in London. He is a past-President of the Royal Society of Medicine (RSM).

Throughout his career, he has helped to develop health care initiatives for children with congenital heart disorders in low- and middle-income countries and, since 1992, has participated in the delivery of surgical missions in a number of countries in Africa, Asia, the Middle East and South America.

At the RSM, he worked with Professor Parveen Kumar to develop a global health programme and he continues to promote global health education for the benefit of UK and overseas health care professionals.

Professor Dame Parveen Kumar
Professor Parveen Kumar was born in India and studied medicine at St Bartholomew's Hospital Medical College, London, where she also trained as a gastroenterologist.

She has held many leading roles in under- and postgraduate medical education. She co-founded and co-edited the world-famous textbook *Kumar & Clark's Clinical Medicine*. This has enabled her to teach, lecture and examine in low- and middle-income countries.

She is a past President of the British Medical Association, the Royal Society of Medicine and past Vice-President and Director for International Education of the Royal College of Physicians.

ACER	Average cost-effectiveness ratio
AMR	Antimicrobial resistance
ARV	Antiretroviral
BMA	British Medical Association
BRICS	Brazil, Russia, India, China, South Africa (example of middle-income countries)
CEWG	Consultative Expert Working Group
DALY	Disability-adjusted life year
EML	Essential medicines list
ENAP	Every Newborn Action Plan
EU	European Union
FAO	Food and Agriculture Organization of the United Nations
GAIN	Global Alliance for Improved Nutrition
GATS	General Agreement on Trade of Services
GATT	General Agreement on Tariffs and Trade
GFATM	Global Fund to Fight Aids, Tuberculosis and Malaria
GHWA	Global Health Workforce Alliance
HiAP	Health in all policies
HIPC	Heavily indebted poor countries
HRBA	Human rights-based approach
HSM	Health social movement
ICCPR	International Covenant on Civil and Political Rights
ICER	Incremental cost-effectiveness ratio
ICESCR	International Covenant on Economic, Social and Cultural Rights
ICPD	International Conference on Population and Development
IFAD	International Fund for Agricultural Development
IFMSA	International Federation of Medical Students' Associations
IGO	Intergovernmental organisation
IHP+	International Health Partnership and related initiatives
ILO	International Labour Organization
IPCC	Intergovernmental Panel on Climate Change
JLI	Joint Learning Initiative
KCMC	Kilimanjaro Christian Medical Centre
LGBT	Lesbian, Gay, Bisexual and Transgender
LIC	Low-income country
LMIC	Lower middle-income country
MCH	Maternal and child health
MDG	Millennium Development Goal
NCD	Noncommunicable disease
NGO	Nongovernmental organisation
NHS	National Health Service
NMP	National Medicines Policy
NTD	Neglected Tropical Disease
OAU	Organisation of African Unity
PHC	Primary Health Care
PHM	People's Health Movement

Pre-WHA	Pre-World Health Assembly
PRSP	Poverty Reduction Strategy Papers
PTO	Person trade-off
PTSD	Posttraumatic Stress Disorder
QALY	Quality-adjusted life year
R & D	Research and Development
RCT	Randomised controlled trial
RSM	Royal Society of Medicine
SARD	Sustainable Agriculture and Rural Development
SBA	Skilled birth attendant
SDG	Sustainable Development Goal
SES	Socioeconomic status
SPM	[Agreement on the Application of] Sanitary and Phytosanitary Measures
TB	Tuberculosis
TBA	Traditional birth attendant
TBT	[Agreement on] Technical Barriers to Trade
TRIPS	[Agreement on] Trade-Related Aspects of Intellectual Property Rights
UDHR	Universal Declaration of Human Rights
UHC	Universal Health Coverage
UN DESA	United Nations Department of Economic and Social Affairs
UNAIDS	Joint United Nations Programme on HIV/AIDS
UNDP	United Nations Development Programme
UNESCO	United Nations Educational, Scientific and Cultural Organization
UNFCCC	United Nations Framework Convention on Climate Change
UNFPA	United Nations Population Fund
UNICEF	United Nations Children's Fund
UNIDO	United Nations Industrial Development Organization
UPU	Universal Postal Union
USAID	United States Agency for International Development
WASH	Water, Sanitation and Hygiene
WHA	World Health Assembly
WHO	World Health Organization
WTO	World Trade Organization
YLD	Years Lived with Disability
YLL	Years of Life Lost

What Is Global Health?

Junior Editor: Freya Langham (Australia)

Introduction

The term *global health* is a relatively new concept. The history of global health demonstrates why and how this new concept is relevant to everybody, wherever they live. *Global health* also encompasses the notion of societal health equity and subscribes to the assertion that health for all is a human right (see Chapter 5.1). Many nonhealth factors, including political and financial issues, determine the well-being of a community; these are also integral to the study of global health. The study of global health demands an appreciation of both scientific methodology and the social sciences. As such, it is a challenging and rewarding area for study and endeavour.

1.1 A History of Global Health

Mike Kalmus Eliasz (UK)

Introduction

'Those who do not remember the past are condemned to repeat it.'

George Santayana

Global health as a discipline for academic study emerged as a distinct entity in the 21st century. It evolved from the study of public health, tropical medicine and international health. More recently, the process of globalisation has shaped the economic environment, national health systems and the health of individuals and nations.

The discipline of public health

The health of a population is determined by the physical and social environment. Much of the study of health has focused on efforts to improve the health of individuals. As the academic discipline of public health emerged, the importance of social and environmental factors on people's health began to be appreciated, and epidemiological tools were used to evaluate these factors.

An early example of a clinical trial related to scurvy, a common illness affecting seafarers. For many years nobody could understand why sailors developed bleeding gums and became unwell whilst at sea. In 1762, in one of the first ever randomised clinical trials, James Lind, a Scottish surgeon, decided to try and identify a treatment for the disease. He divided sailors into separate groups, providing each with different therapies, whilst a control group continued with their usual diet. He discovered that supplying citrus fruits (a source of vitamin C) would prevent scurvy. This method of experimental enquiry, the randomised controlled trial (RCT; see Chapter 4.5), remains a gold standard in the evaluation of therapy.

Early epidemiology

In 1854 hundreds of people died during a raging cholera epidemic of unknown aetiology in Soho, London. An inquisitive physician, John Snow, was sceptical about the prevailing theories regarding the causation of cholera. He noted that most affected patients lived near a water pump in Broad Street (**Fig. 1.1.1**), and that when a padlock was placed on this pump, the number of cholera cases was greatly reduced. This discovery showed the connection between cholera and water supplies. It was one of the first documented uses of 'observational and spatial' epidemiology. Today, in the field of global health, we still look for patterns of disease to better understand the underlying causes and thereby identify potential interventions.

The birth of social medicine

In 1848 a German doctor, Rudolf Virchow, was troubled by what he observed in the coalfields of Silesia. He wrote a long treatise on the theory of social medicine which concluded that the

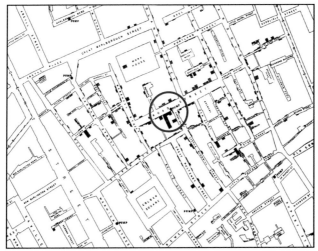

Figure 1.1.1 Original map by John Snow showing the clusters of cholera cases (shown in *black*) in the London epidemic of 1854. The red circle shows the cluster of cases around the pump. Drawn and lithographed by Charles Cheffins. *(Reproduced from Snow J: On the* mode of communication of cholera, *ed 2, London, 1855, John Churchill.)*

greatest determinant of occupational illness was inequality. Much of global health research involves the study of inequality, both local and global. At the peak of the Industrial Revolution, many physicians conflated the ideas of health and well-being with concepts of social justice. The physician Thomas Hodgkin (famous for the discovery of Hodgkin lymphoma) was an early campaigner for public health. At personal detriment, he criticised the Hudson Bay Company for the harm it was causing to the health of Canadian indigenous populations through the supply of alcohol as well as exploitative labour conditions.

Trade versus health—the Opium Wars

The Opium Wars of the 19th century were an early case study of problems posed by the trade of harmful substances which result in conflicting public health and financial imperatives. The lucrative opium trade in Southeast Asia had resulted in widespread drug addiction in China, as a result of which the Chinese administration demanded that British merchants destroy their opium supplies and agree to a 'no opium trade bond'. When the British refused to agree to these demands, a war between the two countries broke out and, following a British victory in this conflict, control of Hong Kong was ceded to Great Britain.

By 1906 approximately 27% of the adult male population in China was regularly using opium.

Today, the forces of trade and globalisation limit potential improvements in health. Legislation restricting the sale of unhealthy products such as alcohol, tobacco and sugar is often opposed by multinational companies (see Chapter 5.2).

Tropical medicine

The movement of people creates exposure to new pathogens and risk behaviours. The discovery of the New World and the Americas by early European settlers exposed local populations to the previously unknown pathogen of smallpox. Malaria and yellow fever killed thousands of European settlers, and control of these and other tropical diseases became an imperative as infections limited the potential for the economic exploitation of newly acquired territories. As a result, new institutions for the study of tropical medicine were established. Today, in the era of jet travel, pathogens have the potential to spread rapidly around the world, and the importance of institutions of tropical health remains undiminished.

Discussion of health on a global stage

The first international negotiations on public health took place in 1851. In response to an ongoing cholera epidemic, the first international sanitary conference was held in Paris to debate how the international community should respond to this public health emergency. Twelve countries participated, each represented by a two-person team of a physician and a diplomat. This conference marked a turning point in the history of global health as it was the first occasion on which pressing health issues were addressed through international cooperation. Later, sanitary conferences throughout the late 19th century and early 20th century were convened on an ad hoc basis up until the birth of the World Health Organization (WHO).

The birth of the World Health Organization

'7 April 1948 is the day WHO was born, and is observed as World Health Day. In an interesting tryst with history, the idea of WHO was conceived over a chance lunch encounter of three medical men at the conference where the United Nations was formalized'.

UN Special, Story of the birth of the World Health Organization
(<http://www.unspecial.org/2014/04/story-of-the-birth-of-the-world-health-organization/>)

In July 1946 all members of the United Nations (UN) signed the constitution of the newly envisioned WHO, and, in doing so, created the first specialised agency of the UN. In 1948 the first World Health Assembly took place, and the agency came into existence. This was the beginning of a new chapter in global health. By the naming of the agency the *World Health Organization* (as opposed to its predecessor under the League of Nations), a more global scope was envisioned for this new body.

Throughout its history, the WHO has been at the forefront of many key global health initiatives. The WHO spearheaded the eradication of smallpox (declared eradicated in 1979), the first time that any disease had been entirely eliminated. The WHO has been a key convening body in drawing the world together to tackle health challenges. It led to the creation of the second-ever legally binding treaty on a global health issue, the Framework Convention on Tobacco Control. WHO guidelines and statistics are used to inform decision making in both high-income countries and low- and middle-income countries. The World Health Assembly is still the only health decision-making space with universal membership where all countries can contribute to collective decision making on measures to improve health (see Chapter 3.1).

Declaration of Alma-Ata and health for all by the year 2000
In 1978 the first-ever international conference on primary care, convened by the World Health Organization and UNICEF, took place in the city of Almaty in Kazakhstan. The meeting was attended by more than 100 national ministers of health, and produced the Declaration of Alma-Ata. This is still seen as a landmark moment in the history of global health. It endorsed the primary care approach to improving health, with a strong emphasis on the need to tackle the social, political and economic determinants of health. It also endorsed a vision of health for all by the year 2000. This was one of the first attempts at setting an ambitious international goal for health.

In the 1980s there was a move away from the broad all-encompassing focus on primary health care. Much of the criticism of the Declaration of Alma-Ata was that it was too broad and vague, and that countries were better off investing in specific interventions or 'best buys'. This was the era of international health, developed against the backdrop of the end of the Cold War. It specifically focused on the burden of disease in developing countries, often neglecting the need for wider social and political change as endorsed by the Declaration of Alma-Ata.

The Millennium Development Goals

Although discussions around health have traditionally taken place in the WHO, the 21st century has seen the emergence of new and a wider range of organisations with a focus on global health issues. In 2000 heads of government convened at the headquarters of the UN in New York to agree on the Millennium Declaration. The subsequent eight Millennium Development Goals (MDGs; see Table 6.1.2) had a strong focus on health issues. For the first time, health was linked with global security as with the UN Security Council resolution on HIV (2000). Subsequently, discussions about global health and poverty became central issues at political forums such as the G8 and G20. Increased financial resources from governments and philanthropists were directed towards challenges in global health by organisations such as Gavi and the Bill & Melinda Gates Foundation. These organisations largely favoured disease-specific interventions to the potential detriment of health system investment and development.

The rise of noncommunicable diseases

Much of the discussion surrounding global health and development until the early 21st century focused on infectious diseases, nutrition and maternal health. Noncommunicable diseases (NCDs) such as heart disease, diabetes and cancer were regarded as diseases of affluence, a problem thought to affect the developed world rather than developing countries. It is now appreciated that many developing countries face a double burden of disease, both communicable and noncommunicable (see Chapters 6.1, 6.3). In 2018 the UN General Assembly will hold its third high-level meeting on NCDs.

Civil society raises its voice

Following the foundation of the International Federation of the Red Cross (IFRC) in 1919, nongovernmental organisations (NGOs) began playing an active role in the health of populations. The IFRC was created to serve the victims of war and conflict, and it advocated successfully for the creation of the Geneva Conventions. These remain the current standards of international law which must be observed during conflict.

In 1970 a group of French doctors serving with the Red Cross in Biafra spoke out against the murder of civilians and attacks on health care personnel by the Nigerian military forces. These experiences led to the creation of Médecins Sans Frontières (MSF, 1971), an NGO which prioritised advocacy for the rights of victims of war over the need for neutrality. Subsequently, MSF came to highlight injustices such as the neglect of women's health by the Taliban in Afghanistan and the lack of research for medicines to treat neglected tropical diseases. Another organisation, International Physicians for the Prevention of Nuclear War, framed nuclear weapons as a public health threat, and was awarded the Nobel Peace Prize for its work on nuclear disarmament. There are now hundreds of NGOs and civil society organisations that seek to hold governments to account whilst working on health issues at the global level (see Chapter 3.4).

Global health in the era of sustainable development

In 2012 the UN Conference on Sustainable Development, known as *Rio+20*, took place. A follow-up to the original Earth Summit held in 1992, it was meant to examine how to work simultaneously on protecting the environment, whilst ensuring economic and social development. Subsequently, 17 Sustainable Development Goals covering the period 2015–30 were agreed at a summit in September 2015 (see Chapters 3.1, 6.7, 7.4). These aim to build upon the achievements of the MDGs and provide more equitable solutions for both health care and associated societal challenges.

Conclusion

The discipline of global health has evolved from that of tropical medicine, and now encompasses efforts by governments and NGOs to address global health needs and inequalities.

KEY POINTS

- Many conferences preceded the emergence of the discipline of tropical medicine.
- The history of the World Health Organization, the Declaration of Alma-Ata and the Millennium Development Goals defines the emergence of global health as an area for study.
- Civil society and nongovernmental organisations have a major role in global health discourse.
- The Sustainable Development Goals for 2015–30 formulated a new strategy for global health development.

Further reading

Declaration of Alma-Ata. International Conference on Primary Health Care, Alma-Ata, USSR, 6-12 September 1978. Available from <http://www.who.int/publications/almaata_declaration_en.pdf>.

United Nations: *United Nations Millennium Declaration.* 2000. <http://www.un.org/millennium/declaration/ares552e.htm>.

United Nations Development Programme: *Sustainable Development Goals.* 2017. <http://www.undp.org/content/undp/en/home/sustainable-development-goals.html>.

World Health Organization: *Constitution of the World Health Organization.* 1948. Available from <http://www.who.int/governance/eb/who_constitution_en.pdf>.

1.2 Key Concepts in Global Health

Salma M. Abdalla (Sudan)   Samuel Ognenis (Australia)

Key definitions

Health

The generally accepted definition of health was set out by the WHO in 1948, and has remained unchanged:

> 'Health is a state of complete physical, mental and social well-being and not merely the absence of disease or infirmity.'
>
> WHO, 2003

Public health

WHO describes public health as organised measures (whether public or private) to prevent disease, promote health, and prolong life among the population as a whole. Its activities aim to provide conditions in which people can be healthy and focus on entire populations, not on individual patients or diseases.

Public health addresses the total system, and is not merely about the eradication of a particular disease. This area of health has three main functions:

- identification of health problems and priorities through the assessment and monitoring of the health of communities and populations at risk;
- formulation of public policies to address these problems and priorities;
- assurance of access to health-promotion and disease-prevention services, in an appropriate and cost-effective manner.

Globalisation

This refers to the 'increased interconnectedness and interdependence of people and countries' (WHO). Globalisation impacts on economic activity, technological change and social and cultural change, all of which are relevant to the provision of health.

Some examples of the effects of globalisation on health include:

- enhanced mobility of health professionals and consumers;
- provision of health services across national borders, by use of new technology;
- increasing prevalence of multinational companies providing private health services and health insurance.

Demographic transition

This important concept in sociology refers to the theory of the stages of demography (**Fig. 1.2.1**), including phases of:

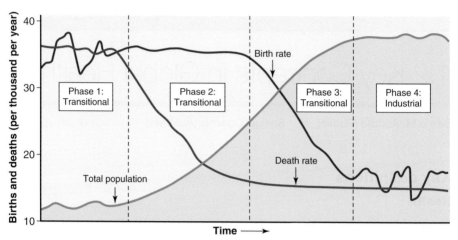

Figure 1.2.1 The stages of demography. *(Redrawn from Marston SA, Knox PL, Liverman DM: World regions in global context: peoples, places and environments, ed 2, Harlow, 2005, Pearson Education.)*

- *High birth rates and high death rates*—and thus a stable population. This is typical of nations before the Industrial Revolution (Phase 1).
- *Reduced death rates* (Phase 2) *and reduced birth rates* (Phase 3)—and thus increased population growth. This is typical of developing or resource-poor nations, where improved public health measures massively reduce death rates. Measures such as contraception and urbanisation are associated with a reduction in birth rates.
- *Low birth rates and (equally) low death rates*—and thus a stable population. This is typical of modern-day 'developed' nations (Phase 4).

Epidemiological transition

This is a theory about the stages of health, from the age of infectious diseases through to increasing prevalence of human-caused disease, and later degenerative diseases (**Fig. 1.2.2**).

Burden of disease

This is a measure to quantify the relative impact of different diseases and injuries in reducing the number of years of *healthy* life. It thus takes into account:
- years of life lost (YLL), through premature death;
- years lived with disability (YLD), through life years with illness, injury or disability. See Chapter 1.3.

Global health

Some commonly used definitions of global health include:
- 'Health issues where the determinants circumvent, undermine or are oblivious to the territorial boundaries of states, and are thus beyond the capacity of individual countries to address through domestic institutions. Global health is focused on people across the whole planet rather than the concerns of particular nations. Global health recognises that health is determined by problems, issues and concerns that transcend national boundaries' (HM Government, 2008).

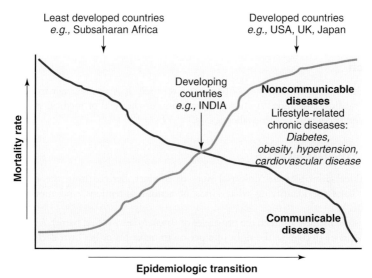

Figure 1.2.2 Changes in mortality rates related to epidemiological transition in countries at different stages of development. *(Modified from Worthman C, Kohrt B: Paradox of success in Public Health. 2013. anthropology.ua.edu)*

- 'An area for study, research, and practice that places a priority on improving health and achieving health equity for all people worldwide' (Koplan et al., 2009).
- 'Health problems, issues, and concerns that transcend national boundaries, may be influenced by circumstances or experiences in other countries, and are best addressed by cooperative actions and solutions' (US Institute of Medicine, 1997).

Global health is an interdisciplinary field which encompasses disciplines such as law, economics, history, social and behavioural sciences, engineering, biomedical and environmental sciences and public policy.

Why is global health relevant?

International clinical placements

Global health is relevant because many health care professionals train and practice both in their country of origin and in foreign lands.

The globalised world

Each year, around 3 billion airline passengers fly within and across borders. Infectious disease epidemics/pandemics and mass migration are all major issues requiring a globalised approach to health policy and leadership. The Internet and the increasing connectivity of individuals across the globe in the 21st century provides a reminder of the importance of being a 'global citizen', and improving the health of everyone in the global, interconnected village.

Diseases do not respect borders

The 21st century has seen the H1N1 influenza pandemic in 2009, the ongoing HIV/AIDS pandemic and the rapid spread of numerous other infectious diseases, such as tuberculosis. An outbreak of a novel *Escherichia coli* strain from Germany in 2011 saw thousands of cases reported in 15 other nations (Centers for Disease Control and Prevention, 2011). The Ebola outbreak of 2014–16 demonstrated how easily diseases can cross national borders.

Research

Global health is an active field for contemporary research. It is also relevant to many aspects of traditional medical education. A strong appreciation of the field of medical ethics is essential when confronting global health challenges.

Global health ethics

Medical ethical principles are 'universal rules of conduct, derived from theories that provide a practical basis for identifying what kinds of actions, intentions, and motives are valued' (Pozgar, 2012).

In a Western medical context, the principles of *nonmaleficence* (avoid harm); *beneficence* (provide benefit); *autonomy* (recognise the right of a person to make his or her own decisions) and *justice* (fair distribution of benefits and harms) are generally applicable, and provide a useful reference point for medical professionals. However, this 'principles-based ethics' approach is often regarded as overly Western-centric, and cannot always be applied in other health contexts. In global health, these general principles of medical ethics apply at an individual level, and transnational issues must take account of variable cultural norms as well as local cultural competency (see Chapter 5.4).

Cultural competency

Cultural competency describes behaviours, attitudes and policies that enable a system to work effectively in cross-cultural situations. It focuses on the capacity of a health system to improve outcomes by integrating culture into health service delivery. It should also be conscious of the dynamics between different cultures, value diversity, and adapt services accordingly.

Global health governance

A concept of growing importance in global health circles is global health governance (GHG). GHG describes the 'rules, norms, and formal institutions that mediate and facilitate international interactions related to health'. These institutions are governments and NGOs (e.g., WHO, World Bank), as well as the laws and agreements that bind these organisations on the international stage. Through GHG frameworks, decisions are made regarding:

- the financing of multiple competing objectives (e.g., provision of HIV/AIDS treatment, efforts to eradicate polio)
- the international regulation governing health policies (e.g., the Framework Convention on Tobacco Control)
- research and statistical surveillance

Externalities

This is an important concept in economics, with broader application in global health. *Externalities* refer to situations where one's production or consumption of a good or service imposes either costs or benefits on others (Organisation for Economic Co-operation and Development, 2002). One example of a *negative* externality is pollution. If a factory dumps waste into a local river as part of its production, it may kill the fish, imposing a cost on local fishermen who need those fish for their income. In contrast, if a new road is built for cars and pedestrians, and then opens up opportunities for business and tourism, this is an example of a *positive* externality.

In health, an individual's health remains primarily of benefit/cost to that person, but there are important externalities to consider. These include:

- The spread of communicable diseases—an infectious individual can put the health of others at risk. On the other hand, preventing and containing infection has external benefits for others in society.
- The effect of ill health on households, and the effect that this has on local and national economies—if an individual is ill for an extended period, that person is less able to work and contribute to wider society.

The social determinants of health

The WHO describes social determinants of health (SDH) (see Chapter 4.1) as 'the circumstances in which people are born, grow, live, work and age, and the systems put in place to deal with illness'.

Externalities with tobacco smoking

The World Health Organization estimates that tobacco smoking causes around 6 million deaths each year. The purchase of a packet of cigarettes incurs a financial cost to the smoker, as well as a benefit in relieving the smoker's nicotine craving. If a smoker sees the price of a packet of cigarettes (the *marginal cost*) as less than or equal to the enjoyment he or she receives from smoking the packet of cigarettes (the *marginal benefit*), then naturally the smoker will buy the packet. However, this looks only at the individual smoker and his or her cost and benefit rather than society as a whole.

The health burden associated with tobacco use is vast. Around 5% of health care expenditure in China and the United States is spent on tobacco-related illness, and 9% of deaths worldwide are attributable to tobacco. These are examples of *negative externalities* of tobacco use as the smoker will not have appreciated the health care costs when purchasing tobacco.

Finally, there is the direct health risk to nonsmokers. Of the 6 million tobacco-attributable deaths, the World Health Organization estimates that more 600,000 are due to nonsmokers being exposed to 'second-hand smoke'. Again, this is not considered by the smoker, and is another *negative externality*.

The packet cost, all things being equal, will take into account the personal net benefit/cost for that smoker. However, there are a number of public/social costs that are not included in the packet cost. Thus the price of tobacco should be higher to include the cost of these **externalities**.

Samuel Ognenis (Australia)

The SDH are decided by a number of factors. Overarching factors are those that cannot be controlled by the individual (*upstream determinants*) but have a significant effect on the individual. Environmental and behavioural factors such as housing and nutrition (*midstream determinants*) have a further impact on the individual's health and mortality (*downstream determinants*). The outcomes of these downstream determinants are strongly influenced by individual behaviour (**Fig. 1.2.3**).

Millennium development goals and sustainable development goals and post-2015 agenda

In 2000, during the UN Millennium Summit, the Millennium Declaration committed nations to eight Millennium Development Goals for the subsequent 15 years (see Chapter 6.1). The

Upstream	Midstream	Downstream

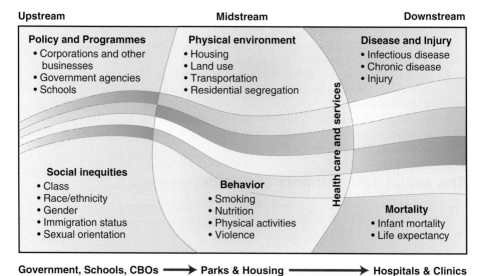

Government, Schools, CBOs ⟶ Parks & Housing ⟶ Hospitals & Clinics

Figure 1.2.3 Interactions determining the social determinants of health. *CBOs,* Community-based organisations. *(Redrawn from <https://nacchocommunique.com/tag/social-determinants-of-health/>.)*

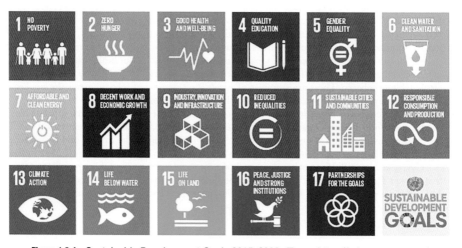

Figure 1.2.4 Sustainable Development Goals 2015–2030. *(From <https://sdgcompass.org>.)*

Sustainable Development Goals (SDG) (**Fig. 1.2.4**) aim to build upon the successes of the Millennium Development Goals in pursuit of health for all as well as many other issues of global importance.

Conclusion

All health care workers should have a strong foundation in key global health concepts. An understanding of the main concepts and definitions pertinent to this area of study facilitates our appreciation of the health inequalities and inequities that exist both within and between nations.

KEY POINTS

- Global health is relevant to health care workers, regardless of nationality.
- Externalities are a key economic concept in the context of public health, health policy and global health.
- Social determinants of health are key concepts which can help explain differences in health outcomes.
- An understanding of the key definitions in global health is becoming increasingly essential for students of health and all associated disciplines.

Further reading

Koplan JP, Bond TC, Merson MH, et al: Towards a common definition of global health, *Lancet* 373:1993–1995, 2009.

Murray CJ: Quantifying the burden of disease: the technical basis for disability-adjusted life years, *Bull World Health Organ* 72:429–445, 1994.

World Health Organization: *Health in 2015: from MDGs to SDGs*, Geneva, 2015, World Health Organization.

1.3 The Global Burden of Disease

Ana Beatriz Lobato (Brazil)   Arthur Mello (Brazil)

Introduction

The Global Burden of Disease Study is a comprehensive regional and global research programme that assesses mortality and disability from major diseases, injuries, and risk factors. It is an analytical, scientific attempt to quantify the comparative significance of health loss caused by diseases, injuries and risk factors by age, sex and geographical location in specific periods. It includes definitions, aggregation across multiple health outcomes and estimations in the setting of sparse and inconsistent data.

In 1990 the World Bank commissioned the original Global Burden of Disease Study, which was published in the *World Development Report 1993: Investing in Health*. This was the first project to produce a comprehensive assessment of the burden of 107 diseases and injuries plus 10 selected risk factors for the world and eight major regions in 1990. It provided a comparable assessment of mortality and loss of health for all regions of the world, and gave a better understanding of the changes in the health of societies. The study was updated by the WHO in 2000–02, and again in 2004 to include a longer analysis of the mortality and burden of disease associated now with 26 global risk factors. These studies use a comprehensive framework and consistent methodology to measure the level of health loss, or 'burden', from all diseases, thus providing a standardised format for comparing different diseases and injuries in a consistent fashion.

They have provided a way of evaluating years of life lost (YLL) from premature death and years of life lived in less than full health. This *health loss* is the gap between the population's current state of health and that of an ideal population in which everyone lives long lives, free from illness or disability. The true health burden can be analysed for each part of the globe, giving a full understanding of the ways in which social and economic changes can influence the health-disease process. These data have been used to inform priorities for research, development, policies and funding. National research institutions and governments have used similar techniques to produce national studies on the burden of disease, allowing further comparisons between countries.

Using data from these studies, it is possible to compare different conditions in a single scenario. For example, a condition that adversely affects the lives of many people but does not usually cause death (e.g., depression) can be compared with a disorder that is less common but often fatal (e.g., brain cancer). It is also possible to compare a condition that causes only a few deaths at a young age (e.g., sudden unexplained deaths in infants) with a condition that causes a large number of deaths at an older age (e.g., coronary heart disease). This approach provides the best estimates of incidence, prevalence and mortality. These consistent and comparative figures on risk factors are very useful for structuring and organising a health system. Countries can now combine this type of evidence with data on policies and their costs to decide how to set their health agendas.

The Institute for Health Metrics and Evaluation and other academic partners collaborated on a new Global Burden of Disease Study in 2010, published in December 2012. This update provides regional estimates of deaths and disability-adjusted life years (DALYs) for the years 1990, 2005 and 2010. This metric provides a standardised quantitative measure of the burden of diseases.

Disability-adjusted life years (DALY)—a measure of disease burden

The Global Burden of Disease Study introduced a new metric—the DALY—as a single measure to quantify the burden of diseases, injuries and risk factors. This combined mortality and morbidity into a more efficient and accurate data set than if only one of the factors had been analysed. DALYs are a big part of global health planning and evaluation; they offer a logical and flexible way to compare disease burden due to mortality and morbidity from different diseases, across populations and with or without interventions.

The DALY measures health gaps as opposed to health expectancies. It measures the difference between a current situation and an ideal situation where everyone lives up to the age of the standard life expectancy, and in perfect health. The DALY is based on YLL from premature death and years of life lived in less than full health. This metric is obtained by the calculation of YLL due to early death and YLD:

$$DALY = YLL + YLD$$

Where:
YLL = years of life lost due to premature mortality.
YLD = years lived with disability.
The YLL metric essentially corresponds to the number of deaths multiplied by the standard life expectancy at the age at which death occurs, and it can be rated according to social preferences. The basic formula for calculating the YLL for a given cause, age or sex, is:

$$YLL = N \times L$$

Where:
N = number of deaths.
L = standard life expectancy at age of death (in years).
In the lexicon of the Global Burden of Disease Study 2010, *disability* is synonymous with any short-term or long-term health loss. YLD was computed as the prevalence of a sequela multiplied by the disability weight for that sequela. To estimate YLD on a population basis, the number of disability cases is multiplied by the average duration of the disease and a weight factor that reflects the severity of the disease on a scale from 0.0 to 1.0, with 0.0 indicating ideal health and 1.0 indicating a state of health equivalent to death. The basic formula (without application of social preferences) for one disabling event is:

$$YLD = I \times DW \times L$$

Where:
YLD = years lived with disability.
I = number of incident cases.
DW = disability weight.
L = average duration of disability (years)
The value of life years is adjusted by:
- the choosing of a particular life expectancy;
- disability weighting (obtained by posing person trade-off [PTO] questions to expert panels, where PTO1 compares life extensions for disabled and healthy people and PTO2 compares cures for illness with extension of life);
- discounting (the value of a life year now is set higher than the value of future life years);
- age weighting (life years of children and old people are counted with less weight) (**Fig. 1.3.1**).

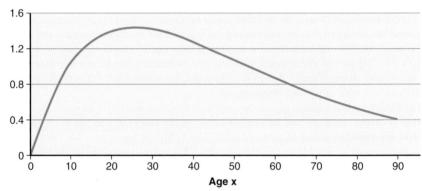

Figure 1.3.1   Relative value of a year of life. *(Redrawn from Fig. 5.1, Chapter 5, Sensitivity and uncertainty analyses for burden of disease and risk factor estimates. In: Lopez AD, Mathers CD, Ezzati M, et al. The global burden of disease and risk factors. The International Bank for Reconstruction and Development/The World Bank; OUP, 2006.)*

Using and criticising the disability-adjusted life year

The DALY metric is largely used in three key areas:

1. Epidemiological surveillance of total disease burden per country or disease (number of DALYs).
2. Measurement of the cost-effectiveness of interventions (cost per avoided DALY).
3. Decisions regarding service provision. This is particularly the case when decisions are being made regarding ensuring there is a package of essential health care services or *core services*. Within a fixed budget, it has been suggested that only the most cost-effective interventions should be included (cost per avoided DALY).

Therefore the DALY is routinely used by clinical staff, health policy advisers, health economists and health leaders when anticipating the needs of their population, trying to design or advocate resources for a new intervention and working to determine the core services on offer by their local or national health system.

Whilst the DALY is a useful measure for the standard comparison of different conditions, it has been criticised with regards to both the validity of the results and the underlying value judgements. The concept of quality of life is difficult to define, and different people and cultures may have very different opinions of what constitutes a good quality of life. It has also been criticised with regards to distributive justice (see Chapter 5.4)—various proponents claim it discriminates against:

- *The elderly and the young.* (The principle of equal worth of people would require equal weight for all ages. However, unequal age weighting implies, for example, that living with a disability (e.g., deafness) at the age of 80 years is considered less bad than living with the same disability at the age of 20 years.
- *Women.* Women have a higher standard life expectancy. By utilising one life expectancy for both sexes, DALYs underestimate the burden of disease for females relative to males, and are less likely to value interventions which aid women.
- *Future generations.* With the DALY, preventative services are given less weight due to discounting. However, it is questionable whether a life year now is of more value than a life year 20 years ahead.
- *The disabled.* The method presupposes that life years of people with disabilities are worth less than life years of people without disabilities.

In *summary*, the DALY combines traditional epidemiological information on mortality with information about loss of quality of life. This approach allows a useful standard comparison of diseases, which is widely used by those managing and designing health services. However, the associated valuc judgements involved in its construction have been criticised.

Major determinants of change in global disease burdens

Many factors can influence global disease burden: demographic changes, urbanisation, consumption patterns, economic growth, climate change, natural disasters, war and conflict, health sector reform, innovation in health care and health technology, intensification of agriculture and management of natural resources.

These major factors are closely related in complex patterns:

- *Demographic change.* An ageing population, with increased life expectancy, modifies the profile of a population and consequently the main causes of morbidity and mortality.
- *Economic growth* is closely linked to many changes that affect health outcomes. These include increases in global trade, better infrastructure and hygiene, higher quality of housing, and altered access to and affordability of food and medical technology. There is a close relationship between poverty and health (see Chapter 4.1). Increased urbanisation and consumption patterns in large geographical regions are usually more pronounced in the less developed areas. Cities have grown exponentially, causing major changes in the habitants' lifestyles.
- *Diet changes*, less physical activity and pollution are all changes associated with urbanisation that can also be related to the increase of NCDs.
- *Intensification of agriculture* can alter living conditions in rural farms and thus alter health burdens.
- *Climate change* affects health in many ways (see Chapter 7.1).
- *War and conflict* (see Chapter 7.3) change living conditions and disrupt many aspects of life. This has a significant impact on health determinants as a result of the increasing numbers of refugees, destruction of infrastructure, particularly of water and sanitation, and collapse of health systems and local economies.
- The effectiveness of the *health sector* depends on planning, accessibility and affordability of services. Poor planning compromises effective implementation of health services, and has a negative effect, especially on vulnerable or marginalised populations (see Chapter 2.2).
- *Innovations in health care and health technology* have wide-ranging effects on diagnostics, investigation, treatment and rehabilitation. Additionally, new technologies enable the spread of health information, allowing greater scope for preventative campaigns and health education.

Important findings from the Global Burden of Disease Study 2010

The 2010 Global Burden of Disease Study investigated 291 types of diseases and injuries and 67 risk factors in 187 countries. The subsequent results have significant policy implications worldwide. Overall, in 1990 there were 2497 million global DALYs, compared with 2482 million DALYs in 2010.

Fig. 1.3.2 shows the leading global causes of DALYs in 2010 compared with the number of DALYs in the previous study in 1990. The leading causes included communicable diseases, NCDs and some injuries. In general, the 2010 study showed that communicable, maternal, neonatal and

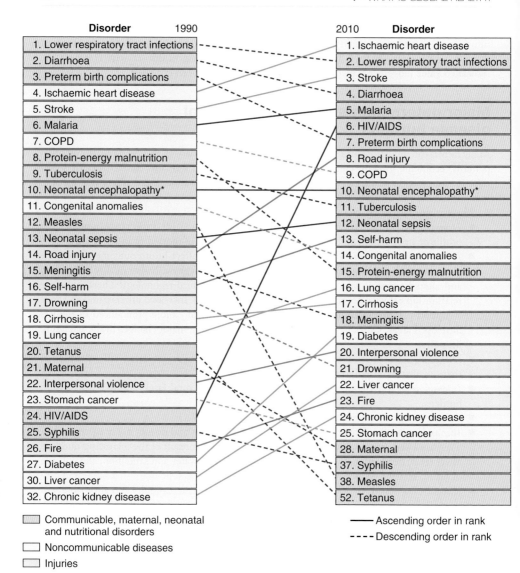

Disorder	1990		2010	Disorder
1. Lower respiratory tract infections				1. Ischaemic heart disease
2. Diarrhoea				2. Lower respiratory tract infections
3. Preterm birth complications				3. Stroke
4. Ischaemic heart disease				4. Diarrhoea
5. Stroke				5. Malaria
6. Malaria				6. HIV/AIDS
7. COPD				7. Preterm birth complications
8. Protein-energy malnutrition				8. Road injury
9. Tuberculosis				9. COPD
10. Neonatal encephalopathy*				10. Neonatal encephalopathy*
11. Congenital anomalies				11. Tuberculosis
12. Measles				12. Neonatal sepsis
13. Neonatal sepsis				13. Self-harm
14. Road injury				14. Congenital anomalies
15. Meningitis				15. Protein-energy malnutrition
16. Self-harm				16. Lung cancer
17. Drowning				17. Cirrhosis
18. Cirrhosis				18. Meningitis
19. Lung cancer				19. Diabetes
20. Tetanus				20. Interpersonal violence
21. Maternal				21. Drowning
22. Interpersonal violence				22. Liver cancer
23. Stomach cancer				23. Fire
24. HIV/AIDS				24. Chronic kidney disease
25. Syphilis				25. Stomach cancer
26. Fire				28. Maternal
27. Diabetes				37. Syphilis
30. Liver cancer				38. Measles
32. Chronic kidney disease				52. Tetanus

Communicable, maternal, neonatal and nutritional disorders

Noncommunicable diseases

Injuries

——— Ascending order in rank

---- Descending order in rank

Figure 1.3.2   Top causes of global disability-adjusted life years in 1990 and 2010. *(Modified with permission from Fig. 10 in GBD 2013 Mortality and Causes of Death Collaborators: Global, regional, and national age–sex specific all-cause and cause-specific mortality for 240 causes of death, 1990–2013: a systematic analysis for the Global Burden of Disease Study 2013. Lancet 385(9963);117–171, 2015.)*

nutritional conditions decreased in absolute terms (both in numbers of DALYs and rates) and relative to NCDs; the notable exceptions were malaria and HIV/AIDS.

The 2010 study was also able to present more specific and relevant data, which has had important policy implications in different countries. The major causes of death in children in low-income countries in 1990 were also among the top 15 causes of DALYs in 2010. These include lower respiratory tract infections, diarrhoea, malaria, complications of preterm birth and

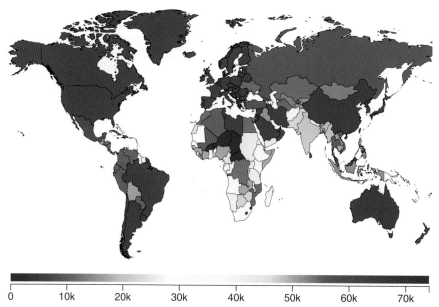

0   10k   20k   30k   40k   50k   60k   70k

Figure 1.3.3 Global distribution of disability-adjusted life years associated with communicable, maternal, neonatal and nutritional disorders in 2010. *(Redrawn from Murray CJ, Vos T, Lozano R, et al: Disability-adjusted life years (DALYs) for 291 diseases and injuries in 21 regions, 1990–2010: a systematic analysis for the Global Burden of Disease Study 2010. Lancet 380(9859):2197–2223, 2012.)*

neonatal encephalopathy. In addition, globally, HIV/AIDS and tuberculosis remained in the top 15 causes of DALYs (**Figs 1.3.3** and **1.3.4**).

NCDs such as ischaemic heart disease, stroke, COPD and diabetes also feature among the top 15 causes of DALYs. The 2010 data show that the burden of NCDs has been increasing in terms of the absolute number of YLL and YLD, and in terms of the share of the total burden over the 2 decades. The largest increases have been associated with diabetes. Some disabling conditions also appeared as leading causes, such as low back pain and major depressive disorder. Low back pain, for example, affects 10% of the world population. Major depressive disorder has also become a strong focus of research, since it carries a significant burden and is related to important causes of death such as self-harm and suicide. The study also found three categories of injury which were among the top 25 causes of DALYs; road traffic injuries, which caused the most DALYs, increased by 33% between 1990 and 2010.

A comparison of data from 1990 with data from 2010 shows some profound shifts in the risk factor analysis. The leading risk factor in 1990 was childhood underweight; however, it was ranked eighth among the risk factors evaluated in the 2010 study, representing an absolute decrease in DALYs of 61%.

The burden of disease attributable to risk factors is shown in **Table 1.3.1**.

The list of leading risk factors includes multiple components of the diet, each of which were evaluated in isolation. Taken together, all components of the diet and physical inactivity accounted for 10.2% of global DALYs in 2010. The burden attributable to tobacco smoking (including exposure to second-hand smoke) remained roughly constant (6.3% of DALYs in 2010) from 1990 to 2010 because of decreased smoking in high-income countries and increased smoking in developing regions.

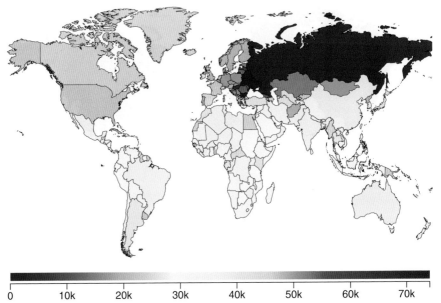

0   10k   20k   30k   40k   50k   60k   70k

Figure 1.3.4   Global distribution of disability-adjusted life years associated with noncommunicable diseases in 2010. *(Redrawn from Murray CJ, Vos T, Lozano R, et al: Disability-adjusted life years (DALYs) for 291 diseases and injuries in 21 regions, 1990–2010: a systematic analysis for the Global Burden of Disease Study 2010. Lancet 380(9859):2197–2223, 2012.)*

Julia's story—risk factors, noncommunicable diseases and disability-adjusted life years (DALYs)

Many patients exhibit risk factors which lead to long-term conditions that significantly reduce their quality of life, and, sometimes, length of life, resulting in a large number of disability-adjusted life years. Julia's story of her experience as a single mother helps to demonstrate the role of public health in tackling systemic challenges.

Julia (a pseudonym) is a 45-year-old single working mother with two jobs, daytime in a supermarket and evenings in a fast food restaurant to earn money to support her family. With these long hours, she does not get much time to cook healthy meals or exercise as it is late when she gets home and she is afraid of going outside after dark in the neighbourhood where she lives. She knows she should exercise and stop smoking.

Recently Julia was diagnosed with hypertension. She tried dieting to lose weight as her family doctor had told her that she might have a stroke. Julia was worried about the care of her family if she became disabled. All her problems and long working hours made her depressed, and she gained more weight.

Hypertension, obesity and depression are extremely common, particularly in the lower socioeconomic groups, such as Julia's. They contribute to a worsening quality of life and a risk of disability and death. These consequences reflected in an associated rise in disability-adjusted life years associated with noncommunicable diseases. This has serious implications for both the health care budgets and the health of the population.

Alexandra Peterson (United States/United Kingdom)

TABLE 1.3.1 ■ Global disability-adjusted life years attributable to the 25 leading risk factors in 1990 and 2010

	Rank	1990 DALYs (95% UI) in thousands[a]	Rank	2010 DALYs (95% UI) in thousands[a]
High blood pressure	4	137,017 (124,360–149,366)	1	173,556 (155,939–189,025)
Tobacco smoking, including exposure to second-hand smoke	3	151,766 (136,367–169,522)	2	156,838 (136,543–173,057)
Household air pollution from solid fuels	2	170,693 (139,087–199,504)	3	108,084 (84,891–132,983)
Diet low in fruit	7	80,453 (63,298–95,763)	4	104,095 (81,833–124,169)
Alcohol use	8	73,715 (66,090–82,089)	5	97,237 (87,087–107,658)
High body mass index	10	51,565 (40,786–62,557)	6	93,609 (77,107–110,600)
High fasting plasma glucose level	9	56,358 (48,720–65,030)	7	89,012 (77,743–101,390)
Childhood underweight	1	197,741 (169,224–238,276)	8	77,316 (64,497–91,943)
Exposure to ambient particulate-matter pollution	6	81,699 (71,012–92,859)	9	76,163 (68,086–85,171)
Physical inactivity or low level of activity	–	–	10	69,318 (58,646–80,182)
Diet high in sodium	12	46,183 (30,363–60,604)	11	61,231 (40,124–80,182)
Diet low in nuts and seeds	13	40,525 (26,308–51,741)	12	61,231 (40,124–80,342)
Iron deficiency	11	51,841 (37,477–71,202)	13	48,225 (33,769–67,592)
Suboptimal breastfeeding	5	110,261 (69,615–153,539)	14	47,537 (29,868–67,518)
High total cholesterol level	14	39,526 (32,704–47,202)	15	40,900 (31,662–50,484)
Diet low in whole grains	18	29,404 (23,097–35,134)	16	40,762 (32,112–48,486)
Diet low in vegetables	16	31,558 (21,349–41,921)	17	38,559 (26,006–51,658)
Diet low in seafood n-3 fatty acids	20	21,740 (15,869–27,537)	18	28,199 (20,624–35,974)
Drug use	25	15,171 (11,714–19,369)	19	23,810 (18,780–29,246)
Occupational risk factors for injuries	21	21,265 (16,644–26,702)	20	23,444 (17,736–30,904)
Occupation-related low back pain	23	17,841 (11,846–24,945)	21	21,750 (14,492–30,533)
Diet high in processed meat	24	17,359 (5137–27,949)	22	20,939 (6982–33,468)
Intimate-partner violence	–	–	23	16,794 (11,373–23,087)
Diet low in fibre	26	13,347 (5970–20,751)	24	16,452 (7401–25,783)
Lead exposure	31	5,365 (4534–6279)	25	13,936 (11,750–16,327)

[a]The 95% uncertainty interval is given in parentheses.

DALYs, Disability-adjusted life years.

Reproduced with permission from Murray CJ, Vos T, Lozano R, et al: Disability-adjusted life years (DALYs) for 291 diseases and injuries in 21 regions, 1990–2010: a systematic analysis for the Global Burden of Disease Study 2010, *Lancet* 380:2197–2223, 2012.

Conclusion

The Global Burden of Disease Study data offer a perspective about the effects of socioeconomic differences between and within countries. As such, the study provides health administrators, public health specialists and clinicians with indications of present and future needs. It also enables cross-regional and international comparison, and helps countries to learn from one another.

Data evaluation with comparable metrics across countries, such as the DALY, identifies the most relevant factors in the change of the burden of diseases globally. These data also provide a focus for health initiatives and health system planning, and enable informed needs-based decision making.

KEY POINTS

- The Global Burden of Disease Study analyses provide an accessible summary of the many global health challenges.
- The Global Burden of Disease Study (2010) introduced a new metric—the disability-adjusted life-year—as a single measure to quantify the burden of diseases, injuries and risk factors.
- The leading causes of morbidity and death include communicable diseases, noncommunicable diseases, and injuries.
- The leading causes of morbidity and death differ greatly between lower-income and higher-income countries.
- The Global Burden of Disease Study helps to highlight the major issues for policymakers so that they can focus on appropriate preventative measures.

Further reading

Lopez AD, Mathers CD: Measuring the global burden of disease and epidemiological transitions: 2002–2030, *Ann Trop Med Parasitol* 100(5–6):481–499, 2006.

Murray CJL, Lopez AD: Measuring the global burden of disease, *N Engl J Med* 369:448–457, 2013.

Murray CJ, Vos T, Lozano R, et al: Disability-adjusted life years (DALYs) for 291 diseases and injuries in 21 regions, 1990–2010: a systematic analysis for the Global Burden of Disease Study 2010, *Lancet* 380:2197–2223, 2012.

1.4 Determinants of Health

Altagracia Mares de Leon (Mexico)

Introduction

Determinants of health are the conditions that shape the health of individuals and populations as a whole, whether positively or negatively, beyond the consequences of genetic factors or biological processes. The WHO has identified key health determinants that deserve special attention.

What makes people healthy and unhealthy?

'Health is created and lived by people within the settings of their everyday life; where they learn, work, play and love. Health is created by caring for oneself and others, by being able to take decisions and have control over one's life circumstances, and by ensuring that the society one lives in creates conditions that allow the attainment of health by all members'.

The Ottawa Charter for Health Promotion, 1986

Access to health services is a big factor in determining health, but many other issues significantly affect the likelihood of good health. The social, political and economic factors, the physical environment, and a person's individual characteristics and behaviours all contribute to whether individuals stay healthy or become ill. A holistic view of health is required so as to be able to identify the determinants of health.

Rudolph Virchow

Rudolf Virchow (1821–1902; Fig. 1.4.1) was a German physician regarded as one of the most brilliant and influential biomedical scientists of the 19th century. He is known as the *"Father of Modern Pathology"*. But he was also a pioneer in social medicine.

In 1848, Virchow was asked by the Minister of Education to help investigate the epidemic of typhus in Upper Silesia. In his *Report on the typhus epidemic prevailing in Upper Silesia*, he emphasised the economic, social and cultural factors involved in its aetiology. Instead of recommending medical changes (i.e. more doctors or hospitals), he outlined a revolutionary programme of social reconstruction including democratic self-government, full employment, higher wages, the establishment of agricultural cooperatives, universal education and the separation of church and state.

Virchow stated that 'disease is not something personal and special, but only a manifestation of life under modified (pathological) conditions'. Arguing 'medicine is a social science and politics is nothing else but medicine on a large scale', Virchow applied ideas on the social causation of disease. He argued that improved health required recognition that 'if medicine is to fulfil her great task, then she must enter the political and social life. Do we not always find the diseases of the populace traceable to defects in society?'

Virchow's legacy has been widely inspirational. He is often credited for being one of the first to make the case for the social origins of illness and the multifactorial cause of epidemics.

Altagracia Mares de Leon (Mexico)

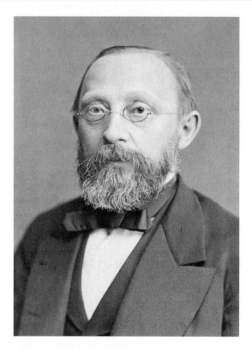

Figure 1.4.1   Rudolf Virchow.

The social, political and economic environment

'The social determinants of health are the conditions in which people are born, grow, live, work and age. These circumstances are shaped by the distribution of money, power and resources at global, national and local levels.'

WHO, 2008

In 2008 the WHO Commission on Social Determinants of Health issued a report that challenged conventional public health thinking on several fronts. The commission found abundant evidence that the true upstream drivers of health inequities reside in the social, economic and political environments. Systematic differences in health between social groups within and between countries, which are avoidable by reasonable means, are health inequities. There is a social gradient in health that runs from top to bottom of the socioeconomic spectrum. Within countries, evidence shows that, in general, the lower an individual's socioeconomic position, the worse that person's health. This is a global phenomenon, seen in low-, middle- and high-income countries.

Socioeconomic status (SES) refers to an individual's social position relative to that of other members of a society. SES is usually measured by determining education, income and occupation. An individual's health is highly correlated with his or her SES. Success in school and the number of years of schooling are major factors in determining health, social and occupational status in adulthood. Low SES alone is one of the strongest predictors of poor health and development. This is not just because material deprivation constrains behaviour and lifestyle choices amongst those living in poverty, but is also because neuroendocrine responses to the stress that SES imposes influence psychosocial well-being (see Chapter 4.1).

- *Education* is strongly linked to health and to determinants of health such as health behaviours and use of preventative services. More years of schooling are clearly associated with improved health outcomes at the individual and population level. Moreover, education helps to promote and sustain healthy lifestyles and positive choices, supporting and nurturing

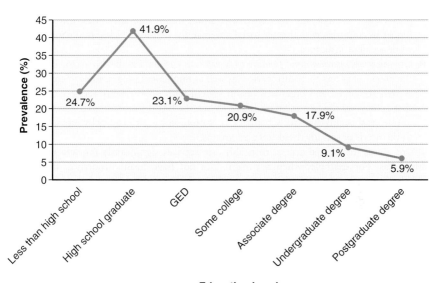

Education Level

Figure 1.4.2 Current cigarette smoking among US adults aged 18 years or older by education level, **2012.** *GED,* General Educational Development credential. *(Redrawn from Jamal A, King BA, Neff LJ, et al: Current cigarette smoking among adults—United States, 2005–2015. MMWR Morb Mortal Wkly Rep 65(44):1205–1211, 2016.)*

human development, human relationships and personal family and community well-being. Improved literacy and health literacy change the intergenerational patterns of disadvantage associated with health inequities. For example, in an African context, simple knowledge and skills such as hand washing can combat a wide range of prevalent diseases. These include vector-borne infections such as malaria, diarrhoeal diseases, neglected tropical diseases (see Chapter 6.2) and nutrition-related conditions (e.g., micronutrient deficiencies). There is a strong relationship between education and health (see Chapter 4.1), illustrated in **Fig. 1.4.2** with respect to smoking.

■ *Social support.* Countries with more generous social protection systems tend to have better population health outcomes, at least across high-income countries for which evidence is available. Social protection can cover a broad range of services and benefits. These include basic income security, entitlements to nonincome transfers (such as food and other basic needs), services such as health care and education, and labour protection and benefits (such as maternity leave, paid leave, childcare and pensions). For example, a United Nations Population Fund report (*The Impact of Social Pensions: Perceptions of Asian Older Persons,* 2008) found that even a small, regular amount of a pension promoted overall well-being in older people, especially in agricultural communities where the older person was now not strong enough to undertake physical work.

'In past days, we used to cultivate. If that income was not enough, we went and worked in other people's land so that we could earn something. Now, we can't do any work. So we are helpless. If we were physically strong, we wouldn't need to ask anybody for help.'

Older woman from Matale, Sri Lanka

■ *Government decisions and policies* have the potential to affect health and health equity. These include finance, education, housing, employment and transport. More generous family policies, for example, are associated with lower infant mortality rates. Life expectancy is higher in countries with greater social coverage for pensions, sickness, unemployment and work accident insurance.

■ *Organisation, operation and funding of health care systems.* The health sector can determine the means of access to health services as well as implement programmes to control diseases. A well-resourced and organised health system with good-quality services offers benefits that go beyond the treatment of illness. When the health care system follows the principle of universal health care (see Chapter 2.1), it promotes health equity by providing attention to the needs of socially disadvantaged groups.

A lack of access (or limited access) to health care services significantly impacts an individual's health status. For example, when a person does not have health insurance, that person is less likely to have a primary health care provider and is more likely to delay medical treatment when needed.

Barriers to accessing health services include:

■ the high cost of the services or medicines
■ lack of insurance (in insurance-based systems)
■ language barriers
■ the availability of infrastructure or medicine
■ lack of a transportation system

Mexico's experience of access to health services in rural areas

Olivia is a 58-year-old woman with multiple sclerosis living in a small, economically disadvantaged location in the northeast of Mexico. Most of the rural population of Mexico are enrolled in a public federal health insurance programme called *Seguro Popular*. This programme reaches the poorest populations who live in the most marginalised areas of Mexico. Unfortunately for Olivia, the coverage does not include all diseases, including multiple sclerosis. Therefore she and her family have to pay out-of-pocket for all of her medical expenses. The nearest hospital is 3 hours away from her community and only attends to emergencies. For routine treatments, medical appointments and medications, she has to travel to a city that is approximately 7 hours from where she lives.

Iza Sánchez-Siller (Mexico)

The physical environment

'Well-designed, accessible housing and adequate services can successfully address fundamental determinants of health for disadvantaged individuals and communities.'

Adelaide Statement on Health in All Policies, 2010

The physical environment has many components relevant to health:

■ The characteristics of the general environment, including the workplace and housing, affect health. These factors are often not considered in a clinical consultation. For example, a child with asthma following treatment in hospital who is sent back to a home with mould and dust mites will soon require readmission.

■ Millions of people struggle every day with poor housing, overcrowding, lack of affordability and lack of basic services. Communities and neighbourhoods promoting good physical and psychological well-being ensure access to basic goods and are socially cohesive. They also protect the natural environment.

■ Health and safety policies and occupational health practices can have a dramatic impact on the well-being of staff. For example, the use of mechanical aids to lift patients substantially reduces the incidence of back problems in health care workers.

- Energy availability is essential for the effective functioning of society. It plays a critical role in all aspects of everyday life. However, despite all the benefits of modern technology, millions of people still live without a reliable source of energy.
- Ecological damage due to the disruption and depletion of natural environmental systems affects the lives of everyone in society. It has the greatest impact on the most vulnerable groups.
- Gender is a determinant for patterns of health and illness. Most care demands for children and care of the elderly and the sick, fall upon women. This limits their ability to contribute to household finances and also affects their personal health.
- Ethnicity refers to the cultural practices and attitudes of a nonhomogeneous community or population that sees themselves as culturally distinct from other groups in society (see Chapter 5.6). This may lead to social inequalities such as limited access to health services (e.g., eligibility for health insurance for immigrants) or a lack of necessary information due to language barriers.

Taking action on determinants of health

Health care workers should be aware of the relevant social, political and economic conditions of the countries they visit. Likewise, policymakers outside the health care arena need to consider the health impacts of their policies and actions. The movement promoting and encouraging all governance departments to work together to maximise health outcomes and health equity is known as *Health in All Policies* (see Chapter 5.1).

Root Out, Reach Out—a global student campaign for health equity

In October 2011, representatives of member states and civil society groups convened in Rio de Janeiro for the World Conference on Social Determinants of Health. Medical students from the International Federation of Medical Students' Associations (IFMSA) organised the *Reach Out, Root Out* global campaign. The campaign put emphasis on the need to 'root out' the causes of global health inequities so as to 'reach out' to those left behind by society, especially in terms of health—the poor, the marginalised, the vulnerable and the underserved.

During the conference, government representatives summarised their agreements through the Rio Political Declaration, which enumerated five areas for action. However, the IFMSA's delegation released an 'alternative declaration', noting the official declaration's inability to explicitly tackle the 'unfair distribution of power, resources and wealth' that drives gross health inequities. The IFMSA called on the global community to ensure the genuine 'inclusion of young people and youth organisations in the movement for action on social determinants of health'.

The IFMSA also declared a *Week of Global Action* on Social Determinants of Health coinciding with the conference and provided a toolkit and other materials to support students around the world in taking action on these issues. It made a firm commitment to make health equity and the social determinants of health a priority of the whole federation. Work in this area continues through the IFMSA Global Health Equity Initiative, which serves as the nerve centre of all advocacy and education activities geared towards health equity and action on the social determinants of health.

Students around the world are increasingly becoming aware of the importance of acting on the broader determinants of health, veering away from a merely biomedical and reductionist approach to addressing health at the individual level and the population level. This commitment is sealed in the last words of **IFMSA's Rio alternative declaration**: '*We medical students commit ourselves to continue engaging with all sectors involved in the work towards global health equity, spreading awareness of the social dimensions of health to our fellow young people, mobilizing them to take action in their respective communities and countries, doing our part, little by little, but with courage, constancy, and conviction.*'

The Root Out, Reach Out campaign video can be viewed at https://www.youtube.com/watch?v=8tqUfq0WIR4.

Renzo Guinto (Philippines)

Conclusion

Health is everyone's business. Good health is a major resource for social, economic and personal development, and a vital dimension of quality of life. Political, economic, social, cultural, environmental, behavioural and biological determinants can all favour health or be harmful to it. If health and health equity are to be improved, a holistic view of the complex interactions of health determinants is essential.

KEY POINTS

- Determinants of health are the conditions that shape the health of individuals and populations as a whole.
- A holistic vision of health is required to be able to identify the determinants of health.
- Health inequities are systematic differences in health between social groups within and between countries, that are avoidable by reasonable means.
- Upstream drivers of health inequities reside in the social, economic and political environments.
- Health is determined by environmental and genetic factors.

Further reading

Commission on Social Determinants of Health: *Closing the gap in a generation: health equity through action on the social determinants of health*, Geneva, 2008, World Health Organization.

Global Health Observatory. 2017. <http://www.who.int/gho/en/>.

Marmot M: Social determinants of health inequalities, *Lancet* 365:1099–1104, 2005.

Marmot M: Universal health coverage and social determinants of health, *Lancet* 382:1227–1228, 2013.

Marmot M: *The health gap: the challenge of an unequal world*, London, 2015, Bloomsbury.

1.5 Evaluation of Health Care

Timothy Martin (Australia)

Introduction

Health care evaluation, in pursuit of quality improvement, is a frequently neglected but critical component of any health system as well as an obligation for all health care professionals. The principles, methodologies and rationale for undertaking evaluation in health care are similar in all environments, and the aim is to improve population health outcomes. This aim can be achieved only through a process of evaluation supported by an organisational culture which encourages active improvement. Effective evaluation requires an appreciation of domains beyond the safety and quality of care. These include cost-effectiveness, service efficiency, access to care, compassionate care and equity.

Health care students and junior medical staff can contribute effectively to patient safety. They should be role models for other colleagues (e.g., by washing hands and by pointing out errors).

Monitoring refers to the regular collection of performance data which then allows an organisation to track improvements (or identify deterioration) in a timely manner. When used in the context of monitoring, *evaluation* may instead refer to the intermittent collection of data, perhaps through audits. *Inquests, inquiries and commissions* may be instigated at local or governmental level in response to an event. These are also valid forms of evaluation, as is *academic research*, ultimately undertaken to improve clinical outcomes. The processes of evaluation should be regarded as a form of social accountability. The health system exists to serve both patients and society as services are often publicly funded (see Chapter 2.2). All health professionals, as public servants, have an obligation to promote efficient, safe and cost-effective health care.

Measures for evaluation

The indicators used for undertaking evaluation must be appropriate to the area under scrutiny. Judgements regarding clinical efficacy may conflict with evaluations focused on financial efficiency.

When hospitals and national health systems are being evaluated, information about factors such as efficient working practices, accessibility, safety and patient satisfaction must be provided in addition to data regarding patient mortality and morbidity.

Measuring health/disease

Measuring health is a key component in any kind of health evaluation, whether at an individual intervention level or at a systems level. 'Health' is notoriously difficult to measure. *Mortality* (rate of death), *morbidity* (rate of disease/disability), *incidence* (the occurrence or frequency of a disease) and *prevalence* (the commonness or number of patients with a disease at any one time) are indicators commonly used to assess the impact that a disease has on society, or the efficacy of an intervention. In some cases a single indicator may produce a reliable assessment of health. The mortality rate in the 2014 Ebola outbreak was 50%, and given the acute nature and high fatality rate of this illness, the mortality rate was likely to represent an adequate indicator of the efficacy of the available treatments.

Evaluation of long-term morbidity presents a different challenge when trying to assess health. The DALY (see Chapter 1.3), as used in the Global Burden of Disease Study, addresses this challenge in an ingenious way.

Tackling sepsis at Mulago Hospital

Mulago Hospital in Uganda is the national referral hospital with an inpatient capacity of 1600 beds, currently serving a population of 36 million people. Recently, patient turnover has more than doubled, and the wards are crowded, enabling easy transmission of infections. Sepsis and related complications, secondary to increased infection rates, are one of the commonest causes of death. Staff and students realised the need to measure the extent of the problem, and to evaluate the impact of possible interventions. A multidisciplinary team was formed, and resident students from the Department of Microbiology conducted laboratory studies on the prevalence and associated factors of nosocomial infections. Samples were also collected from sites across the hospital and analysed for culture and sensitivity. Patient records were examined to determine the prevalence of different types of infections. Drug charts were analysed to determine antibiotic use.

The investigators found that urinary tract infections represented the most common (34%) type of nosocomial infections. Seventeen percent of nosocomial infections occurred in surgical wounds, and these were the second most commonly acquired hospital infection. Fifty-nine to eighty-eight percent of the MRSA isolated was resistant to commonly used antibiotics, and more than 60% of patients received an antibiotic on admission without any documented evidence of infection. This irrational antibiotic use is likely to have been a key cause of the increased resistance patterns against commonly used antibiotics, and policies were subsequently developed to address this problem.

Jack Turyahikayo (Uganda)

Measuring interventions

The gold standard technique for evaluating a new intervention is the *randomised controlled trial* (RCT). The RCT aims to compare two identical groups of individuals: one exposed to the intervention and the other not exposed. It is commonly used for clinical trials of new pharmaceutical products, and it is important to understand the detail of what is being compared in the two groups so as to know whether the use of an RCT is the most appropriate tool for evaluation. The measure of comparison depends on the desired outcome. An intervention might be designed to prolong life (decrease mortality), improve quality of life (decrease morbidity) or prevent the development of the disease (lower incidence and subsequent prevalence). For example, nonsteroidal antiinflammatory drugs (NSAIDs) provide pain relief, and generally do not prolong a patient's life; therefore measuring the mortality impact of NSAIDs in an RCT would be inappropriate. Similarly, antihypertensive agents generally prolong life but do not alter the quality of life. In this instance, measuring the impact on morbidity using an RCT would also be inappropriate.

When an intervention is directed at the prolongation of life as well as improving the quality of life, one of the most common measures used for evaluation is the *quality-adjusted life year* (QALY). The QALY is similar to the DALY in that it is a measure of both mortality and morbidity. However, whereas the DALY is a health gap measure, the QALY is a health gain measure. One QALY gained represents the addition of the equivalent of 1 year of full health as a result of the intervention.

Cost-effectiveness analysis

'*Cost effectiveness analysis compares the cost and health benefits of an intervention to assess the extent to which it can be regarded as providing value for money. This informs decision-makers who have to determine where to allocate limited health care resources.*'

Ceri Phillips, health economist

Cost-effective analyses are crucial when limited budgets mean that health care needs to be rationed. Every aspect of the health system, whether a discrete intervention or a hospital or a government policy, requires careful and considered cost evaluation. Evaluation is a form of social accountability, and it may be unethical to prioritise the least economical treatments in the context of limited health financing.

The *average cost-effectiveness ratio* (ACER) is a common way to determine the cost-effectiveness of an intervention:

$$ACER = \frac{\text{Cost of intervention}}{\text{Benefit (often in QALYs)}}.$$

The unit of benefit depends on what the intervention is designed to achieve. For instance, the ACER for a condom distribution programme might be US$3 per STI prevented. The most common benefit measure is the QALY. Another common cost-effectiveness measure is the *incremental cost-effectiveness ratio* (ICER). This compares the cost/benefit of two different interventions or scenarios. As an example, two new vaccines are introduced to the market: a group B *Neisseria meningitides* vaccine and a new rotavirus vaccine. The ICER is US$45,000–75,000/QALY for the meningococcal vaccine, meaning that the intervention costs between US$45,000 and US$75,000 to gain 1 year of life at full health. In comparison, the ICER for the rotavirus vaccine is substantially lower at less than US$15,000/QALY. In this example, it would be logical to subsidise the rotavirus vaccine but not the meningococcal vaccine.

Other commonly used indicators

Life expectancy is a commonly used surrogate measure of the overall health of a country's health care system, or its level of development. Although a crude measure, it is also useful to track long-term improvement especially with regard to particular diseases within a country, or within subpopulations.

Common key performance indicators used in the evaluation of health care institutions include the hospital standardised mortality ratio, mortality rates for particular/common diseases, unplanned hospital readmission, rate of hospital-acquired infection, preventable adverse drug reactions and patient satisfaction.

Areas commonly analysed at a health systems level include access and equity, efficacy/quality, efficiency and cost-effectiveness. All indicators are vulnerable to bias and manipulation, and no single indicator, in isolation, can offer a complete picture of the health status of a population. An understanding of the limitations of each indicator is essential as it is human nature to 'game' the system in an attempt to artificially improve appearances. This may result in the inappropriate use of health resources.

Quality and safety

Clinical staff have been shown to focus largely on the technical aspects of care, whereas patients often focus on compassion and communication issues. A key aspect of quality health care is the minimisation of error. Medical errors occur in 10%–30% of patients. Common avoidable errors include falls, pressure ulcers, medication errors, hospital-acquired infection and venous thromboembolism. It is important to evaluate the following elements of care:

- How could this event have happened?
- What were the processes that led up to the event?
- Were any other errors made?

- Were there policies in place to prevent such an error and were they followed?
- How can we prevent such an event from occurring in the future?

The response to these questions is part of the process of evaluation.

A patient transfusion reaction

Catastrophic events occur rarely in health care. How could such an event occur and how can we prevent a similar one from occurring again?

You are a locum doctor called in late at night to cover for a sick doctor. It is a quiet night until you are called to a patient with cardiac arrest in the cardiac care unit. You rush to the patient and find her unresponsive, with no signs of life. Advanced life support is commenced and you read through her records to try and find out the background. To your horror, you find that although the patient is blood type A positive and a unit of O-positive blood was ordered, the blood transfused was type B positive. Thus the patient has likely died of a severe transfusion reaction. To make matters worse, the blood was transfused at 7 p.m. the night before, however there was no record of any checks on the patient for 10 hours.

Timothy Martin (Australia)   (Based on a true story.)

In this case study, multiple errors were identified including the failure to follow policies concerning blood transfusions by staff as well as ineffective clinical governance. This is known as a *systems error*, an event that has occurred as a result of multiple cracks in the system in addition to any mistakes by individuals. The Swiss cheese model (**Fig. 1.5.1**) is a commonly used representation of these errors. The holes in the cheese must align for the error to occur. In other words, multiple organisational safeguards must fail for the event to have occurred.

The area of patient safety, a domain of clinical governance, is a relatively recent area of focus. In the United Kingdom the issue of *medical or iatrogenic error* was highlighted in the Bristol Royal Infirmary Inquiry following the revelation of poor outcomes in congenital heart surgery for a group of babies. The formal reporting of clinical outcomes was initiated in a number of speciality areas, especially in surgery, in an attempt to reduce the incidence of medical error, thereby improving the quality of patient care.

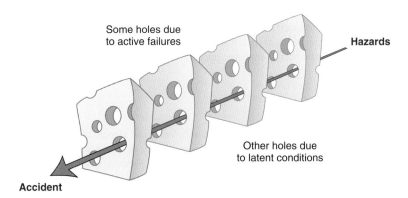

Successive layers of defences

Figure 1.5.1 **The Swiss cheese model.** *(Redrawn from Reason J: Human error: models and management. BMJ 320(7237):768–770, 2000.)*

Clinical governance

The process of *clinical governance* (**Fig. 1.5.2**) has been implemented in many countries. Responsibility for patient safety and quality control lies with the entire health care team as well as with the leadership. Health care workers are often overworked in an underresourced setting, and so those people with more time, including health care students, should also identify deficiencies and bring them to the attention of colleagues.

Effective clinical governance requires a diverse number of inputs to improve the quality of patient care.

A number of common tools are used to identify, evaluate and implement care in the local health care setting. A common template is the *plan–do–study–act* structure. This is a four-stage process entailing:

- *Plan*: Research the issue, develop objectives and plan the intervention.
- *Do*: Implement the intervention.
- *Study*: Monitor and evaluate the intervention.
- *Act*: Integrate the lessons learnt from the first three stages to improve the intervention.
- *Repeat*!

The instruments commonly used to identify issues or learn from an acute incident include root cause analyses and critical incident reports. For more complex scenarios, a method used regularly is the *theory of change*. This is an outcomes-based framework designed to facilitate the mapping of short-term and medium-term achievements to reach a long-term goal. Connections between objectives must be reasoned and testable.

A salient feature of all evaluation tools is that they are designed to promote logical, structured analysis of the issue and how to go about fixing it. The tool most universally used to evaluate performance in health care is the clinical audit.

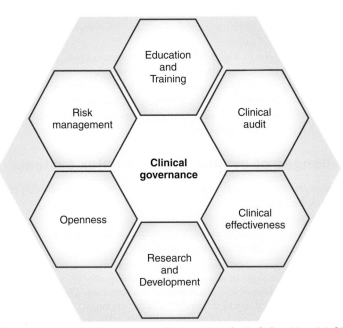

Figure 1.5.2   The domains of clinical governance. *(Redrawn from Scally G, Donaldson LJ: Clinical governance and the drive for quality improvement in the new NHS in England. BMJ 317:61–65, 1998.)*

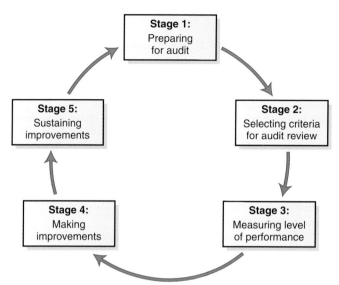

Figure 1.5.3 **The audit cycle.** *(Redrawn from Scally G, Donaldson LJ: Clinical governance and the drive for quality improvement in the new NHS in England. BMJ 317:61–65, 1998.)*

The audit cycle

An audit is a process that aims to compare what occurs in practice with the standards set by a particular organisation, with the end goal of improving care. A key difference between research and audit is that the purpose of an audit is to measure performance against current best practice, whereas the purpose of research is to identify best practice (in other words, the addition of new knowledge). The process of auditing is continuous, and improvements must be sustained and reanalysed through repeated audits.

The audit cycle is shown in **Fig. 1.5.3**. As an example, a hospital might have a policy that outlines a target of 90% of patients in hospital longer than 4 days should be receiving deep vein thrombosis prophylaxis. An audit designed to assess practice might involve the retrospective review of patients' records to find out what percentage of patients received care in line with the policy. As a result, changes might be made to improve practice. To complete the audit cycle, the effects of these changes must be further audited.

The challenges of evaluation in complex systems

As health systems are complex, large, unwieldy and unpredictable, any evaluation of health system performance is challenging.

Managing emergency departments in Australia

Overcrowding in emergency departments (EDs) is a common phenomenon. It has been shown to cause a significant increase in mortality, reduction in quality of care, increase in adverse events and errors, and delayed investigations and interventions. There are multiple ways of evaluating this problem and its impacts as shown in this example.

The causes of ED overcrowding are complex. Overcrowding occurs when the number of patients presenting is consistently greater than the number discharged from the ED or admitted to hospital. In Australia, the reasons for increasing presentation include an ageing population, complex medical needs, reduced access to after-hours family doctors and the increased community recognition of mental illness. Funding arrangements that might favour simple elective surgical procedures over complex care may also contribute.

The solution to this problem does not necessarily require an increase in the number of EDs as any subsequent increase in capacity may lead to a further increase in demand. The fundamental problem in this example is access block: patients who need to be admitted to hospital are kept in the ED because of a lack of free acute inpatient beds. This is a problem of ward occupancy, a symptom of hospital-wide overcrowding/dysfunction rather than one focused on EDs.

Timothy Martin (Australia)

Leadership and evaluation

'If your actions inspire others to dream more, learn more, do more and become more, you are a leader.'

John Quincy Adams

Most health care organisations aim to continually develop and improve the care they provide. However, episodes of poor care still occur, and inefficient, costly or ineffective interventions are still used in the absence of an institutional culture of regular self-evaluation. A disengaged leadership exacerbates this scenario. A leadership team that operates with integrity and transparency, whilst fostering an environment that supports positive change, is likely to develop happier staff and lead to improved outcomes. To be effective, performance evaluation must be conducted in a nonjudge-mental and generally blame-free way. In such a constructive environment, the focus is on the patient and ensuring the patient receives the best care possible.

Conclusion

Appropriate monitoring and evaluation of all health strategies is essential if the quality of patient care is to be improved. The ability to direct limited resources in an appropriate manner is facilitated by a detailed appreciation of the tools available to evaluate the variety of factors which affect health care provision.

KEY POINTS

- Appreciate the importance of health care evaluation in improving patient outcomes and as a form of social accountability
- Consider the varied domains which are required for effective evaluation
- Understand the strengths, weaknesses, bias and consequences of some common indicators and consider the challenges of selecting indicators
- Appreciate the difficulty of implementing change in complex systems
- Recognise the crucial role of leadership and organisational culture in promoting an efficient and effective system that values continued improvement

Further reading

Bauman A, Nutbeam D: *Evaluation in a nutshell: a practical guide to the evaluation of health promotion programs*, ed 2, Sydney, 2014, McGraw-Hill Education.

Berwick DM: Continuous improvement as an ideal in health care, *N Engl J Med* 320:53–56, 1989.

World Health Organization: *Patient safety*, 2017. <http://www.who.int/topics/patient_safety/en/>.

Health Care Provision

Junior Editor: Renzo Guinto (Philippines)

Introduction

Access to basic health care services remains a huge challenge in many parts of the world. It is estimated that nearly 1 billion people *never* see a health worker in their lives, whilst a third of the world's population lacks access to essential medicines. Each year, 150 million people suffer financial catastrophe, and about 100 million are pushed into poverty because of out-of-pocket payments for medical care. Poorly designed health systems can be drivers of health inequities and injustice.

Health care provision, whilst very technical and practical, is also deeply political. The way services are designed, funded and delivered is shaped by policies that are dictated by the larger social, political and economic context. This makes health care systems potentially vulnerable to personal interests and changing agendas.

Health is not solely determined by health care systems. However, transforming the provision of health care remains a fundamental aspect of improving global health. Health systems, if they are to meet the emerging health needs of a rapidly changing world, require innovation and imagination as well as a firm commitment to the principles of human rights, equity and social justice.

2.1 Health Systems

Xiaoxiao Jiang (China)　■　Sebastian Schmidt (Germany)

'The health of a mother and child is a more telling measure of a nation's state than economic indicators.'

Harjit Gill, CEO, Philips ASEAN and Pacific

The World Health Organization (WHO) defines a health system as *'the sum total of all the organizations, institutions and resources whose primary purpose is to improve health.'* The scope of this definition is extremely broad, encompassing initiatives relating to the underlying determinants of health (see Chapter 4.1) as well as to more direct health-related interventions. The importance of health systems is being increasingly recognised. The tendency to favour vertical, disease-specific interventions is being replaced by initiatives which broadly strengthen health systems.

A number of models have been postulated in an attempt to monitor the efficacy of health systems. Two models of particular interest are those developed by the WHO and by the Harvard School of Public Health. The WHO model (**Fig. 2.1.1**) divides health systems into six building blocks.

The components of a health system

The WHO definition mandates that many organisations and institutions must work together to create effective health systems. At a global level, the WHO, health-oriented international non-governmental organisations (NGOs) and various bilateral aid agencies cite health promotion as their main mission. At national level, the ministry of health is a primary player, although private sector initiatives, including pharmaceutical companies, may contribute significantly to health care. Other sectors closely interact with the health system; for example, agriculture (food production), transport (access to health care, spread of infection) and education (dissemination of knowledge about health). Their primary purpose is not health care but, nevertheless, as recognised in the WHO 'six building blocks model', they should be considered when health issues are being analysed and addressed.

The Harvard School of Public Health model further emphasises the major interactions within a health system and defines so-called control knobs. These elements (finance, payment controls, organisational issues, regulatory issues and behaviours) significantly affect the ability of a health system to deliver quality, efficiency and access to patients.

World Health Organization model (Fig. 2.1.1)

Goals of a well-functioning health system

The goals in the WHO model are improved health, responsiveness, social and financial risk protection and improved efficiency:

- ■ *Improved health* incorporates an improved overall level of health, as demonstrated by measures of premature death and morbidity. A well-functioning health system ensures that

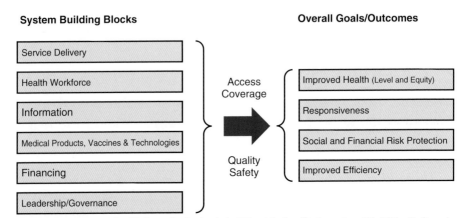

Figure 2.1.1   The World Health Organization's six building blocks. *(Redrawn from World Health Organization: Everybody's business: strengthening health systems to improve health outcomes; WHO's framework for action, Geneva, 2017, World Health Organization. Available from <http://www.who.int/healthsystems/strategy/everybodys_business.pdf>.)*

health benefits are shared equitably across the population, minimising the ever-increasing gap between rich and poor.

■ *Responsiveness* refers to the way in which the health system responds to the reasonable expectations of the population. It discounts the public expectation for improved health, as that is covered in the first goal. It focuses more on patient/service user satisfaction in areas such as personal respect and patient-centred care. Ethical considerations such as confidentiality, dignity, autonomy and patient choice are integral to this goal.

■ *Social and financial risk protection* targets the risk of causing poverty or destitution as a result of health care expenditure. Protection may be achieved through the pooling of financial risk in a number of different ways (see Chapter 2.2).

■ *Improved efficiency* involves facilitation of the progress towards health system goals within the given resources. It is important that efficiency outcomes are not achieved at the expense of other goals such as equity.

Health systems can also be measured against *cross–system goals*, where the effect of the health system on education, economic productivity or democratic participation is considered. Increased investment in health leads to increased economic productivity.

System building blocks

■ *Service delivery*

Health services need to be delivered in ways that are accessible to the population wherever they live. To make a positive contribution to the health of individuals and populations, services must be effective, efficient, appropriate and timely. If a service does not fulfil these criteria, patients are unlikely to accept or to access it. A good health care service delivery system needs to understand the demand for the service, have the appropriate packages of integrated service, have a well-functioning network of providers, ensure good management and supervision, and establish and maintain effective infrastructure and logistics.

■ *Health workforce*

Human resources are the backbone of a health system. The health workforce comprises all whose primary intent is to provide, protect and improve health. The critical shortage of health care workers makes the strengthening of this health system building block particularly important.

■ *Information*
Access to information, both for professionals and for patients, is a critical component of effective health systems. Health policies and interventions need to be based on sound evidence, especially when new technologies are being adopted. The WHO has an important surveillance role in global health. It provides contemporary data on the global burden of disease which can be used to evaluate health system performance (see Chapter 1.3).

■ *Medical products, vaccines and technologies*
Medical products (drugs, medical devices and vaccines) all play vital roles in prevention, diagnosis, treatment and palliation. An effective health system needs to ensure safe and efficient use of these products by establishing norms, regulating procurement processes, and providing financial support in the research and development (R & D), production, transportation and use of all medical products.

Mobile and new technologies play important and innovative roles in health care delivery, both in resource-rich settings and in remote and poor communities where human resources are scarce.

■ *Health system financing*
Health care provision is expensive, and a health system will inevitably be dysfunctional in the absence of appropriate funding. There are different funding models (see Chapter 2.2).

■ *Leadership and governance*
A system with good leadership continually innovates and strives for quality in all areas of health care. Effective organisations and systems empower all staff to be leaders and to bring about positive change.

Health in UK general practice
This experience describes how a small UK general practice made use of mobile technology to improve the efficiency of its service delivery, and some of the challenges it encountered.

'Through use of mobile messaging (SMS) we sent appointments to patients, and established an online access forum through which patients can register, book or cancel appointments and request repeat medication.'

Some patients preferred to speak to a doctor rather than use mobile technology, whilst some patients without Internet access were disadvantaged. Overall, clinic attendance and patient experience improved.

Elizabeth Tomlinson (UK)

Measuring health system performance

The measurement of health system performance is complex but the WHO has produced standard tools to facilitate this exercise. *The World Health Report 2000* was a seminal document in which the health systems of most countries were ranked. Unfortunately, inaccuracies and deficiencies of national datasets discredited this document and caused particular offence to countries such as Brazil (which is ranked 125th in the world). More recently, increasing health demands and economic austerity have led to a resurgence of interest in attempts to measure health system performance. The Organisation for Economic Co-operation and Development has measured 40 health quality indicators and noted that quality-led governance of health systems is an essential feature of high-performing systems. Additionally, the Council of the European Union (2013) has recommended that health system performance assessment should be implemented for 'policymaking, accountability and transparency'.

World Health Organization's *The World Health Report 2000*

The World Health Report 2000: Health Systems: Improving Performance, was delivered by the World Health Organization and compared 191 health systems around the world using key performance measures. Variations between countries resulted in key policy changes.

The five performance measures were population health, health inequalities, health system responsiveness, distribution of responsiveness within the population and distribution of the health system's financial burden.

Countries with similar characteristics in terms of income and health expenditure demonstrated major variation in health system performance. The USA, a country with the highest spending on health care expenditure (as a proportion of GDP), had a lower life expectancy than Japan and Cuba, both of which spent significantly less of their GDP on health care.

Problems in health systems resulted in inappropriate or inadequate utilisation of resources. The poor were particularly disadvantaged when health systems were inefficient. The report recommended that more people should be covered by health insurance in order to share the financial risk and increase access to health care. Some health systems, for example those in China and Mexico, implemented reforms including a huge expansion of insurance coverage. This improved equity of public health expenditure and access to health care.

Alexandra Peterson (USA/UK)

External influences on health systems

Health systems do not function in isolation, and complex nonhealth factors can result in failure. It is estimated that health ministers can only influence about 20% of the population's health—the remaining 80% is dependent on other factors, which include finance, agriculture, education and private sector influence. Global challenges, such as climate change, conflict and terrorism, migration and trade inequities, all place significant pressures on health systems. The health systems under greatest pressure are the most vulnerable and therefore the most sensitive to such external forces.

Conclusion

Health systems are increasingly becoming the focus of global health development initiatives. The interplay between the different building blocks of a health system is complex. Innovation is essential: many of the world's health systems are failing (on many levels) to meet the basic needs of their population.

KEY POINTS

- Health systems aim to improve the health of individuals and populations.
- Analysis of the building blocks and interdependencies within health systems facilitates the optimal allocation and use of resources.
- It is essential to measure health system performance and innovate accordingly.

Further reading

EuroREACH: *Controls knobs*, 2010–2013. <http://www.healthdatanavigator.eu/performance/frameworks/control-knobs>.

Reich MR, Takemi K, Roberts MJ, Hsiao WC: Global action on health systems: a proposal for the Toyako G8 summit, *Lancet* 371:865–869, 2008.

World Health Organization: *Everybody's business: strengthening health systems to improve health outcomes: WHO's framework for action*, Geneva, 2007, World Health Organization. Available from: <http://www.who.int/healthsystems/strategy/everybodys_business.pdf>.

World Health Organization: *Monitoring the building blocks of health systems: a handbook of indicators and their measurements strategies*, Geneva, 2010, World Health Organization. Available from: <http://www.who.int/healthinfo/systems/WHO_MBHSS_2010_full_web.pdf?ua=1>.

2.2 Health Sectors

Gerald Makuka (Tanzania) ■ Vita Sinclair (UK)

> 'You can't have public health without working with the public sector. You can't have public education without working with the public sector in education.'
> **Paul Farmer, Cofounder and Chief Strategist, Partners in Health**

Health sectors group together organisations concerned with the design and delivery of health care services. They encompass public and private sectors as well as NGOs and patient groups. These sectors differ in financing, philosophy and accountability.

Public sector

The *public sector* refers to health care provision delivered by the state (**Table 2.2.1**). The responsibility for publicly provided health care lies with the government. This system aims to provide the maximum benefit to most people, including vulnerable groups (children, the elderly and the unemployed). Common criticism levied at state-delivered health care is that it can be inefficient and slow to respond to changing demands. It also may prioritise the needs of the population over those of the individual. State involvement in health care, though controversial, places health as a 'public good'. All individuals, when healthy, can work and contribute to society for the benefit of all.

The public sector provides health care through general taxation or public insurance. As payment is compulsory, tax-based systems are more efficient than some of the voluntary insurance markets, which may be expensive to administer. The amount of funding allocated to the national health budget from general taxation is a political decision; this may not be adequate for the true health needs of the population.

Some countries (e.g., France, Germany, Switzerland, Indonesia) have a social health insurance system whereby the public make regular contributions to a government insurance fund which is exclusively allocated for health care provision. Individuals with low incomes are provided with health cover free of charge.

In these systems, individuals are reimbursed by the fund for previously agreed services. An advantage of this approach is that the operation of the insurance fund tends to be in line with government health policy goals, yet it maintains a degree of independence from the politics of government. Proponents of such systems argue that they are more efficient than tax-based systems. Money is allocated to health regardless of actual expenditure, so any residual profit can be invested to grow the fund. Disadvantages of this system include higher administrative costs and problems reaching disenfranchised individuals. Some lower middle-income countries (LMICs), for example India, use community-based health insurance schemes based on smaller pools of individuals. These may prove to be precursors of national social health insurance schemes.

Entirely publicly funded health systems are uncommon. Cuba is a rare example of a country with such a system. All health services have been delivered by the state since the revolution in

TABLE 2.2.1 ■ **Public sector summary**

Provider	Financing	Accountability	Population served	Examples
The state	Taxation, public insurance	The electorate	Typically high percentage of population	UK, Canada, Cuba, Tanzania, Ghana, France, Germany, Sweden, Malaysia, Brazil

1959. Patients have reduced choice about where they access services, but all citizens can obtain free health care. Surprisingly, health outcomes are significantly better than in other countries in the region. As an example, infant mortality is lower than in the USA (4.2 versus 6.0 per 1000).

Cuba has achieved these outcomes through substantial investment in medical training. It has the second highest doctor-to-patient ratio in the world, and concentrates on training doctors for primary health care (PHC). It is mandatory for most doctors to spend at least 1 year in a rural health post. Cuba has exported large numbers of doctors to other low-income countries (LICs), for example Venezuela and Mozambique, and its health system is much admired internationally for exceptional health outcomes and value for money.

Private sector

Private providers of health care deliver services for profit (**Table 2.2.2**). Patients pay for services using either point-of-service out-of-pocket payments or by taking out private health insurance. In private health insurance schemes, premiums are based on the estimated future costs of providing health services to them; those with increased medical needs pay more. In contrast to social health insurance schemes, premiums are related to an individual's ability to pay.

The private sector in India

India has a population of about 1.32 billion, and 60%–70% of people are urban and rural poor. The main provider of health care is the private sector. Health care needs to be affordable and accessible.

These aspirations are addressed through a 'hub-and-spoke' distribution of services. Rural outposts form the spokes, and tertiary hospitals the hubs. Rural hubs see a high volume of cases at low cost, and tertiary centres become very efficient at performing complex health care interventions. Pricing structures mean that profits from wealthy patients can be used to subsidise the care of poorer ones.

The efficacy of the hub-and-spoke mechanism hinges in large part on innovative use of resources. The concept of *task sharing*, whereby lay and mid-level health care professionals undertake clinical tasks previously allocated to more expensive medical staff, contributes to improved clinical and financial productivity.

Life expectancy in India increased from 63.7 years in 2004 to 68.5 years in 2016, with a concomitant reduction in infant mortality from 57.9 to 40.5 per 1000 births. Some of the principles implemented in the Indian health care system may facilitate the journey towards universal health coverage.

Vita Sinclair (UK) and Gerald Makuka (Tanzania)

TABLE 2.2.2 ■ **Private sector summary**

Provider	Financing	Accountability	Population served	Examples
Private industry	Point of service, private insurance	CEO/shareholders	Typically small percentage of population	USA, many countries have partial private provision

In many high-income countries, the private health sector supplements an established public sector. Individuals opt for private care to obtain shorter waiting times and more personalised care. In less economically developed countries, the private sector may be the mainstay of health care provision. Private health care provision is primarily available to individuals who can afford direct payments or insurance premiums. Many uninsured patients either forgo access to health care or face catastrophic health expenditure. A criticism of private insurance schemes is that they may promote inappropriate investigations and price escalation.

> *'The need to pay out-of-pocket can also mean that households do not seek care when they need it. An analysis of 108 surveys in 86 countries has revealed that catastrophic payments are incurred by less than 1% of households in some countries and up to 13% in others. Up to 5% of households are pushed into poverty as a result of costs associated with illness'*

WHO, 2015

In the USA, where the private health care system is funded primarily by private insurance, 17.1% of GDP was spent on health care in 2014, compared with 9.1% in the UK and 11.1% in Cuba (World Bank data). High health care expenditure is commonly seen in systems based on private insurance payments as neither clinicians nor patients are directly responsible for health care costs.

Nongovernmental organisations

NGOs may be small local charities or large international organisations (**Table 2.2.3**). They typically function in LICs where there are unmet health needs, for example in rural or poor urban areas, following natural disasters and in war zones. NGOs normally provide free or highly subsidised health care. Critics of NGOs, especially of some larger international organisations, allege that their goals are not always aligned with local health care needs (**Table 2.2.4**). Donors often demand short-term answers, and funding may disproportionally favour the treatment of certain diseases (e.g., malaria, HIV infection) to the detriment of others. An example of an effective NGO which operates in 37 countries is Marie Stopes International. This delivers sexual and reproductive health interventions, and has become an established and *integrated* part of health systems in high-income countries and LMICs.

TABLE 2.2.3 ■ **Summary of nongovernmental organisations**

Provider	Financing	Accountability	Population served	Examples
Nongovernmental organisations	Donations from individuals, government, industry	Trustees	Often target underserved groups	Marie Stopes, Macmillan Cancer nurses, Médecins Sans Frontières, Tropical Health and Education Trust

TABLE 2.2.4 ■ Benefits and criticisms of nongovernmental organisations

	Public sector	Private sector	Nongovernmental organisations
Benefits	Provision for vulnerable populations More able to pool risk	Can lead to more innovation through competition and response to market forces May be more cost-efficient	Serve those unable to pay Fill gaps in services
Criticisms	Inefficient Slow to change	Typically serves a smaller portion of the population Can compound inequality	Not democratically elected Can skew funding

Patient groups

Improved access to communications technology and changing attitudes towards patient involvement in health care are responsible for the significant growth of the patient sector. Patient and client groups can provide clinical services, educate patients, change policy and support research. The role of patient groups is often informal, although increasingly, formalised channels are emerging which enable patient groups to contribute to service design. In Brazil, for example, it is mandatory for 50% of seats on health councils to be held by representatives of patient groups or NGOs. The following case study details patient involvement in health care in Botswana.

Public health care in Botswana: involving the community

Botswana is an example of an upper middle income country which has made great strides in delivering publicly provided primary health care, accessible to all, with particular emphasis on community involvement.

Botswana covers 225,000 square miles, nearly 70% of which is rural desert. Health care is delivered almost exclusively at the village level through small government-run clinics. The country's health strategy focuses primarily on prevention through services such as HIV testing and high blood pressure screening.

Crucial to this strategy is the encouragement of health-seeking behaviour. The government has developed structures to increase community participation in health care delivery, integrating the patient and public sectors. Botswana also has a parallel system of traditional health practitioners who operate outside the government services.

Attached to each clinic is a village health committee which comprises local residents who liaise between villagers, clinic workers and politicians. Mobile clinics visit patients living more than 8 km from a clinic on a monthly basis. Patients can raise issues through suggestion boxes available at the clinics or at committee meetings. Similar structures exist for the district as well as nationally. This encourages responsive service design at all levels.

Vita Sinclair (UK) and Gerald Makuka (Tanzania)

Patient groups provide a personal connection to the experience of ill health and can thereby help to influence health care policies Patients and their families contribute actively to care delivery, for instance by changing dressings and contributing to nursing care.

Interactions between sectors

Most countries use a mixture of public, private and nongovernmental sectors in health care provision. These sectors have begun to interact in new ways in response to evolving challenges. Public–private partnerships combine the private sector's ability to respond to changing market forces more efficiently and the public sector's drive to ensure equality of access.

GAVI, the Vaccine Alliance, is arguably the largest public–private partnership created to date. It is responsible for an estimated 370 million childhood vaccinations since its inception. GAVI combines the WHO, the World Bank, the Bill & Melinda Gates Foundation and many more industry and governmental stakeholders. It uses public and charitable financing to provide a market for private sector expertise in vaccine development and distribution.

Conclusion

The health sector landscape is complex. The contrasting political ideologies lead national governments to place differing emphasis on attributes such as equity, efficiency, access and innovation. Consequently, no two countries have the same health care system. The interaction between different health care sectors differs between countries, and therefore an international uniform approach to health care provision is unrealistic.

KEY POINTS

* Health care can be delivered and funded in many different ways.
* Delivery of health care is improved when the various health care sectors work collaboratively.
* Patient groups may facilitate equity of access to local and national health care needs.

Further reading

Boslaugh SE: *Healthcare systems around the world, a comparative guide*, Thousand Oaks, 2013, Sage Publications.

Wood C, Ngatia P, Nyakwana T, et al: *Community health*, ed 3, Nairobi, 2008, African Medical and Research Foundation.

World Health Organization: *Country cooperation strategy 2014-2020: Botswana*, Brazzaville, 2014, World Health Organization, Regional Office for Africa. Available from: <http://apps.who.int/iris/handle/10665/246289>.

2.3 Universal Health Coverage

John Jefferson Besa (Philippines)　　Renzo Guinto (Philippines)

'I regard universal health coverage as the single most powerful concept that public health has to offer. It is inclusive. It unifies services and delivers them in a comprehensive and integrated way, based on primary health care.'

Margaret Chan, former WHO Director General

Introduction

The goal of universal health coverage (UHC) is to ensure that all people obtain the health services they need without suffering financial hardship. The WHO constitution declares that the 'highest attainable standard of health' is a fundamental human right. Equity of access to health care, regardless of financial background or geographical location, is a fundamental goal of health care provision. Progress towards UHC is still slow, and inequities exist in most health care systems. Barriers to achieving UHC include out-of-pocket payments, unaffordable transport costs and an inability to take paid leave from work to attend health care facilities.

History of universal health coverage

The beginnings of UHC can be traced back to the 'sickness funds' established in Germany in the 1880s under Otto von Bismarck. Employers and employees were required to contribute to a sick fund which made agreements with doctors and hospitals for the provision of services; however, not everyone was covered. A number of countries (Austria, Hungary, Norway, Denmark, Sweden, Russia, Chile, Spain, Portugal, Greece, France, Sweden, Finland and Australia) followed this path. In these countries, health care provision evolved mechanisms to ensure a certain level of access for the whole population—either by taxation or by part-financing by social insurance (see Chapter 2.2). Countries with significant progress towards UHC are depicted in **Fig. 2.3.1**.

Dimensions of universal health coverage

When considering UHC, three fundamental questions arise (**Fig. 2.3.2**):

1. *Who is covered?* Are all individuals covered or just those enrolled in a national insurance scheme? What about spouses and children?
2. *Which services are covered?* Are only a few selected *'essential'* services covered? Is *comprehensive* health care provision delivered?
3. *What proportion of the cost is covered?* Is only a small proportion of the cost covered? Are a wide range of or only a select few services covered?

Fig. 2.3.2 demonstrates the inevitable compromises that governments must consider between the three dimensions when working towards UHC. No high-income countries that are commonly

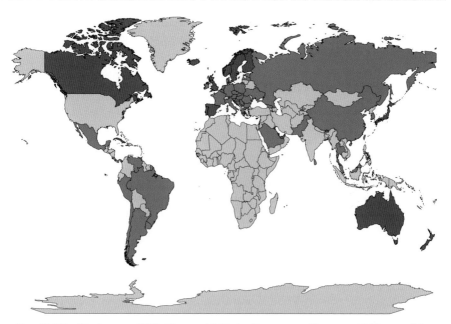

Key: BLUE = Single payer UHC, Green = UHC via other means, Grey = no UHC or no data.

Figure 2.3.1 Universal health coverage *(UHC)*. *(Redrawn from Fig. 1 in Garrett L, Chowdhury A, Pablos-Méndez A: All for universal health coverage, Lancet 2009, 374(9697):1294–1299, 2009.)*

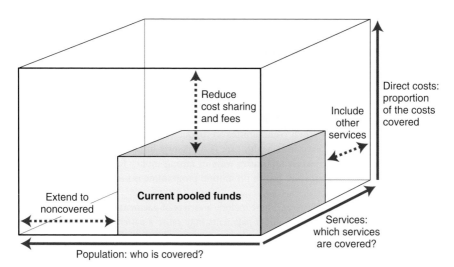

Three dimensions to consider when moving towards universal coverage

Figure 2.3.2 The three dimensions of universal health care. *(Redrawn from Fig. 1 in Waddington C, Sambo C: Financing health care for adolescents: a necessary part of universal health coverage, Bull World Health Organ 93:57–59, 2015.)*

said to have achieved UHC have covered 100% of the population for 100% of the possible health services for 100% of the cost. Attainment of UHC requires working towards improvements in each of the three dimensions.

Strategies for universal health coverage

The WHO definition of UHC incorporates the objectives of equity of access to health services, quality and effective health services, and financial-risk protection. For countries striving to achieve UHC, these objectives can be related to the following common core principles:

- *Reduced out-of-pocket spending.* Also known as *direct payments*, this refers to the exchange of money between the patient and the health care provider at the point of care. These may be official payments such as co-payments or deductibles, or unofficial under-the-table payments where health care providers demand an additional bribe to deliver care. UHC aims to reduce these kinds of payments so that people can access health services when needed, regardless of their ability to pay at the point of care.
- *Increased prepayment.* In a prepayment system, funds to pay for health care services are collected in advance of care being accessed. In general, resources are collected from households, organisations and companies. Funds may also be obtained from outside the country (external sources). Financial resources can be received via taxation (general or specific) or by compulsory or voluntary health insurance contributions. In this way, health care is free or subsidised at the point of access. This delivers a more progressive system whereby wealthier individuals support those who otherwise could not afford health care.
- *Risk pooling (fund pooling).* This refers to the management of financial resources in such a way that financial risk is shared amongst the population. Personal bankruptcy can therefore be avoided in those individuals who might otherwise not access essential medical care. Fund pooling requires a prepayment system and thus provides a service to all, free at the point of access.

Barriers to universal health coverage

Progress in achieving UHC in many parts of the world is slow. *The World Health Report* from 2010 on health systems financing identified three fundamental, interconnected problems impeding progress:

- *Availability of resources.* Health resources encompass medicines, health technologies and health care providers. Rural communities are frequently unable to access these resources, and the provision of accessible health care is frequently limited as a result of inadequate funding. Some countries use innovative ways of raising money for health care. For example, in Thailand a progressive health promotion programme is funded by high taxation on alcohol and tobacco.
- *Overreliance on direct payments.* These include a variety of payments additional to any health insurance co-payments. Such direct payments may cause a patient to delay a consultation or lead to catastrophic expenditure in order to procure treatment. They may inappropriately force an individual to choose between health expenditure and other essentials such as food or education.
- *Inefficient and inequitable use of resources.* It is estimated that 20%–40% of health resources are wasted. Examples of wastage and inefficiencies include the use of expensive medicines when cheaper alternatives are available, and irrational antibiotic prescription. Other inefficiencies are listed in **Box 2.3.1**.

Reducing waste and improving efficiency increases the quality of care provided and also allows ministries of health to lobby more effectively for health care funding.

BOX 2.3.1 ■ Inefficiencies in resource utilisation

Improper storage of medicines
Provision of unnecessary services
Underutilisation of available technologies
Inefficient systems in health care institutions
Lack of motivation of health care workers due to poor salary
Medical errors of health care professionals

The role of health financing in universal health coverage

Health financing involves the mobilisation, accumulation and allocation of money for health care. This ensures the health needs of individuals and, at the same time, creates financial incentives for providers.

Effective system organisation and resource allocation is fundamental to the advancement of UHC. Health care may be directly provided by the government, purchased from a separate agency (known as *purchaser–provider split*), or paid for directly by the individual (out-of-pocket spending). To protect people from financial catastrophe in the event of unexpected illness, payment for health services must be made in advance. In practice, this means that public sector provision (either through taxation or through social/community insurance systems) is an essential component if UHC is to be achieved. Private insurance can also contribute to this goal, but this relies on the ability of individuals to afford premiums. Direct payment systems leave those unable to pay at serious risk of being unable to access essential health care.

The notion of equity of access to health care lies at the core of UHC. Public sector health care provision is most successful at achieving equity. However, critics of such provision argue that it is inefficient and does not incentivise innovation and high-quality care. Governments have attempted to engage market forces so as to improve efficiency and promote innovation in the provision of health care. Private providers may be more effective at incentivising health care workers, thereby retaining staff and reducing health worker migration. Private health care providers may face a conflict of interest potentially resulting in overinvestigation and treatment of patients for financial gain. As a result, various countries have evolved safeguards designed to promote equity and avoid inappropriate expenditure:

- *Price scheduling*: the government, or other regulatory body, stipulates both a maximum price and a minimum price that can be charged for a particular service. This helps to protect individuals from excessive charges.
- *Capitation*: all providers receive a predetermined fee for patients which may vary according to age, sex or area of residence. Patients are free to change their nominated provider on an annual basis. However, the quality of care may be compromised as the provider is already guaranteed payment for each registered individual.
- *Case payment*: a fee is received for each case treated. Case payments can be based either on a single flat rate per case (independent of diagnosis) or on case classification. The most popular case classification approach is the *diagnosis-related groups* system, with around 470 diagnostic groups. Diagnosis is recorded on discharge, after results of tests and interventions are known. Fees vary, and are based on the average treatment cost of the condition.
- *Global budget*: the provider receives a nominated sum of money for all of the health services it provides to eligible recipients during a given period. The budget may be fixed, or may vary depending on differences in morbidity. If the actual cost of health care delivery is higher than the allocated budget, the provider shoulders the shortfall, and if it is lower, the provider

keeps the profit. Providers may be tempted to substitute cheaper less effective interventions for higher-cost interventions. This concern is in part addressed by flexible budgets based on morbidity, implementation of quality control measures and promotion of competition between providers.

Tackling inequity in Cambodia

Cambodia's health equity fund is an example of an innovative way of ensuring health care provision for those who could not otherwise afford it.

Cambodia has lowered the burden of health costs on the poor and improved access to health services by promoting a number of health reforms:

1. establishment of official user fees
2. development of community-based health insurance
3. subcontracting of government health service delivery to nongovernmental providers

However, fee exemption systems were failing to protect the vulnerable poor, who were excluded from access to health services because of cost. In response to this, a health equity fund was established. This is a financing package, funded by a combination of government, communities and development partners, to purchase health care for those who cannot otherwise afford it. It has been efficient and effective in reducing inequalities and expanding health service coverage.

John Jefferson Besa and Renzo Guinto (Philippines)

Primary health care and universal health coverage

'Primary health care is essential health care based on practical, scientifically sound and socially acceptable methods and technology made universally accessible to individuals and families in the community through their full participation and at a cost that the community and country can afford to maintain at every stage of their development in the spirit of self-reliance and self-determination.'

Declaration of Alma-Ata, 1978

UHC grew out of the concept of primary health care (PHC)—a term which was coined in the Declaration of Alma-Ata. PHC emerged in response to growing global health inequities. It moved the focus away from biomedical discovery towards community-based health care. PHC included basic public health interventions, immunisation programmes and the treatment and prevention of common illnesses. The Declaration of Alma-Ata set out PHC as a *multisectoral* issue. This extended beyond classical health care boundaries to include community and national issues. It grew out of a recognition that huge inequities exist in health status within and between countries. There was a significant emphasis on enabling communities to become self-reliant. The declaration called strongly for international collaboration in working towards PHC, recognising that improved health of other communities and nations has a positive impact on local health outcomes.

Grassroots social movements played a key role in the rise of PHC. Activists were instrumental in advocating health as a human right. Although the declaration set an ambitious agenda, the goals were specific, measurable, achievable, realistic and timely. However, by 2000, PHC was weakened by the growing strength of market influences, vertical (disease-specific) health care programs and corporate interests.

Subsequently, the People's Health Movement (PHM) was formed as a global network of health activists, civil society organisations and academic institutions, particularly from LMICs. The PHM still aims to achieve comprehensive PHC whilst addressing the social, environmental and economic determinants of health. The movement works at the local, national and global levels through networks, coalitions, organisations and individuals focusing on specific campaigns in line with the People's Health Charter (formulated by the PHM).

Whilst the fundamental aims of UHC and PHC are very similar, it is possible that some UHC initiatives focused on hospital-based care for formal sector workers have led to underutilisation of PHC facilities. As UHC seems to be taking an increasingly prominent position in the post-2015 development agenda, it remains important that the two movements progress towards common goals.

A multisectoral approach to achieving universal health coverage

To achieve UHC, domestic sectors must collaborate with support from the international community. National governments have the most significant roles. They can make positive contributions by prioritising health and committing to appropriate health expenditure. Additionally, they can legislate, execute, monitor and evaluate programs, policies and laws that deal with the grassroots causes of health inequity. Governments also influence private health insurance provision through tax and regulatory policies. Ultimately, governments can direct other agencies to address the social determinants of health in pursuit of the goal of UHC.

The role of the private sector in achieving UHC is being increasingly recognised. Public and private sector collaborations harness the ability of the private sector to finance and provide health services, particularly in LICs and LMICs.

Civil society organisations are emerging key players in UHC. They incorporate a wide array of NGOs and not-for-profit organisations. Civil society organisations are advocates for the interests and values of their members or others, based on ethical, cultural, political, scientific, religious and philanthropic considerations. They help to promote accountability by government. They may advance UHC by lobbying the government at public events and through media campaigns and press conferences.

Social media for social justice

Social media offer a new and powerful advocacy tool in the 21st century. This example shows how civil society can harness social media to effect positive change towards universal health coverage.

In 2012 the Canadian Government, in an attempt to cut costs, announced a health service reform that would discontinue health care provision for a significant number of refugees and asylum seekers, forcing them to attend emergency departments. This led to huge costs for emergency department visits for uninsured individuals. In response, the Canadian Doctors for Refugee Care was established. It organised a public rally and a grassroots social media advocacy campaign to coincide with the 2013 National Day of Action. This enabled organisers to harness the provider-to-public reach of social media, broadcast factual information about what these policy changes meant for refugees and refugee claimants, and, ultimately, put pressure on policymakers to reverse the government's decision.

The impact of this campaign was profound as a result of widespread dissemination via social media. It garnered international attention in more than 30 countries and the message (#IFHjune17) reached millions of people. As a result of this campaign, the Ontario provincial government committed to reinstate appropriate coverage. This was an impressive demonstration of the power of civil society, acting through social media to campaign for universal health coverage.

Naheed Dosani, Latif Murji and Anjum Sultana (Canada)

Despite the efforts of governments, the private sector and local civil society organisations, poor countries are often unable to finance UHC. Thus support from the international community is essential. External partners must increase contributions to meet previously agreed international commitments. They may also be able to assist in the development and application of financial tools and systems, foster capacity building, support the establishment of reliable information and accounting systems, and share best practice in terms of revenue raising, risk pooling and purchasing systems. Support from the international community must be sustainable (thereby allowing developing partners to become reliably self-sufficient) before external support is reduced.

Conclusion

As countries recognise the links between unattainable health care costs and poverty, UHC has increasingly become an international priority. UHC is a prominent goal in the post-2015 development agenda, emphasised by strong support from the WHO for this aspiration.

KEY POINTS

- Health should be regarded as a universal human right.
- Personal (out-of-pocket) health care expenditure heightens the risk of poverty.
- Universal health coverage seeks to promote equity and quality in health care delivery.

Further reading

Declaration of Alma-Ata. International Conference on Primary Health Care, Alma-Ata, USSR, 6-12 September 1978. Available from: <http://www.who.int/publications/almaata_declaration_en.pdf>.

Kleinert S, Horton R: From universal health coverage to right care for health, *Lancet* 390(10090):101–102, 2017.

World Health Organization: *WHO | World Health Organization*, 2017. <http://www.who.int/>.

property legislation allows drug companies to retain exclusive patents for drug production for up to 25 years.

Diseases primarily affecting LICs and LMICs receive a disproportionately small amount of global R & D investment. Only 10% of investment is focused on diseases that affect 90% of people. In contrast, lifestyle ailments that affect wealthy populations attract far greater R & D investment. Ten times as much was spent on developing a cure for male baldness when compared with the cost of developing a cure for malaria. There is little investment in adapting medicines and technologies for resource-limited settings (e.g., lack of refrigeration causes vaccines to degrade in hot environments).

Alternative models

The Consultative Expert Working Group (CEWG) on Research and Development: Financing and Coordination was established by the WHO in 2010. It was tasked to analyse the current situation of R & D for health needs in developing countries as well as providing recommendations for better financing and coordination. This group recommended an alternative model based on the concept of *delinkage*: the costs of researching and developing a new drug were no longer to be directly retrieved through patented sales of that drug. In this model, governments would invest at least 0.01% of GDP in a pooled fund for global public goods, including medicines R & D. Incentives to promote innovation included prizes to be offered at different milestones in the R & D process.

A further financing strategy suggested the establishment of a health impact fund. Rewards were to be awarded to researchers on the basis of the health impact of the medicines that they developed. Both models seek to promote equity in access to affordable medicines whilst promoting innovation by manufacturers.

The CEWG report also proposed a new global health R & D observatory to improve cooperation, participation and coordination of health and biomedical R & D, thus avoiding unnecessary duplication of research initiatives.

The role of universities

Universities are institutions which create and disseminate knowledge for public benefit. They have a significant role to play in R & D, and account for between 25% and 33% of new medicines. They may be well placed to invest in R & D for challenges which appear to be unattractive to commercial entities.

As universities may lack the resources to undertake large-scale clinical trials or the manufacturing facilities necessary to commercialise promising therapies, they often license their medicine patents to pharmaceutical companies. The university then usually receives royalties from sales and can take steps to ensure that the fruits of research are accessible to those who are most in need. These include the adoption of socially responsible licensing policies, especially applicable to product sales in LICs and LMICs.

Universities Allied for Essential Medicines

Students have been at the forefront of improving access to the fruits of university-based medical research.

In 2001, inspired by the stark contrast in access to medicines amongst attendees at the World AIDS Conference in Durban, South Africa, a first-year law student returned to university and with others decided to take on a challenge that would set a precedent for placing health access above drug development. They led efforts that resulted in Yale University and Bristol-Myers Squibb permitting generic competition in sub-Saharan Africa (**Fig. 2.4.2**). This resulted in steep price reductions (30-fold) for stavudine (d4T), and supported the first HIV treatment clinic in sub-Saharan Africa. This catalysed

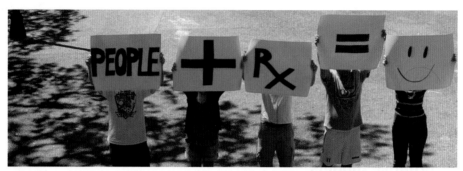

Figure 2.4.2 Universities Allied for Essential Medicines members promoting their message through effective use of symbols. © *Universities Allied for Essential Medicines.*

the profound transformation in the market for antiretroviral medications from high price, low volume to universal access. The campaign demonstrated the potency of students as agents of social change as well as the value of working within universities to influence change. Some of these student activists, went on to cofound the Universities Allied for Essential Medicines, a nongovernmental organisation that strives to promote the role of universities in contributing to greater global access to essential medicines through innovation and research.

Roopa Dhatt (USA)

Conclusion

Much progress has been made through the widespread adoption of the concept of *essential medicines*. The HIV/AIDS epidemic focused attention on issues of access, and unprecedented activism helped to dramatically reduce prices of antiretroviral medicines. Policy work and technical support by the WHO has created clear guidance for governments seeking best practice in the processes which improve access to essential medicines. Implementation of this guidance remains incomplete and, in some countries, access to essential medicines remains an elusive goal on the path to UHC on account of the double burden of communicable and noncommunicable diseases.

KEY POINTS

- The essential medicines list promotes the availability of appropriate treatments in low-income countries and lower middle-income countries.
- The development of medicines and their delivery to patients is an expensive and complex process.
- Improvements for underserved populations and health disorders can be achieved as a result of active lobbying by students, health workers and the public.
- The appropriate use of antibiotics is critically important.

Further reading

Antezana F, Seuba X: *Thirty years of essential medicines: the challenge*, Valencia, 2007, Farma Mundi.

't Hoen EFM: *The global politics of pharmaceutical monopoly power*, Diemen, 2009, AMB.

University of Manchester: *Who owns science? The Manchester manifesto*, 2009. Available from <http://www.isei.manchester.ac.uk/TheManchesterManifesto.pdf>.

World Health Organization: *The world medicines situation report 2011*, Geneva, 2011, World Health Organization.

World Health Organization: *Research and development to meet health needs in developing countries: strengthening global financing and coordination*, Geneva, 2012, World Health Organization. Available from: <http://www.who.int/phi/CEWG_Report_5_April_2012.pdf>.

2.5 The Health Workforce

Robbert Duvivier (Netherlands)

> *'We have to work together to ensure access to a motivated, skilled, and supported health worker by every person in every village everywhere.'*
>
> **Jong-Wook Lee, Former WHO Director General**

Introduction

The WHO defines the health workforce as 'all people engaged in actions whose primary intent is to enhance health'. This includes those who provide health services directly, (dentists, nurses, midwives and physicians) as well as allied health professions (including community health workers and social workers). It also includes those who help make the health system function (including health managers and support personnel). It may be referred to as *health human resources* or *human resources for health*. This area includes planning, development, performance, management, retention, information and research on human resources in the health care sector.

The health workforce crisis

Two reports were instrumental in putting the health workforce high on the global health agenda. Both emphasised a crisis—a shortage of health workers to deliver essential health services. In 2004 the Joint Learning Initiative (JLI)—a consortium of more than 100 health leaders—analysed the global health workforce and raised awareness about the importance of the health workforce in combating health disparities. *Working Together for Health* (WHO, 2006) suggested strategies to overcome the crisis at community, country and global levels.

Following the publication of these two reports, the Global Health Workforce Alliance (GHWA) was created in 2006. The GHWA is a partnership of national governments, civil society, international agencies, finance institutions, researchers, educators and professional associations. It serves as a common platform for action to address the workforce crisis through identifying, advocating and implementing solutions. Since its inception, the GHWA has convened three global forums (2008, 2011, 2013). The third global forum resulted in the report *A Universal Truth: No Health Without a Workforce* (2014), which is essential reading for clarification of the contemporary challenges in this area.

In 2013 the WHO estimated that there was a global shortage of 17.4 million health workers (WHO, 2016), with 83 countries facing a major shortage; this was most acute in sub-Saharan Africa. The health worker crisis was further accentuated by the rise in chronic health problems with comorbidities in the ageing population. Such pressures are further compounded by a lack of health care workers in rural areas and poor working conditions which encourage them to emigrate overseas. It is estimated that there will still be a vast shortage of healthcare workers in 2030 of about 14 million.

Addressing the challenges posed by deficiencies in the health workforce is now regarded as critical if health systems are to be strengthened and population health outcomes improved. 'Human resources are the most important of the health system's inputs. The performance of health care systems depends ultimately on the knowledge, skills and motivation of persons responsible for delivering services' (WHO).

Crisis due to undersupply and migration of health care workers

Counting health workers

The measurement of the numbers in the health care workforce is inconsistent across countries due to inadequate data collection and confusion regarding the definition of *health care workers*. There is no universal classification system for *health workers*. The WHO definition is given in **Table 2.5.1**.

Other professionals contribute to the protection and advancement of societal health, but their primary goal is not necessarily the improvement of health. These include police officers and primary school teachers as well as similar professional groups who are not included in the definition of the health workforce.

Other classifications of health care workers, for instance the International Standard Classification of Occupations, also used by the WHO via the Global Health Observatory, simplify the grouping of different workforce components for ease of data collection but fail to address major shortcomings of these data. WHO data are most complete for nurses and physicians, but there is little information about other health service providers.

The 2014 report *A Universal Truth: No Health Without a Health Worker* provides the following summary on the quality of the data sources used for the Global Health Observatory:

'Few countries have a comprehensive and valid information base on available health workers. The WHO Global Health Observatory reports workforce data for 186 countries, but 53% of these countries have fewer than seven annual data points on midwives, nurses and physicians across the past 20 years. Further, of the 57 countries identified in 2006 with low human resources for health density and low service coverage, 17 countries have no data point in the past five years.'

In 2013 there was a shortage of 7.2 million skilled health care workers, and this is predicted to rise to 12.9 million workers by 2035. A crisis in health worker provision may arise for many reasons, including the migration of trained staff to more affluent countries. In the United Kingdom and Ireland, around one-third of doctors were trained abroad, and this compares with 23% in Australia and 26% in the USA.

There are many economic, social and physical reasons for why people emigrate. Common threads in this process may be classified into 'push' and 'pull' factors. Push factors are those related to their country of origin, whereas pull factors are related to their destination of travel (**Table 2.5.2**).

The WHO Global Code of Practice on the International Recruitment of Health Personnel (2010) promotes principles and practices for ethical recruitment. It has been adopted by many

TABLE 2.5.1 ■ **World Health Organization health workforce**

Doctors	Health educators
Nurses	Family carers
Pharmacists	Dentists
Laboratory technicians	Physiotherapists
Traditional healers	Community health workers
Support workers (e.g,. catering and maintenance staff)	Management and clerical staff
Public health personnel	Health sector volunteers

Modified from WHO technical data on Global Health Workforce Statistics (2016). www.who.int.

TABLE 2.5.2 ■ Summary of push and pull factors that influence health worker migration

Push	Pull
Low pay (absolute or relative)	Higher pay
Poor working conditions	Opportunities for remittances
Lack of resources to work effectively	Better working conditions
Limited career opportunities	Better resourced health systems
Limited educational opportunities	Career opportunities
Impact of HIV/AIDS	Aid work
Unstable work environment	Political stability
Economic instability	Travel opportunities

Reproduced with permission from Buchan J, Sochalski J: Nurse migration: trends and policy options, Bull World Health Organ *82:587–594, 2004.*

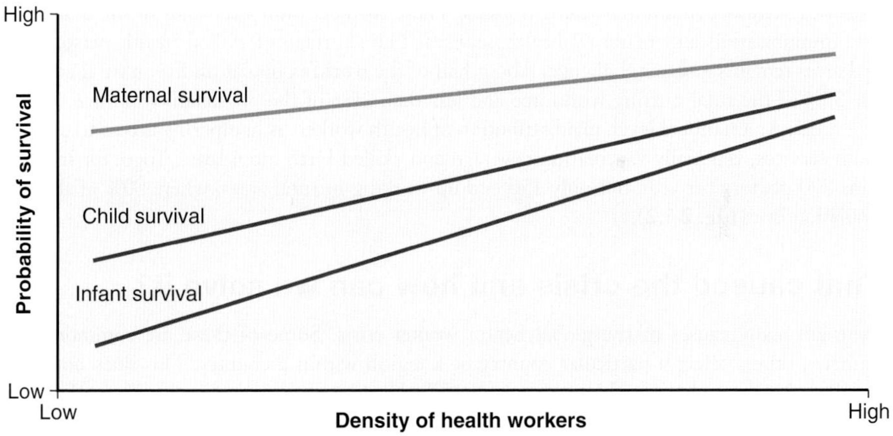

Figure 2.5.1   Density of health workers and health outcomes. *(Redrawn from Anyangwe SCE, Mtonga C: Inequities in the global health workforce: the greatest impediment to health in sub-Saharan Africa,* Int J Environ Res Public Health *4(2):93–100, 2007.)*

countries, and serves as a framework to identify countries from which recruitment could be harmful because of their critical staffing shortages.

Crisis due to mismatch in skill mix

Deficit in numbers

Data from *The World Health Report 2006* have demonstrated that there is a direct correlation between health worker density and health outcomes (**Fig. 2.5.1**). Poor staffing may lead to worsening mortality rates, increased infection rates or higher rates of occupational accidents.

A more precise analysis of the state of the health workforce in different countries can be found in the 2014 GHWA report. This document compares the 'current health' workforce with an established threshold of the number and types of health workers that are needed in any given country to meet its health needs. The gap between this *threshold* level of health worker availability and the *current* level constitutes the degree of 'shortage'.

Thresholds are difficult to define as, despite a growing evidence base, there is no single global norm or standard for health worker density. This means that there is no set rule for the number and mix of health workers (so-called 'skill mix') that must be present to enable a health system to work effectively. The JLI noted that health workers are essential in the delivery of basic health interventions needed to attain the Millennium Development Goals for health, such as skilled birth attendance and child immunisation rates. Thus the JLI estimated that a minimum of 2.5 health workers (midwife, nurses or physicians) per 1000 of population is required. The WHO sets a level of 2.28 skilled health professionals (midwives, nurses or physicians) per 1000 of population to ensure that 80% of births are attended by a skilled birth attendant. This may still be a conservative staffing requirement as the International Labour Organization and the GHWA reports suggest that a threshold of 3.45–5.94 skilled health professionals per 1000 of population is required. In 2014, 83 countries fell below the WHO threshold.

Skill mix imbalance and distribution

The thresholds in defining these health worker shortages fail to include many occupational categories such as community health workers. These workers fulfil vital roles in the delivery of basic immunisation and maternal health services. The shortage of skilled health personnel in rural areas remains a major challenge. About half of the world's population live in rural areas but only 38% of the total nursing workforce and less than 25% of the physician workforce work in these areas. At a national level, maldistribution of health workers is hampering access to essential health services, especially vaccination coverage and skilled birth attendants. Togo, for instance, trains 890 doctors per year, but only 150 end up working in rural areas, where 80% of the total population live (**Fig. 2.5.2**).

What caused the crisis and how can we solve it?

There are many causes of the global health worker crisis. Some of these are common to all countries, others affect a particular country or a region within a country. This does not imply that the solutions to local problems are, necessarily, local interventions. The health worker crisis is, at its core, a global crisis as countries are interdependent and interconnected by the flow of goods, services, capital, knowledge and people.

The Milbank report (2011) formulated three hypotheses for the underlying causes of the health workforce crisis:

- *inadequacies in the health workforce* due to a failure to train an adequate number of health workers;
- *lack of health workers* who, despite being trained, are ready and willing to serve in the health system;
- *lack of employment opportunities* for health workers.

A possible solution to the first hypothesis involves the creation of a pipeline of health workers. This can be achieved by an increase in the number of enrolled students, the establishment of new training institutions, and the transformation of existing curricula. It is essential to guarantee the quality of the health workforce (*fitness for purpose*) as well as the quality and safety of the care they provide (*fitness for practice*). This can be achieved by reviewing educational programmes, standards and processes to ensure that they meet population health needs.

The second hypothesis covers health workforce planning, and addresses human resource challenges on a national scale. This requires political and financial commitment.

The third hypothesis focuses on the lack of employment opportunities, which affects the sustainability of the workforce. Succession planning, reduction of migration through improved education and welfare, and ethical recruitment processes may help to address this challenge.

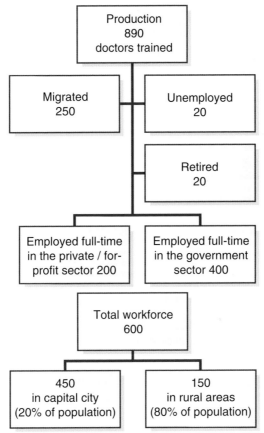

Figure 2.5.2 **Example of health workforce dynamics in Togo.** *(Derived from Global Health Workforce Alliance, World Health Organization: A universal truth: no health without a workforce, Geneva, 2014, World Health Organization.)*

Health care workers as advocates in Colombia

Health professionals, including health care students, have an important role as advocates for policy change.

In 2013 a flood of marching white coats passed through the streets of Colombia's capital city, Bogota. Thousands of protesters engaged the nation with the biggest professional mobilisation seen in the last 30 years of Colombia's history in a single voice of protest against proposed new health reforms.

The remarkable thing about this movement was its strong leadership from health care workers themselves. Of the *white coat mobilisation*, as it was termed by the national media, most were medical students, interns or residents. Empathy towards their patients and fellow doctors (who were forced to remain at work) motivated them to make a difference. It was, in large part, a student movement. Suddenly, in a country where nongovernmental organisations lack influential power, students gathered to make a stand.

The outcome of this protest was the official recognition of the human right to health as a statutory law and the abandonment of the previously proposed reforms.

Sebastian Fonseca (Colombia)

Conclusion

The health workforce is at the core of any health system. There is a current and ongoing global health workforce crisis. The causes of this crisis are complex, and include the undersupply, migration and mismatch of health care workers as well as an imbalance in skill mix. Any solution to the crisis depends on sufficient and appropriately directed investment in human resources for health.

KEY POINTS

- There is a global shortage of approximately 17.4 million health care workers.
- Political, economic and working conditions influence migration of health care workers.
- A solution to the global health workforce crisis is essential if universal health coverage is to be achieved.

Further reading

Global Health Workforce Alliance, World Health Organization: *A universal truth: no health without a work-force*, Geneva, 2014, World Health Organization. Available from: <http://www.who.int/workforcealliance/knowledge/resources/GHWA-a_universal_truth_report.pdf?ua=1>.

O'Brien P, Gostin LO: *Health worker shortages and global justice*, New York, 2011, Milbank Memorial Fund. Available from: <https://www.milbank.org/wp-content/files/documents/healthworkershortages.pdf>.

World Health Organization: *The world health report 2006: working together for health*, Geneva, 2006, World Health Organization. Available from: <http://www.who.int/whr/2006/>.

World Health Organization: *Global strategy on human resources for health: workforce 2030*, Geneva, 2016, World Health Organization. Available from: <http://www.who.int/hrh/resources/globstrathrh-2030/en/>.

World Health Organization: *WHO | Global Health Observatory (GHO) data*. 2017. <http://www.who.int/gho>.

Global Health Actors

Junior Editor: Waruguru Wanjau (Kenya)

Introduction

This section provides a brief overview of the main global health institutions and their specific roles and the contexts within which they function. The messages in this section are encapsulated in the history of the Global Polio Eradication Initiative. Between 1988 and 2000 the global incidence of polio decreased by 99% as a result of the unique collaboration between the partners in the Global Polio Eradication Initiative.

3.1 The United Nations and the World Health Organization

Kelly Thompson (USA)

Health is 'a state of complete physical, mental and social well-being and not merely the absence of disease or infirmity.'
Word Health Organization (1948)

Introduction

The World Health Organization (WHO), established in 1948, is currently undergoing reform as it seeks to maintain its role as a leader in global health. The United Nations is taking an ever-increasing role in global health governance, as the link between health and economic development is better recognised.

Global health cooperation

The origins of the WHO date from the 1851 International Sanitary Conference. At that time, there was an ambition to harmonise maritime quarantine requirements on cholera, plague and yellow fever in Europe. Subsequently, the International Office of Public Hygiene, established in 1907, was succeeded by the Health Organisation of the League of Nations (1920). Following discussions at the UN Conference on International Organization in 1945, it was agreed that an international health organisation should be created. This entity led to the establishment of the WHO in April 1948.

At its outset the WHO's top priorities were malaria, women's and children's health, tuberculosis, venereal disease, nutrition and environmental sanitation. The World Health Assembly (WHA) agenda items (1970–2012) contained the following five categories: communicable diseases (25.3%), health systems (19.1%), noncommunicable diseases (13.9%), preparedness surveillance response (13.7%) and health through the life course (8.5%). The WHO and global health cooperation has developed as a result of health needs and evolving political agendas (**Table 3.1.1**).

The World Health Organization: the who, what and how

Now in its 48th edition (2014), the WHO constitution, ratified in 1948, is still the main guiding document of the WHO. The functions of the WHO are wide-ranging, and include the following broad mandates:

- act as a directing and co-ordinating authority in international health work;
- collaborate with other UN agencies and actors on health issues;
- assist governments in strengthening health services;
- provide standardised technical services, diagnostic procedures and public health responses;

TABLE 3.1.1 ■ **Timeline of global health cooperation**

1948	**The Constitution of the World Health Organization** (WHO) comes into effect
1948	The WHO takes over the **International Classification of Diseases**
1948	The first World Health Assembly (WHA) is held in Geneva, with 53 delegations from 55 member states
1952	**The yaws eradication programme** began—by 1964 the number of cases had been reduced by 95%
1955	The **malaria eradication programme** was launched
1969	The International Health Regulations (originally *International Sanitary Regulations*) are renamed and cover cholera, plague, smallpox and yellow fever
1972	**Dr Albert Sabin donates the oral polio vaccine** to the WHO for universal use
1975	The Special Programme for Research and Training in Tropical Diseases is established to address the global response to neglected tropical diseases
1977	**The first Essential Medicines List** is released for the first time. The list has been updated every 2 years since 1977, and serves as a guide for national governments and institutions on what medicines are essential to include in their formularies.
1978	**The goal of 'health for all' is set** at the International Conference on Primary Health Care in Alma-Ata
1979	**Smallpox is certified as eradicated** following the development of the smallpox eradication programme in 1967
1986	**The Global Programme on AIDS** is created
1986	The first International Conference on Health Promotion is held, leading to the Ottawa Charter for Health Promotion setting out an action plan to achieve health for all by 2000
1988	**The Global Polio Eradication Initiative** is established. Since its establishment, the number of polio cases has dropped by 99%, and only three countries in the world have never stopped polio
1990	*The Global Burden of Disease* **report** is released, and the disability-adjusted life year is introduced as a new metric
1996	The Joint United Nations Programme on **HIV/AIDS (UNAIDS)** is created
2000	The UN Security Council discusses AIDS, leading to the adoption of Resolution 1308—the first time health is discussed there
2000	The Commission on Macroeconomics and Health is created to assess the links between health and development
2000	**The Millennium Declaration**—leading to the Millennium Development Goals—is adopted at the UN. Three of the eight goals are health related: goal 4 to reduce child mortality; goal 5 to improve maternal health; and goal 6 to combat HIV/AIDS, malaria and other diseases
2001	The UN General Assembly Special Session on HIV/AIDS leads to the Declaration of Commitment on HIV/AIDS
2002	**The Global Fund to Fight AIDS, Tuberculosis and Malaria** is established
2003	**The Framework Convention on Tobacco Control** is adopted by the WHA—the first international treaty adopted by the WHA
2004	**The Global Strategy on Diet, Physical Activity and Health** is adopted
2005	**The Commission on Social Determinants of Health** is launched to help countries address the social and political factors affecting health
2005	**The Partnership for Maternal, Newborn and Child Health is launched** to serve as a strategic partnership between member organisations in academia, research and teaching, donors and foundations, health care professional associations, multilateral organisations, nongovernmental organisations, partner countries and the private sector to advance the achievement of Millennium Development Goals 4 and 5
2008	The WHO begins to advocate to **protect health from the effects of climate change**
2010	**The UN Secretary General's Global Strategy for Women's and Children's Health** is launched at the Millennium Development Goals Summit

Continued on following page

TABLE 3.1.1 ■ **Timeline of global health cooperation** (Continued)

2010	The WHA adopts the **Global Strategy to Reduce Harmful Use of Alcohol**
2011	The WHO **Pandemic Influenza Preparedness Framework** is adopted
2011	A political declaration is adopted by the high-level meeting of the General Assembly on the prevention and control of noncommunicable diseases
2012	The UN General Assembly adopts Resolution A/67/L.36 (global health and foreign policy), which outlined the importance of **2012 Universal Health Coverage**
2014	The UN Security Council adopts Resolution 2177 on the exceptional and vigorous response to the Ebola outbreak
2016	**The Sustainable Development Goals** are established (2016–30). Goal 3 relates to health issues

(Data from World Health Organization: *WHO in 60 years: a chronology of public health milestones*, 2008. Available from <http://www.who.int/features/history/WHO_60th_anniversary_chronology.pdf>)

- eradicate epidemic, endemic and other diseases, address injuries and address environmental health;
- ensure cooperation among scientific and professional groups;
- negotiate conventions, agreements and regulations;
- improve maternal and child health;
- initiate health research;
- improve training and teaching of health professionals;
- standardise scientific nomenclature.

This list attempts to connect both technical and political aspects of health, and is often regarded a cause for the perceived ineffectiveness of the WHO.

To achieve its mandate, the work of the WHO is directed at the global level by three main bodies: WHA, WHO Executive Board and WHO Secretariat. The WHO is a membership-based organisation, and therefore countries (member states) are required to accept its constitution. New members must be approved by a simple majority vote of the WHA.

The *WHA*, which consists of health ministers of all member states, meets annually. It is the main force driving WHO policy. It elects Executive Board members, appoints the Director General, supervises financial policies and approves the budget.

The *Executive Board* is composed of 34 individuals from different states who are technically qualified in the field of health. Their role is to implement the decisions and policies of the WHA. The board proposes the WHA agenda and the programme of work for the WHO, and meets at least twice a year.

The *Secretariat* drives the work of the WHO at a global level. It reports to the Director General and the technical and administrative staff of the WHO. It is responsible for carrying out the day-to-day operations of the WHO. Additionally, the Director General's Office is responsible for preparing the WHO budget and strategic direction, which must then be approved by the WHA. Member states provide annual reports on actions taken and progress made, laws and policies impacting health outcomes and epidemiological reports. These are then collated by the Secretariat and progress reports are presented to the WHA.

The WHO also has a complex regional and national structure. Work is divided amongst six regions (with their own regional headquarters, elected regional directors and regional sessions), each of which operate and function similarly to the WHA. The regions are divided on a sociopolitical and geographical basis into the following: Africa, Americas (Pan American Health Organization), eastern Mediterranean, Europe, Southeast Asia and western Pacific. The WHO also has national offices in 150 countries to provide technical and other support to meet local needs. Regional offices are led by directors elected by the local ministers of health. As a result, there may be conflict between regional politics and the policies established by the WHA.

There is reciprocity of representation between the WHO and the United Nations. Representatives from the United Nations are invited as nonvoting observers to the WHA, Executive Board meetings and other WHO meetings. In turn, the WHO is invited to meetings of a number of UN committees to provide advice and feedback on agenda items related to health. The WHO has official constitutional agreements with organisations within the UN system, including the International Labour Organization (ILO), the Food and Agriculture Organization of the United Nations (FAO), the United Nations Educational, Scientific and Cultural Organization (UNESCO), International Fund for Agricultural Development (IFAD), the United Nations Industrial Development Organization (UNIDO) and the Universal Postal Union (UPU). The WHO also has constitutional agreements with nonstate actors such as nongovernmental organisations (NGOs) and the private sector.

The Pre-World Health Assembly for Youth

The Pre-World Health Assembly (Pre-WHA) for Youth is a 3-day workshop for young people, organised by young people. Those attending include medical and other health care students, public health students and practitioners, economists and lawyers.

The Pre-WHA seeks to upskill and train youth advocates and health leaders on global health diplomacy and governance. It also aims to educate and empower future health leaders with an enhanced understanding of global health. Workshops provide an understanding of the function of the World Health Organization and the inner workings of the World Health Assembly (WHA). Participants develop an advocacy strategy to address key agenda items in the subsequent WHA meeting. The Pre-WHA, led by the International Federation of Medical Students' Associations, has initiated youth engagement at the WHA.

These Pre-WHA meetings provide knowledge about global health, global health diplomacy and the Sustainable Development Goals development process.

Meggie Mwoka (Kenya)

The changing role of the World Health Organization and the United Nations in global governance for health

'The WHO remains the only actor in the global health system that is built on the universal membership of all recognized sovereign nation states'

Frenk and Moon, 2013

An increasing number of agencies have been developed to address global health needs in recent years. This has been portrayed by some as a failure of the WHO in the context of its original remit (1948). However, others argue that the WHO was never meant to address *all* global health needs.

WHO reform was initiated in 2010 in response to the deficiencies in funding combined with the dependence of the WHO on voluntary contributions from member states. The WHO has always struggled to balance its roles both as a standard-setter and as a provider of technical and other support to developing countries. Key roles identified include the production of global public goods (e.g., the International Classification of Diseases and the WHO Model List of Essential Medicines) and stewardship, by providing strategic direction for the global health system (e.g., by developing the Framework Convention on Tobacco Control).

WHO staff are largely health care professionals who are not trained or prepared to address the broader social or economic aspects of health. The growing recognition that health is more than a disease process has forced the WHO and also the UN system as a whole to address the broader dimensions of health. UN bodies that have staff members and departments dedicated to health include the Joint United Nations Programme on HIV/AIDS (UNAIDS), the United Nations Department of Economic and Social Affairs (UN DESA), the United Nations Children's Fund (UNICEF), the United Nations Population Fund (UNFPA), the United Nations Development Programme (UNDP), the ILO, the United Nations Environment Programme (UNEP), and the World Bank.

The decentralisation from the World Health Organization of the AIDS response

The development of the Joint United Nations Programme on HIV/AIDS (UNAIDS) is an example of decentralisation from the World Health Organization (WHO) of health governance within the UN system.

When the WHO began annual reporting on AIDS cases in 1981, there was only one person in the whole organisation working on sexually transmitted infections. The organisation was not prepared for the growing AIDS epidemic, and it was also hesitant to mount a larger response because many cases were in wealthy countries.

The Control Programme on AIDS was created in 1986 (later renamed the Global Programme on AIDS in 1987). Its Director, Dr Jonathan Mann, subsequently described the components of the AIDS epidemic to the UN General Assembly for the first time. He recognised three components of this epidemic: the AIDS virus, the AIDS diseases, and 'the third epidemic, of social, cultural, economic and political reaction to AIDS'. As a result, the international response moved from a solely medical-centric approach to a broader and inclusive movement.

The WHO, as the lead agency in the global response to AIDS, was expected to coordinate its activities with other UN agencies, but this integrated response was not delivered. An external review also noted these inefficiencies, and a task force was developed, which led to the establishment of UNAIDS.

UNAIDS was tasked with the following roles:
- to coordinate leadership
- to create consensus on programming and policy
- to ensure monitoring and reporting
- to build capacity of national governments on developing national strategies on HIV

UNAIDS has advanced global governance and has shown that an effective response to health challenges must address nonhealth, as well as health, issues.

Kelly Thompson (USA)

Following the development of UNAIDS, the UN has continued to become more involved in health outside the WHO. The UN General Assembly has also passed a resolution on global health and foreign policy promoting universal health coverage. A resolution on noncommunicable diseases was adopted at the High-Level Meeting on Non-communicable Diseases (2014). Health has also played a key role in the UN development agendas, featuring in three of the eight Millennium Development Goals and goal 3 of the Sustainable Development Goals in the post-2015 agenda.

Conclusion

The UN system is a complex system of member states and agencies. International health considerations extend beyond the direct remit of the WHO and necessitate an appreciation of political as well as health care imperatives. Health and its determinants are inextricably linked to development, peace and stability and other global sociopolitical issues.

KEY POINTS

- The World Health Organization (WHO) is a member state-driven organisation addressing global health issues.
- The WHO consists of three main bodies: the World Health Assembly, the WHO Executive Board and the WHO Secretariat.
- The global health landscape is changing. The WHO and the UN system are currently redefining themselves to address issues of governance.
- The global AIDS response exemplifies the expansion of global and public health responses from a singular to a broader socioeconomic and political approach.

Further reading

Clift C: *What's the World Health Organization for? Final report from the Centre on Global Health Security Working Group on Health Governance*, London, 2014, Royal Institute of International Affairs.

Frenk J, Moon S: Governance challenges in global health, *N Engl J Med* 368:936–942, 2013.

Joint United Nations Programme on HIV/AIDS: *UNAIDS: The first 10 years*, Geneva, 2008, Joint United Nations Programme on HIV/AIDS. Available from: <http://data.unaids.org/pub/report/2008/jc1579_first_10_years_en.pdf>.

Mann JM: Statement at an informal briefing on AIDS to the 42nd session of the UNGA, *J R Stat Soc [Ser A]* 151(1):131–136, 1988.

3.2 International Organisations

Charlotte Holm-Hansen (Denmark)

Introduction

An international organisation is an organisation that operates in at least two countries, at a regional level or on a global scale. Such organisations can be intergovernmental organisations (IGOs) or NGOs, which include nonprofit organisations. They play a significant part in discussions about the development agenda, foreign and health policies and the distribution of international aid. States may engage in unilateral (one-way), bilateral (two-way) and multilateral (many partners involved) agreements. Factors such as history, culture, religion, ethics, political orientation, national priorities and trade agreements may influence the decision-making processes regarding aid allocation. These anthropological aspects must be appreciated when trying to understand the reasoning and priorities of donor (and recipient) countries.

An IGO is an entity created by treaty between two or more nations, working in good faith on issues of common interest. As an example, the UN Charter, the treaty establishing the United Nations in 1945, and the Constitution of the World Health Organization led to the formation of the WHO in 1948. A treaty lists the main purposes of the organisation; for example, maintaining international peace and security (United Nations) or attainment by all people of the highest possible level of health (WHO). An IGO is subject to international law, and possesses the ability to legally enforce agreements.

Aid is often ineffective, and projects with a good intention might have only short-term or very little impact. The Paris Declaration for Aid Effectiveness recognised that aid can and should be 'producing better impacts'. This concept was further refined in the Accra Agenda for Action (2008) and in the Busan Partnership (2011).

International Organisations and aid for health

The WHO has been the leading agency in the field of health aid and development, but many new global health partnerships, both public and private, have also evolved. As no single organisation coordinates all health care initiatives, there is significant potential for duplication within the aid agenda. The Ebola outbreak (2014) revealed significant deficiencies in the international response to a global disease threat; however, some initiatives, such as the Global Polio Eradication Initiative, have met with significant success and provide a rationale for the effectiveness of multilateral projects.

Multilateral initiatives bring together different organisations (e.g., governments, private institutions, philanthropic organisations) to pool funds so as to address disease-specific causes. An example of this is the Global Fund To Fight Aids, Tuberculosis and Malaria (GFATM) founded in 2002. This was formed by governments, civil society, the private sector and the people affected by these diseases. Its annual budget is almost US$4 billion, and the fund operates in 140 countries. The GFATM signed the Paris Declaration in 2005, and operates from a set of key principles: country ownership, performance-based funding and partnerships. The collaborative working of the GFATM with other international, national and local stakeholders has led to an effective and widely accessible treatment programme for malaria (e.g., in South Sudan).

The work of the Global Fund To Fight Aids, Tuberculosis and Malaria: a community rises in South Sudan

A network of community-based distributors (CBD) was formed with the support from international non-governmental organisations, including Population Services International, the Ministry of Health in South Sudan and the Global Fund To Fight Aids, Tuberculosis and Malaria. Through the CBD network, anti-malarials were made available free of charge. A select group of villagers were trained in the diagnosis and treatment of malaria and other childhood diseases, thus vastly enhancing access to health care in remote communities. CBDs do not receive a salary but are provided with quarterly rations of basic food items and necessities. They have the satisfaction and sense of fulfilment from knowing that they are saving lives every day.

A large number of philanthropic, religious, and civil society organisations (NGOs) work in global health. These organisations offer a wide range of experience, skills and knowledge as well as access to local communities. They often address gaps in health service delivery but are sometimes criticised for preferring their own agendas to other critical local needs. Philanthropy has made a great contribution to development, and many of the biggest health-related projects are funded by private funds and foundations such as the Bill & Melinda Gates Foundation and the Clinton Foundation. There is an increasing recognition that health programmes need to invest in tackling the determinants of health, such as social, economic and environmental factors. This is essential if aid is to be effective.

Regional organisations

Countries often operate and negotiate in political blocks. These blocks determine health priorities and plans for reform, for example, of the WHO. Examples of regional organisations include the European Union (EU), the African Union, the Arab League and the Association of Southeast Asian Nations. These can be financial or nonfinancial institutions and are membership organisations which operate as one nation geopolitically.

The EU was founded in 1948 after World War II by six countries with the aim of ending the frequent and bloody wars between neighbours. There are currently 28 member states, and the EU functions as a politico-economic union. All decisions are negotiated by its member states. It operates through supranational institutions: the Commission, the Council, the Court and the Parliament. The Presidency of the European Council rotates amongst its member states every sixth month and the Presidency has the role of agenda setting, management of the Council and coordinating national policies. In relation to the WHO, the EU member states, led by the Presidency, coordinate their views on different global health issues in a joint statement. At WHO governing bodies, the EU requests, and is usually granted, a special observer role. On most issues, the EU can agree on a common policy, but where this is not the case, countries or smaller groups of countries can choose to stress their views as a separate entity. For instance, on the issue of reproductive health, the Scandinavian countries (Norway, Denmark, Finland, Iceland and Sweden), tend to have much more liberal views than some of the more Catholic countries.

The *African Union* is another regional organisation, consisting of 53 member states (all the African states with the exception of Morocco). It was formed in 2001 as a transition from the former Organisation of African Unity (OAU) and its motto is 'A United and Strong Africa'. The main objective of the OAU was to get rid of the remains of colonisation and apartheid, promote unity and solidarity, and coordinate development and international cooperation. There is a heavy disease burden in Africa, and it is therefore beneficial for countries to collaborate on key issues as a group.

Development banks

Development banks are institutions dedicated to the funding of economic development, at a national level for both medium-term and long-term projects. Multilateral development banks are usually formed by a group of both donor and borrowing nations to provide advice (largely financial) on development programmes. The World Bank (*Working for a World Free of Poverty*) is an example of this form of bank. It provides low-interest loans, interest-free credits and grants to developing countries. Its original purpose was to foster development and economic growth after World War II, and today it has two ambitious goals, to be attained by 2030:

- end extreme poverty within a generation by decreasing the percentage of people living on less than US$1.90 a day to less than 3%;
- promote shared prosperity by fostering income growth by the bottom 40% for every country.

The World Bank's investments have a wide remit, including the environment, agriculture, education, infrastructure and health.

Partnerships (see Chapter 3.5) are crucial to the mission of the World Bank for scaling up and intensifying programmes and outreach as well as providing expertise. An example of the World Bank's work is the International Health Partnerships and related initiatives (IHP+). The IHP+ was founded in 2007 by the World Bank, the WHO and many states as a global compact for achieving the Millennium Development Goals. This was seen as a key step in putting the Paris Declaration on aid effectiveness and development cooperation into practice within the health sector. The IHP+ achieves results by the mobilisation of national governments, civil society organisations and development agencies. It promotes a country-driven health strategy with support from the international community, and is currently focused on delivering the health-related goals within the Sustainable Development Goals. In 2016 there were 66 signatories.

External debt management of heavily indebted poor countries and the impact on health

The World Bank defines heavily indebted poor countries (HIPC) as those countries facing an unsustainable debt burden even after application of existing debt management strategies. The HIPC Initiative was launched in 1996 as a joint cooperation between the World Bank and the International Monetary Fund with the aim of helping such countries face the burden of their debt. By 2015 36 countries had completed a programme resulting in the cancellation of their external debt in full by the International Monetary Fund, World Bank and other creditors.

One of the goals of this programme is to increase spending on social programs such as health by formulating sustainable payment strategies with the help of other institutions. Debt relief, combined with poverty reduction strategy papers (PRSP) outlining actions needed, decreases the financial pressure on the state. A reduction amounting to 1.9% of GDP is equivalent to an average of 90% of public spending on health in heavily indebted poor countries. The allocation of funds to action-oriented public health measures outlined in the PRSP and adopted by the HIPC is already a major step in pursuit of better health care. However, this does not always translate into tangible results throughout the population. For instance, there are still inequities in the benefits provided by public health spending: the poorest often experience fewer gains than their richer counterparts.

Chérine Zaim (Canada)

Conclusion

International organisations, in addition to the WHO and other traditional UN agencies, have a key role in global health. Bilateral donors provide key funding, and influence global health policy. There are an increasing number of international institutional players, such as International Monetary Fund and the World Bank. Health is being addressed by the broader development community and global health-related issues are now encompassed in documents such as the Paris Declaration. Political entities such as the EU and the African Union also address global health issues in their work.

KEY POINTS

- Anthropological aspects must be accommodated when one is evaluating aid and aid for health.
- The Paris Declaration and the Accra Agenda for Action have challenged and improved the health sector architecture.
- Although the World Health Organization continues to play a significant role in health aid and development programmes, global health partnerships and a variety of international organisations are taking an increasing role in health.
- The role of the development banks is expanding: for example the World Bank and the International Health Partnership.

Further reading

Gupta S, Clements B, Guin-Siu MT, Lerouth L: Debt relief and public health spending in heavily indebted poor countries, *Bull World Health Organ* 80:151–157, 2002.
Organisation for Economic Co-operation and Development: *Paris Declaration and Accra Agenda for Action*, 2017. <http://www.oecd.org/dac/effectiveness/parisdeclarationandaccraagendaforaction.htm>.

3.3 National Governments

Ivan Lumu (Uganda)

'If they are to deal effectively with the challenges posed by globalization, global health actors must solve two paradoxes. The first one is the sovereignty paradox. This paradox states that in a world of sovereign nation-states, health continues to be primarily a national responsibility, yet the determinants of health and the means to fulfil that responsibility are increasingly global.'

Julio Frenk, 2010

Introduction

Despite growing appreciation of the global dimensions of health, national governments retain the sole primary responsibility for the provision of health for their citizens and decision making in multilateral institutions. Considerations regarding national sovereignty frequently override global priorities. Multilateral institutions, such as UN organisations, are not directly accountable to the people whose health governments are meant to ensure. The aims of these institutions may conflict with the priorities of national governments and result in inequitable provision of essential health care.

Sovereignty

Sovereignty is defined as the independent authority of a country and the right to govern itself. Although this concept is central to the current global health governance system, global determinants of health challenge this traditional view. The Ebola crisis of 2014 illustrated the inability of the governments of Sierra Leone, Guinea and Liberia to control an Ebola virus outbreak which could have affected the entire world. The global community was not tasked with the provision of health to the national populations in these three states; it did, however, engage with an obligation to intervene to protect the global population from an infectious disease with a high mortality. The responsibility to combat Ebola was beyond the control of any *one* of the affected nation states. In the context of sovereignty and global health, sovereignty is dualistic. Sovereignty is both a challenge and a necessity. It is a necessity in protecting the health and well-being of a state's citizens. It is, however, a challenge when national and global interests compete with each other, especially when global decisions limit the policy space of the state (**Box 3.3.1**).

Sovereignty may also compromise the representation of minority groups within nation states. In most global health structures, it is assumed that national governments represent the needs and interests of all people within their borders. The voice of minorities or marginalised groups may be poorly represented. Although such groups may be represented by NGOs, they may be unable to effectively represent their specific concerns beyond national boundaries. In poorer countries a lack of coordination between health care initiatives may compromise the ability of the state to deliver effective care to its citizens.

BOX 3.3.1 ■ Tension between national and global policies

- Compulsory licenses and reforms in patent law so as to expand access to medicines
- Plain packaging and other tobacco control policies
- Domestic courts' enforcement of the right to health-related human rights as laid out in national constitutions
- Stricter regulation of the marketing of unhealthy food items so as to contain the obesity epidemic
- More rigorous environmental standards
- Improved labour rights and minimum wages
- Domestic responses to infectious disease (e.g., quarantine, isolation and trade restrictions)

Reproduced with permission from Lancet–University of Oslo Global Governance for Health Youth Report (2014).

Patan Hospital, Nepal

Global health actors motivated by religious altruism bring their own agendas and are often criticised for prescriptive and paternalistic approaches which do not harmonise with the local government's agendas.

Alice Cozens spent 2 months during her medical elective as a student at Patan Hospital, Nepal. She found that this hospital exhibited how a religious organisation had instigated a high-quality health care project alongside the government and then relinquished its role to the government health care system.

Patan Hospital is now a highly regarded major acute care city hospital with excellent facilities, exceeding the expectations of a government district hospital. Although it is autonomous, its policies are in keeping with those of the Government of Nepal. This allows Patan Hospital to effectively work closely with the Nepali health system and be active in advocating appropriate health policies and programmes for the rural population at national government level.

Alice Cozens (UK)

National governments as national policymakers

Governments contribute to global health care policy as members of multinational organisations. Policies deriving from universal populations needs include the Declaration of Alma-Ata, Millennium Development Goals and Sustainable Development Goals (see Chapters 1.1, 3.1, 3.5, 6.7, 7.6). Global health policies are made with the intention that they should be adapted to local situations through the implementation of national health policies.

The social determinants of health (see Chapter 4.1), which play a large part in determining individual health, are influenced by government policies outside the remit of 'health'. These include transport, food, welfare and work policies. Governments that take a 'health in all policy' approach are likely to have a profound beneficial effect on population health.

Healthy eating issues: tackling a national challenge right from the start

Obesity and poor eating habits evolve in early childhood. This is a significant issue in many countries, including Austria. The Austrian Department of Health has attempted to tackle this through the establishment of a national action plan for nutrition. The case of a 12-year-old called Mark demonstrates the relevance that national policies such as these can have for individual patients.

A mother came to our clinic with her 12-year-old son, Mark, whose performance at school had deteriorated. He was constantly tired and thirsty. On examination, he was severely obese for his age, and type 2 diabetes was subsequently diagnosed. This condition is increasingly common amongst children, mainly due to increasing childhood obesity, and places a considerable burden on the health care system. Further discussion with Mark and his family demonstrated poor understanding of the need for healthy eating.

A number of national government policies have been launched to tackle this issue (e.g., 'Healthy Eating from the Start' and 'Nutritional Guidelines for Schools'). The plans recommend that Mark should consume three servings of vegetables and two servings of fruit each day.

Maria van Hove (Austria)

The structures of national health systems also determine access to health, particularly the division of public versus private and the availability of publicly funded health care. In most countries, national governments determine health priorities as well as the health system structure. When health expenditure is a very small percentage of gross domestic product (GDP), health care may be largely privately or donor funded. In these situations, national policies tend to be biased by the wishes of donors.

The impact of national policies is affected by the processes which lead to their adoption. Governments which engage with all stakeholders and members of civil society formulate more practical and effective policies. Civil organisations, representing specific sectors of society, can be effective in mobilising grassroots involvement with national challenges. They may highlight key issues and develop solutions through the development of appropriate policies. Many national governments organise stakeholder meetings to consult on policies and strategies before implementation.

The generation of an advisory council on youth for policy and health

Youth health (adolescent and young adult health) is often neglected in the formulation of national policy. Medical students have argued the case for the inclusion of youth health in national policies.

The Advisory Council on Youth, a Croatian governmental body, was formed to review previous strategies on youth through the Ministry of Social Affairs and Youth. Youth-led organisations, with members from varied backgrounds, were invited to join the council with the mandate to review previous strategies, gather youth opinions, give input about the needs of youth and, with the support of experts, propose a new strategy on youth.

Medical students from the Croatian Medical Students' International Committee served on the Advisory Council to advocate compulsory health education in primary and secondary schools. This resulted in a change in policy to ensure education around a wide range of health issues, including mental health, sexual health and the prevention of drug abuse. Students contributed to other chapters of the strategy, including social protection and employment, thereby facilitating knowledge exchange and competency building for young people.

Ljiljana Lukic (Croatia)

National governments decide the proportion of national income allocated to health. The percentage of total health spending differs significantly, ranging from 17.4% of GDP in the United States to 1.8% in Myanmar in 2016 (**Fig. 3.3.1**). A health system is unlikely to be able to provide a good level of service when funding is poor, but population health is not necessarily improved solely by major increases in funding. However the per capita spending on health determines the health options available to individual citizens and the need for out-of-pocket expenditure, which, itself, can promote poverty.

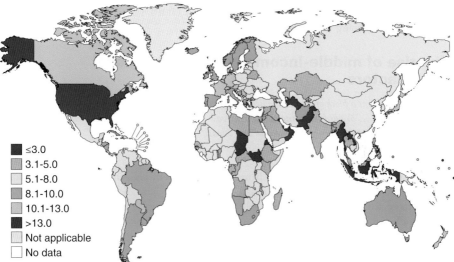

**Total expenditure on health
as a percentage of the gross domestic product, 2012***

Legend:
- ≤3.0
- 3.1-5.0
- 5.1-8.0
- 8.1-10.0
- 10.1-13.0
- >13.0
- Not applicable
- No data

Figure 3.3.1 Total expenditure on health as a percentage of gross domestic product (2014). *(Redrawn from World Health Organization: Total expenditure on health as a percentage of gross domestic product (US$), 2017. <http://www.who.int/gho/health_financing/total_expenditure/en/>.)*

National governments as member states in multilateral institutions

The membership of the UN system is based on 193 recognised member states. In the WHO, member states constitute policy which is ratified through the WHA. National governments receive input on health issues from various UN bodies. It is often difficult for them to develop coordinated local policies, given that UN agencies work within health from different perspectives. As an example, different elements of maternal and child health are under the responsibility of UN Women, UNFPA, UNAIDS, UNICEF and the WHO. It can therefore be extremely challenging for national governments to integrate the different country programmes. National ownership and oversight is key for the effective coordination and implementation of multilateral health care initiatives.

Decisions related to health care in multilateral institutions, such as the WHO, are influenced by various actors (e.g., civil society movements and NGOs). The governance of multilateral relationships may be compromised when a national health agenda is unduly influenced by wealthier states or donor institutions. Additionally, the legitimacy of IGOs can be questioned as these bodies are not directly accountable to the people whose universal human rights they are meant to protect.

National governments as bilateral donors

Donor national governments play a multifaceted role in global health through their donor agencies, by working directly with other national governments (bilateral agreements) and by contributing to multilateral initiatives such as Gavi. By wielding influence on different levels, a single national government plays a greater role in the larger global health picture. In absolute terms, the United States Agency for International Development is the biggest development agency, followed by the United Kingdom's Department for International Development. As a percentage of GDP, Norway is the biggest contributor to international aid (1.07% of GDP), followed by Sweden (1.02% of GDP) and Luxembourg (1.0% of GDP).

The rise of middle-income countries as global health actors

> 'BRICS represent a block of countries with a … great potential to move global public health in the right direction … towards reducing the current vast gaps in health outcomes and introducing greater fairness in the way the benefits of medical and scientific progress are distributed.'
>
> **Margaret Chan, former WHO Director General, 2011**

Although global health aid was previously mainly dominated by high-income countries, middle-income countries such as the BRICS (Brazil, Russia, India, China, South Africa) have recently become more active as key actors. They help to shape global health policy by jointly promoting access to affordable medical products through the World Trade Organization (WTO) Agreement on Trade-Related Aspects of Intellectual Property Rights. Other examples of leadership by BRICS countries include Brazil's leadership in the Framework Convention on Tobacco Control, India's production of most generic drugs and South Africa and Brazil's engagement with the WHO and multilateral initiatives such as Gavi.

Conclusion

The concept of sovereignty is central to the formulation of policy in global health. National governments play a multifaceted role in global health as national policymakers, members of multilateral institutions and bilateral donors. One of the major determinants of a population's health is national health policy, spending and structure.

KEY POINTS

- National governments are responsible for national health policy and the provision of national health services.
- National governments represent their populations in multilateral institutions, including the UN system and multilateral initiatives such as Gavi.
- Decisions in the multilateral system, especially the UN system, are made by member states.

Further reading

Frenk J, Moon S: Governance challenges in global health, *N Engl J Med* 368(10):936–942, 2013.

Frenk J, Gómez-Dantés O, Moon S: From sovereignty to solidarity: a renewed concept of global health for an era of complex interdependence, *Lancet* 383(9911):94–97, 2014.

Kickbusch I: BRICS? Contributions to the global health agenda, *Bull World Health Organ* 92(6):463–464, 2014.

Reid R: *The healing of America: a global quest for better, cheaper, and fairer health care*, London, 2010, Penguin.

3.4 Nongovernmental Organisations and Social Movements

Roopa Dhatt (USA)

'In South Africa, we could not have achieved our freedom and just peace without the help of people around the world, who through the use of non-violent means, such as boycotts and divestment, encouraged their governments and other corporate actors to reverse decades-long support for the Apartheid regime.'
Desmond Tutu

Introduction

Health activism is needed more than ever before. Health issues, for instance the prohibition of smoking in public areas, are both a part of the public discourse and a vital aspect of the changing landscape of society. As the global community aspires towards a world with greater equity and well-being, collective action through social movements and NGOs are two key vehicles for achieving social change. NGOs are non-profit-making, nonviolent organisations which seek to influence the policy of governments and international organisations and/or to complement government services (such as health and education). NGOs, working hand-in-hand with social movements, can lead to transformation in health care.

Social movements

Social movements include many groups and individuals acting towards a common goal to change society in a particular way. They enable people to voice grievances, raise concerns and demand action. They also provide a context for learning and inspiration for people to share experiences and create strategic frameworks for action. Three key ingredients are required for this: political opportunity, organisation capacity and framing and packaging ability.

Participants in a social movement are often called *activists*. They may be front line (e.g., physical protesters), direct action (e.g., writers of campaign letters) or supporters (e.g., fundraisers).

The African American Civil Rights Movement

The African American Civil Rights Movement was a social movement which demonstrated the importance of each of the three key ingredients required for the development of a social movement.

Societal stratification based on race gave rise to a struggle over civil rights as discrimination against African Americans and other ethnically disadvantaged groups had resulted in socio-economic, political and personal marginalisation. Community leaders developed a strategy of

81

nonviolent resistance (civil disobedience) at local, state and federal level. This culminated in the March on Washington for Jobs and Freedom, where Martin Luther King Jr gave his 'I Have a Dream' speech (1963). The United States was now amidst the largest societal transformation driven by a social movement. The changes that were enacted (Voting Rights Act 1965, Civil Rights Act 1968) as a result of the Civil Rights Movement affected all aspects of social and political life. It resulted in increased education and training opportunities in health as well as access to health care for all minorities in the United States.

Political opportunity: a landscape for change

Collective action requires political opportunity to have an impact on policy. This often occurs during a period of uncertainty when there are significant political shifts in power (e.g., leadership changes associated with sociopolitical turmoil).

Linked to such opportunity are factors that impact the landscape for change:

- *Window of opportunity*: an ideological space (in time and place) that has favourable circumstances for change.
- *Resources*: a source or supply of financial, social, cultural, structural, political or intellectual capital.
- *Capable leadership*: leaders who have the sociopolitical abilities to inspire and organise people.
- *Infrastructure*: an underlying foundation or framework.
- *Concentration*: a critical mass of like-minded people.
- *Identity*: people with identical characteristics or commonalities.

Organisation capacity: network reach and resilient infrastructure

Social movements encompass organisations which arise from various sections of society. These groups may be based, for instance, on the community, student societies, religions, professions or specific interests. NGOs can be catalysts for the development of social movements by providing the infrastructure for sustainability. They thus assist with vision building, capacity building and network building. In general, the wider the diversity of participating groups, the stronger the movement. The roles of social movements are:

- *capacity building*, the process through which skills, abilities and knowledge are transmitted;
- *coalition and network building*, the process through which collaborative relations are created;
- *team building*, the process through which people working together create connections and bonds;
- *spirit building*, the process through which emotional inspiration is created;
- *movement building*, the process through which action for a particular cause expands.

Framing and packaging ability

A social movement is united by its vision. The aim is to convince the target audiences of the validity and credibility of the messages; effective *framing* and *packing* of messages is essential. The aim is to convince 'the target audiences of the validity and credibility' of the message—therefore framing and packing messages effectively is essential. They should be focused and inspirational whilst resonating with the audience. Messages are a call to action, and should be supported by a *goal* (**Box 3.4.1**).

> **BOX 3.4.1 ■ Building an effective core message**
>
> - *Framing:* the process through which a message is constructed and contextualised.
> - *Packaging:* the means through which a message is shared and transmitted.
> - *Cultural:* the beliefs, social practices and characteristics of ethnicity, class, religious and other social groups shared by people in a specific space.
> - *Goal:* a specific, measurable, achievable, relevant and time-bound objective.

Health social movements

Social movements often impact health. Health social movements (HSMs) focus specifically on health issues. These are defined as 'collective challenges to medical policy, public health policy and politics, belief systems, research and practice which include an array of formal and informal organisations, supporters, networks of cooperation and media.'

Health social movements framework

The People's Health Movement is a global network bringing together grassroots health activists, civil society organisations from academic institutions from around the world, particularly from low and middle income countries.

> *'Equity, ecologically-sustainable development and peace are at the heart of our vision of a better world – a world in which a healthy life for all is a reality'.*
>
> **From the Charter of the People's Health Movement, an equity-focused example of a health social movement (2000)**

HSMs arose because of the adverse working conditions during the Industrial Revolution in the 19th century. During the 20th century, the emergence of the Feminist Movement led to a particular focus on women's health, and reproductive rights. Other examples of HSMs in this century include the Global Polio Eradication Campaign and the global commitment to primary health care (Declaration of Alma-Ata, 1978). The importance of ethics and research practices in medicine was highlighted following the Nuremberg trials (1945–9). The commonality in these movements is that they addressed specific areas of health:

1. access to or provision of health care services
2. disease, illness experience, disability and contested illness
3. health inequality and inequity based on race, ethnicity, sex, class and/or sexuality

HSMs have had a huge impact. For example, the HSM in 1987 transformed the AIDS epidemic with the development of antiretroviral therapy. The dialogue shifted from testing to treatment to advocacy for access to health care for the most marginalised populations globally. Antiretroviral treatment for one person for 1 year was priced at US$15,000. In response to this price tag, civil society organisations and NGOs created global, national and local coalitions to thwart the corporate dominance of pharmaceutical companies on moral, political and economic grounds.

There are three main forms of HSMs:

- The *constituency-based health movements* (most classic type). They 'address health inequality and health inequity based on race, ethnicity, gender, class and/or sexuality differences.' Some of the constituency-based movements include women's health, sustainable development movement and the social movement that transformed the trajectory of the HIV/AIDS epidemic.
- *Embodied health movements.* These 'address disease, disability or illness experience by challenging science on etiology, diagnosis, treatment and prevention' (Brown et al, 2004).

■ *Health access movements* seeking equitable access to health care and improved provision of health care services. These focus on health system reforms, including improving access to treatments and therapies. They also emphasise the rights of marginalised people.

Emerging diseases; what medical students can achieve: #KickEbolaOut

The Ebola epidemic that emerged in 2014 hit West Africa with full force, further crippling the already weakened health systems. While global organisations, especially, the World Health Organization (WHO), were slow to respond, civil society in affected countries organised to increase awareness, to promote preventive public health measures and to provide care to those affected, including student groups. Students from the International Federation of Medical Students' Associations, through the local Sierra Leone Medical Students' Association, launched #Kick-EbolaOut. The students entered communities to provide education and support, distributed leaflets, held radio programmes and also brought disinfectant supplies to remote communities. They built rapport before giving guidelines. Their work has been recognised by health ministries and the WHO as it showcased the role young people have in public health, especially in emerging diseases.

Nongovernmental organisations

Examples of NGOs in the health sector include professional organisations, patient interest groups and disease or issue-based groups (**Table 3.4.1**). The numbers of NGOs have grown substantially in the past century, with estimates of as many as 1.2 million organisations of this type in the United States. These NGOs employ an estimated 10.9 million individuals, with revenues of nearly US$680 billion. They hold a significant amount of financial capital for social work, and receive approximately one-quarter of governmental humanitarian spending; for example Denmark channels 36% of its humanitarian funding through (Danish) NGOs.

NGOs create an identity based on shared values and ethical and socially responsible practices. Their vision and mission places them in a position of moral authority. Through engagement as advocates, advisors, activists, facilitators and supporters, they can mobilise communities, thereby gaining more political capital. Their formal structure enables them to bring extreme focus to their work, and the publication of annual reports enhances their public accountability.

However, these formal structures may promote unnecessary bureaucracy. This can be frustrating for activists. Their special areas of focus may disregard wider societal needs and may, on occasion, conflict with other local imperatives. An interesting example of an effective NGO coalition is the G4 Alliance, a global alliance for surgical, obstetric, trauma and anaesthesia care. The G4 Alliance is an advocacy-based organisation dedicated to the building of political priority for surgical care as part of the global development agenda. At the 68th WHA (2015), it launched its global campaign and engaged with members through the use of digital technology, #WeAreG4Surgery.

TABLE 3.4.1 ■ Nongovernmental organisation federation profiles

Organisation	No. of countries of operation	Founding member	Year founded
CARE	94	United States	1945
MSF	72	France	1971
Oxfam	>90	United Kingdom	1942
Save the Children	68	United Kingdom	1919
World Vision	92	United States	1950

CARE, Cooperative for Assistance and Relief Everywhere; *MSF,* Médecins Sans Frontières
Data from Agency annual reports for 2001.

The impact of digital technologies on social movements

Social media and the digital space are integral in connecting people. For example, Twitter and Facebook enable the public to participate in every aspect of society, including health care. The impact of these technologies remains unclear, and people are still limited by their geosociopolitical constraints. The digital space has enabled HSMs to interact with policymakers more effectively.

An example of this is the World We Want After 2015 campaign, where more than 1 million participants from all over the world contributed to discussions on the sustainable development agenda.

Women's leadership in global health: Twitter campaign highlights top women in global health

Gender inequality, especially in leadership, is a disconcerting reality. Women in global health leadership roles are rarely given the podium. In an effort to publicise the discussion following numerous sessions with predominantly male-only panels, Ilona Kickbush launched a provocative social media campaign asking people to nominate leading women in global health.

'I started this after one of those meetings where I was listening to men all day and I thought what can I do?' she (Ilona Kickbush) said. 'I thought I must showcase women and I sent out tweets asking others to come up with names. Very quickly people were getting messages of congratulations for making it on to the list and others were saying how proud they were to be on it.' In what began as an effort of to highlight 100 women, the list has now grown to more than 300 women (#wgh100).

Following the social media spark #WGH300, Women in Global Health launched a gender equity in health leadership campaign at the 68th World Health Assembly in May 2015.

Roopa Dhatt (USA)

'As healthcare students it is our responsibility to raise awareness about health issues and fight for our patients and societies. There are so many social movements to help us do this. For example, students interested in public health within Hawler Medical College in Kurdistan joined the World Malaria Day campaign. We took photos and wrote on our hands saying "I raise my hand to #defeatmalaria". Will you raise your hand for a cause you care about?'

Chra Abdulla, medical student (Kurdistan)

Conclusion

Social movements and NGOs play an important role in advancing social change. Individuals can engage effectively in health issues as informed advocates. HSMs are an effective means of promoting health and well-being for all.

KEY POINTS

- Social movements are integral to the creation of societal balance and transformation.
- Social movements require three main ingredients: political opportunity, organisation capacity and framing ability.
- Nongovernmental organisations provide the opportunity for concentrating masses, capacity and coalition building and rallying the masses to lead social change. However, they function under distinct constraints, primarily related to transparency, representation and accountability.
- The digital age has transformed social movements, redefining and creating new space for organisation and activism.

Further reading

Advocacy toolkit: influencing the post-2015 development agenda. <http://www.sustainabledevelopment2015.org/index.php/news/284-news-sdgs/1544-advocacy-toolkit-influencing-the-post-2015-development-agenda>.

Brown P, Zavestoski S: Social movements in health: an introduction, *Sociol Health Illn* 26(6):679–694, 2004.

Brown P, Zavestoski S, McCormick S, et al: Embodied health movements: new approaches to social movements in health, *Sociol Health Illn* 26(1):50–80, 2004.

Laverack G: *Health activism: foundations and strategies*, London, 2013, Sage Publications.

3.5 Building Equitable Partnerships

Mustapha Kamara (Sierra Leone) ▓ Jake Newcomb (USA)

> *'If we are together nothing is impossible. If we are divided all will fail.'*
>
> Winston Churchill

Introduction

Collaborative working is essential in a complex and diverse global health arena. A variety of partnerships facilitate this collaborative approach. Examples of partnerships in global health include country-level financing in aid coordination, global international partnerships, academia–industry partnerships, and public–private partnerships.

The principles of trust, openness, equality and mutual respect lie at the core of successful partnerships. An effective partnership requires equitable collaboration with mutually agreed goals and objectives. Partnerships may benefit member organisations and partners by allowing them to share information and expertise, human and material resources, or intangibles such as reputation, trust and visibility. Partnerships may allow organisations to combine operations and realise economies of scope and scale in the provision of public health services. They should underpin the coordinated delivery of programmes and services, thereby improving population health.

Structures and types of partnerships

Partnerships develop at individual, institutional, national and international levels. They may involve IGOs, NGOs and academic and commercial institutions.

The Northumbria Healthcare NHS Foundation Trust (United Kingdom) and Kilimanjaro Christian Medical Centre Institutional Health Institution Partnership

Health partnerships between institutions in the United Kingdom and low or lower middle-income countries are an increasingly important model of development. These relationships provide mutual benefits through facilitating capacity building, education and training for both partners as well as staff exchange between the two institutions.

Inaugurated in 2001, the link between Kilimanjaro Christian Medical Centre (KCMC) and Northumbria Healthcare NHS Foundation Trust was launched as a training link between the two establishments. With focus on clinical coding, occupational therapy, physiotherapy and tissue viability, the collaboration has expanded to involve an increasing number of hospital departments. Surgical practice at KCMC focused on theatre nursing, sterile supplies, ultrasound-guided and laparoscopic surgery. A real-time telecommunications link allowed surgeons to observe and support their Tanzanian counterparts. In 2014 the project was awarded the Karen Woo Surgical Team of the Year Award by the *British Medical Journal*.

In a further project on the management of burns, training courses were developed that led to an improvement in the clinical and nonclinical competencies of health care workers in both institutions. Further research led to the development of a toolkit to provide evidence of the benefit of this partnership to both the NHS and professionals at KCMC.

Mubashir Jusabani and Sakina Rashid (Tanzania)

BOX 3.5.1 ■ Hardy's six partnership principles

Recognise and accept the need for partnership.
- Identify need and goals for partnership
- Identify potential partners
- Engage
- Evaluate and select partners.

Develop clarity and realism of purpose.
- Agree on the goals, objective and principles of partnership
- Define roles and responsibilities
- Create work-plan
- Set target for success
- Build internal support in each organisation

Ensure commitment and ownership.
- Set structure for managing project
- Define process for decision-making and dispute resolution
- Identify and mobilise resources
- Implement!

Develop and maintain trust.
Create clear and robust partnership arrangements.
- Agree an MOU (Memorandum of Understanding)

Monitor, measure and learn.
- Ensure sustainability of project/benefits
- Decide whether to continue or disband the partnership
- Institutionalise the partnership or execute exit strategy
- Conduct final evaluation and share learning from project and partnership

---

Reproduced with permission from the Office of the Deputy Prime Minister. Hardy B, Hudson R, Waddington E. Assessing strategic development – the partnership assessment tool. ODPM free literature. Product code: 03LRGG01269.

Partnerships are social networks. The following three aspects of social networks help define the structure of partnerships:

- *Network breadth:* This reflects the array of different actors (partners), which determines the amount and type of organisational resources that may be contributed.
- *Network density:* This measures the amount of interconnectedness between organisations/sectors, which facilitates their ability to work together.
- *Network centrality:* This reflects the relative influence of a single organisation within a partnership, which can be important for coordinating and focusing collaborative actions.

Building partnerships

The process of building partnerships is complex and requires several stages. These are illustrated in Hardy's six partnership principles (**Box 3.5.1**).

Factors affecting partnership working

Factors to be considered when building and maintaining a partnership include:

- *Individual factors*: personal expectations and perceived benefits. In building partnerships, there must be trust and mutual respect, with compromise between partners where necessary. The lack of certain skills can make individuals feel disempowered but this may also represent an opportunity for learning.

- ■ *Organisational factors*: governance structures and decision-approval procedures. The degree of formalisation, the responsibility of each partner, internal structure and operating procedures are important issues in partnership development. These should be clearly stated in a memorandum of understanding. Transparency and joint decision making by all involved parties as well as a mechanism for conflict resolution are essential.
- ■ *Contextual factors*: political environment or composition of the health system. These are factors that can either help or destroy the partnership, and include the political environment and the degree of health system decentralisation.

Global health partnerships

Global health partnerships include public–private partnerships, service provider–patient interactions, thematic partnerships, country-level financing/aid partnerships, global or international partnerships, academia–industry partnerships, academic–community partnerships, and intersectoral partnerships. These are not mutually exclusive and examples of some of these categories include:

Large international global health partnerships between major stakeholders are useful when programmes are being scaled up. An example of is the GFATM (see Chapter 3.2). Between 75 and 100 global health partnerships have mobilised important and new resources against major global health threats. Recipient countries are forced to demonstrate transparency and accountability. Key indicators and targets must be monitored as continued funding is dependent on review of performance. Major challenges for global health partnerships include effective coordination and long-term sustainability. However, a global health partnership targeting a very limited and narrow area (e.g., a single disease) does not necessarily respond to the dominant health concerns of an individual country. As there is no single organisation with the mandate to coordinate all these various partnerships, inefficiencies and duplication are inevitable. These issues were highlighted in the Paris Declaration (2005), which provided a road map to improve the quality of aid and its impact on development.

A public–private partnership is a government service or private business venture funded and operated through a partnership between government and one or more private sector companies. These include academia–industry partnerships. Although public–private partnerships have existed at a national level for many years, interaction between the public and private sectors within the UN system developed only following reforms instituted by Secretary-General Kofi Annan. There is evidence to suggest that areas within the United Nations in which private companies have large stakes (e.g., much of health care) are better funded than areas where there are few private interests (e.g., education). Additionally, private philanthropic initiatives may adversely affect the coordination of development efforts through duplication. There are also concerns that many initiatives prioritise short-term results to the detriment of longer-term improvement.

Examples of public–private partnerships include:

- ■ *Product development partnerships*. These are public–private partnerships that focus on pharmaceutical product development for diseases of the resource-poor world. These include preventative medicines such as vaccines and microbicides, as well as treatments for otherwise neglected diseases. International product development partnerships accelerate research and development of pharmaceutical products for underserved populations and do not profit private companies.
- ■ The *Roll Back Malaria* Partnership (1998). This is the global framework for coordinated action against malaria. It forges consensus among key actors in malaria control, harmonises action and mobilises resources to fight malaria in endemic countries.

- The *Aeras Global TB Vaccine Foundation* is a product development partnership dedicated to the development of effective tuberculosis vaccine regimens. This will prevent tuberculosis in all age groups, and will be affordable, available and adopted worldwide.
- *The WHO.* The WHO collaborates with NGOs, the pharmaceutical industry, and foundations such as the Bill & Melinda Gates Foundation and the Rockefeller Foundation. Some of these collaborations can be regarded as global public–private partnerships; 15% of WHO's total revenue in 2012 was financed by private foundations.

Pharmaceutical industry partnerships: Pfizer and AIDS medication in South Africa

The partnership between Pfizer, local governments, nongovernmental organisations (NGOs) and other international actors demonstrates some of the benefits and challenges of this form of partnership. In 2015 about 7 million South African citizens had HIV, with a prevalence of 19.2% in adults aged between 15 and 49 years. Pfizer (a leading pharmaceutical company) developed many of the antiretroviral drugs and drugs against opportunistic infections that affect AIDS patients, including fluconazole (Diflucan).

Following several complaints that fluconazole was expensive, Pfizer launched an initiative to distribute it free of charge in South Africa. It worked in partnership with NGOs, local governments and international partners, including Axios International, IMA World Health, and the International Dispensary Association. Through this partnership, Pfizer supported 63 developing countries in Africa, Asia, the Caribbean and Latin America, and provided training and education materials to 20,000 health care professionals.

However, critics of this partnership suggested that the fact that antiretroviral drugs were excluded in this initiative meant that impoverished patients had to become extremely unwell to benefit from the world's most profitable pharmaceutical company. As public–private partnerships become increasingly common, there remains a challenge to ensure equity in health care.

Ismail El-Kharbotly (Egypt)

Service provider–patient interactions are relationships between medical practitioners/hospitals and individuals seeking their services. The nature of these services may be influenced by the wishes of the people seeking them.

Intersectoral partnering is the process of creating joint interorganisational initiatives across two or more sectors. These partnerships involve collaboration between organisations from various sectors: the state (government), the market (business) and civil society (NGOs).

An academic–community partnership is a related form of partnership: for example, a relationship between an academic institution and a community at risk of a particular health problem. Such relationships are generally facilitated by one or more dedicated academics (e.g., the Blantyre Malaria Project in Blantyre, Malawi, which focuses on the research and eradication of paediatric malaria within the community).

Conclusion

As recognised by Millennium Development Goal 8 (Global Partnership for Development) and Sustainable Development Goal 17 (Partnerships for the Goals), working in partnerships is a critical challenge in the current era of global health development. The diversity of partnerships illustrates the potential benefits of working together with a variety of stakeholders. Effective collaboration and equity within a partnership is a central tenet for success.

KEY POINTS

- There are many examples of partnership and collaborative working in global health. These constitute a key mode for the delivery of global health interventions.
- Partnership structures depend on network breadth, density and centrality.
- The types of partnership include collaborative, comprehensive and limited forms of partnership.
- Partnership working depends on factors at the individual, organisational and contextual levels. They are enhanced if partners have similar principles.

Further reading

Lorenz N: Effectiveness of global health partnerships: will the past repeat itself?, *Bull World Health Organ* 85(7):567–568, 2007.

Millennium Project: *Millennium Development Goal 8*, 2006. Available from <http://www.unmillenniumproject.org/goals/gti.htm#goal8>.

Politics, Economics and Education

Junior Editor: Eleanor Turner-Moss (UK)

Introduction

Fundamental influences determine how countries and their populations work and live. Political debates and decisions often fail to recognise the implications for health, yet discussions continue in the name of health to maintain political and economic power. This political agenda can adversely affect social determinants of health, and has wider implications for the morale and general well-being of a country.

4.1 Poverty, Social Inequality and Health

Nicolas Blondel (Spain)　　Alice Clarke (UK)　　Baher Mohamed (Egypt)
Basem Mohamed (Egypt)

Introduction

'Everyone has the right to a standard of living adequate for the health and well-being of himself and of his family, including food, clothing, housing, and medical care and necessary social services, and the right to security in the event of unemployment, sickness, disability, widowhood, old age or other lack of livelihood in circumstances beyond his control.'

Article 25(1) of Universal Declaration of Human Rights

When one is examining the complex interplay between poverty and health, there are two major questions. Firstly, do people have enough food, medicines, shelter and finance? A deficiency of these can lead to *absolute* poverty. Secondly, how are these resources distributed within society? Inequitable distribution of resources can be a cause of *relative* poverty. An integrated economic, political and health care agenda is a fundamental requirement for good individual health as well as population health.

Poverty and health

Wealth and poverty are basic indicators of health and life expectancy, and are key determinants of health (**Fig. 4.1.1**). The World Bank defines *extreme poverty* when individuals live on less than US$1.25 a day. This is an absolute measure, and today roughly 1.2 billion people worldwide meet this definition. A third of the world's overall population live on less than US$2.50 a day and 80% live on less than US$10 a day. These crude metrics do not account for issues such as female empowerment, education and literacy rates. However, when resources such as housing and medicine are provided free of charge by, for example, the state, extreme poverty can be compatible with a good quality of life.

More recently, there has been increasing interest in the health impacts of *relative poverty*. Here, poverty is measured with reference to others in the same nation or society. In the United States, despite being one of the wealthiest world economies, a lack of health insurance makes health-related expenses a leading cause of bankruptcy. In the United Kingdom, another affluent country, the rate of child poverty correlates with life expectancy (**Fig. 4.1.2**).

Discussions on poverty have always focused on the lack of access to food, fuel, medicines and water. Each day 22,000 children die because of a lack of these basic resources (UNICEF). Approximately 850 million people worldwide lack access to clean water and do not have enough to eat. This situation is likely to worsen with the deleterious effects of climate change. More than a third of deaths in children younger than 5 years are related to malnutrition, and life expectancy is shortened by more than 2 decades in deprived communities.

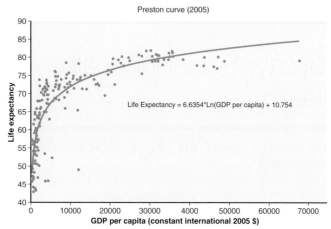

Figure 4.1.1 The Preston curve. Life expectancy (years) correlated with GDP per capita. *(Redrawn from Preston SH: The changing relation between mortality and level of economic development, Int J Epidemiol 36(3):484–490, 2007.)*

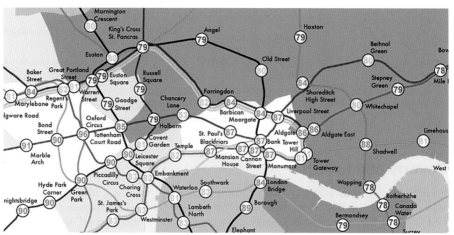

Figure 4.1.2 Life expectancy (years) changes across tube stops in London, and correlation with rates of child poverty. *(For complete data on London underground lines, see Cheshire J: Lives on the line: mapping life expectancy along the London tube network, Environ Plan A (2012) 44(7):1525–1528.)*

The impact of poverty on access to treatment

Safina's story demonstrates how patients in low-income countries with preventable conditions can be deprived of appropriate medical treatment because of lack of financial capability.

Safina is a 2-year-old girl who was admitted with high temperature, flaccid lower limb paralysis, loss of sphincter control and tonic–clonic seizures. This presentation was in stark contrast to her previously excellent neurological development and sphincter control. Because of lack of finances, Safina's mother— a single parent—was unable to afford a CT scan (~US$75). Her condition did not respond significantly to medical therapy in the following 5 weeks. Eventually, a CT scan was performed which demonstrated dermal sinus, a congenital spinal condition amenable to surgical treatment. Sadly, because of financial pressures, this treatment was delayed for many months, and Safina was ultimately left paraplegic. It is likely that this sad outcome could have been minimalised had her family been able to access the necessary financial resources.

Sakina Rashid (Tanzania) and Marieke Dekker (Tanzania)

Social inequality and health

Social inequality has been shown to be linked to poorer health outcomes. Poverty also contributes to social marginalisation and is linked to other determinants of health, such as social class, race or caste. Assessing health inequality is complex, and reduction in inequality may require active redistribution of wealth. High levels of inequality adversely affect economic growth, and reduce a country's ability to alleviate poverty. The state can play an important role through its ability to implement progressive taxation to fund social programmes:

- *Progressive* taxation systems are those which redistribute money from the wealthy to the poor. Taxing wealthier populations can fund investment in social spending.
- *Regressive* taxation systems, which include those taxes which affect basic requirements, are those which affect the poor as much as, or more than, the wealthiest. These taxes disproportionately affect the poor because they spend a higher percentage of their overall income on basic necessities.

The global financial crisis of 2008 provided an opportunity to appraise the impact of recession and subsequent allocation of social resources on health. It also showed how inequalities and political and social policies can affect health outcomes.

Health in Greece following the financial crisis

Social spending and progressive welfare programmes were cut in many countries following the financial crisis. This can have disastrous effects on health as demonstrated by experience in Greece.

In Greece, cuts to public spending following the financial crisis removed many of the social safety nets which previously protected vulnerable people. Twenty-two percent of the population reported living in material deprivation, not being able to heat their homes or pay their rent, and by 2011 the proportion had risen to 28%.

Reduction in social insurance excluded a third of the population from health coverage, and 70% of people were unable to afford the costs of prescription drugs. The cost of maternity care resulted in a 21% rise in the number of stillbirths between 2008 and 2011. HIV infection rates rose from less than 20 per year in 2010 to nearly 500 per year by 2013.

Reduced investment in health infrastructure also had a profound impact. The closure of mental health clinics, with the reduction of trained staff and services, coincided with an increase in mental health needs. As a consequence, there was a rise in suicide by 45% between 2007 and 2011, mainly affecting men of working age who had been made redundant.

These examples show some of the diverse impacts of social policies affecting both poverty and health, and highlight the complexity of the interplay between these issues in times of financial trouble.

Nicolas Blondel (Spain)

At times of economic crisis, governments can minimise adverse effects by the redistribution of available resources to social programmes including those for mental health. For example, Iceland, with similar economic challenges to Greece, avoided an increase in the rate of suicides by increased investment in this area of health care.

A disease perspective on poverty

Poverty is linked to burden of disease for many communicable and noncommunicable diseases. Each year, infectious diseases kill 3.5 million people—mostly the poor and young children who live in lower middle-income countries (LMIC). Poverty increases vulnerability to communicable diseases, and lack of access to medical care. The poorest suffer a double burden of medical costs and loss of income from a previously productive family member. LMIC are more vulnerable to outbreaks and epidemics. Haiti, following a major earthquake in 2010 experienced a cholera epidemic of 91,770 cases with 2071 deaths. The lack of basic resources such as oral rehydration solutions contributed significantly to these poor outcomes.

Apart from infectious diseases, those living in poverty are also subject to other diseases seen in higher-income environments. These include noncommunicable diseases (NCDs) and mental health disorders. Neglected tropical diseases are an additional burden in many countries with extreme poverty.

A life course perspective on poverty

Socioeconomic status affects health throughout all stages of life. Malnutrition, resulting from poverty, adversely affects child development and contributes to increased levels of morbidity and mortality. Growth delay resulting in stunting is a common finding in low-income countries and LMIC. This situation is compounded by an increased susceptibility to infections and a lack of access to health care facilities.

The health of older people is also compromised by poverty in high-income countries as well as low-income countries. Ten percent of older Americans live below official poverty thresholds. The quality of life in ageing populations is closely linked to socioeconomic status.

Fuel poverty in the United Kingdom

Fuel poverty is an example of relative poverty which affects vulnerable groups.

Fuel poverty occurs when a household spends a tenth or more of its income on energy. It can be caused by high fuel costs, low incomes and poorly insulated homes. Forty-four percent of households in Northern Ireland experience fuel poverty. This has a direct effect on physical and mental health, and can cause excess deaths during winter. Those particularly affected are young children, the elderly and those with preexisting medical conditions. Improved insulation in houses reduces fuel consumption, with associated environmental and health benefits.

Alice Clarke (UK)

Tackling poverty

'The ill or the poor cannot be treated only by medications and doctors, but by ensuring freedom, education and prosperity for the whole population.'

Attributed to Rudolph Virchow

In 1978 the Declaration of Alma-Ata at the International Conference on Primary Health Care recognised that robust population health could be attained only when a comprehensive and universally accessible primary health service coordinated its actions with related sectors of national and community development.

Population health improved dramatically with the introduction of clean drinking water, better sanitation and hygiene, and improved nutrition. Female education, higher wages, and labour legislation transformed hitherto squalid living and exploitative work conditions. In the meantime, many resource-poor countries have adopted intersectoral health programmes that directly combine poverty reduction strategies with health promotion strategies.

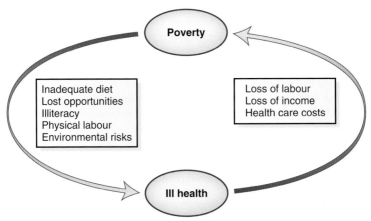

Figure 4.1.3   The vicious cycle of poverty and health. *(Redrawn from <http://vwordpress.stmarys-ca.edu/ nadiabellafronte/files/2014/05/poverty-and-health-2l67sgi.gif>.)*

Many programmes attempting to tackle poverty (**Fig. 4.1.3**) aim to stop the vicious cycle of poverty and health. Examples of innovative and successful programmes tackling poverty to improve health include:

- The Pan American Health Organization's prevention and primary health services programme tailored for producers, agricultural workers and livestock producers.
- BRAC's (formerly Bangladesh Advancement Committee) microfinance organisation for the poor that has developed a sustainable livelihood initiative for ultrapoor women.
- Brazil's programme to eradicate poverty and hunger. In 9 years this achieved a 61% decrease in child malnutrition, as well as a 15% decrease in rural poverty. The initiative 'Zero Hunger' adopted in 2003 made Brazil a world-famous site as it succeeded in raising 23 million of 192 million citizens out of poverty.
- The Hungarian special unit for tuberculosis treatment targeting homeless and alcoholic tuberculosis patients. This addressed the most intractable determinants of the disease— substance misuse and homelessness.

A global perspective on poverty

'These days there is a lot of poverty in the world, and that's a scandal when we have so many riches and resources to give everyone. We all have to think about how we can become a little poorer.'

Pope Francis

The target of Millennium Development Goal (MDG) 1 was to eradicate extreme poverty and hunger. Extreme poverty rates were reduced by half (target 1A) 5 years ahead of the 2015 deadline. Although the MDG 1 target 1C to reduce hunger by 50% was almost met by 2015, an estimated 15.5% of the world population still suffers from hunger. MDG 1 may have been partially achieved, but improvements should be balanced against the effects of increasing social inequality. The World Bank *Global Monitoring Report 2014/2015* stated that 'the average income of the richest 10 percent of the population is now about 9.5 times that of the poorest 10 percent, as opposed to 7 times 25 years ago.' (<http://pubdocs.worldbank.org/en/637391444058280425/GMR-2014-Full-Report.pdf>). The World Bank therefore continues to prioritise ending poverty *and* inequality. The Sustainable Development Goals (SDGs) continue to prioritise the abolition of poverty and hunger.

Conclusion

Poverty and health are closely interrelated. The uneven distribution of global resources has negative implications for the health of society. Absolute poverty has long-term consequences throughout life, and relative poverty is also linked to poor health outcomes. Sustainable intersectoral interventions targeting the social determinants of health are essential for a more equal society. Health care professionals have a key role to play in tackling the causes of poverty and ill health, and in championing equitable access and treatment, regardless of socioeconomic status.

KEY POINTS

- Poverty and good health are intricately interconnected.
- Poverty can be extreme or relative.
- The effects of poverty can be reduced though political interventions.
- The eradication of poverty remains the target of Sustainable Development Goal 1.

Further reading

Kim JY, Millen J, Irwin A, Gershman J, editors: *Dying for growth: global inequality and the health of the poor*, Monroe, 2000, Common Courage Press.

Sachs J: *The end of poverty: economic possibilities for our time*, New York, 2006, Penguin.

Stuckler D, Basu S: *The body economic: why austerity kills*, London, 2013, Basic Books, London.

Wilkinson RG, Pickett K: *The spirit level: why more equal societies almost always do better*, London, 2009, Allen Lane.

4.2 Trade and Health

Benjamin Ebeling (Denmark)   Jesper Kjær (Denmark)

Introduction

'Before you finish eating your breakfast this morning you've depended on half the world. This is the way our universe is structured. We aren't going to have peace on earth until we recognise this basic fact.'

Martin Luther King Jr

Trade fuels global economies, and trade agreements are influenced by and depend on global politics and power balances. Trade affects health through numerous social determinants. Health issues can be affected by trade arrangements both directly and indirectly. For example, a direct effect is the cost of medical products, which are often subject to commercial patents. High prices of drugs may be prohibitive. An indirect effect occurs when trade agreements promoting foreign investment strengthen local health systems.

The importance of trade for health

Aspects of globalisation can be disadvantageous for the poorest countries. This occurs for three main reasons:

- Most trade and trade relationships are concentrated in the wealthiest parts of the world. The exchange of resources and wealth between these stakeholders alone enriches them further whilst excluding poorer countries. For example, in 2006 the African region contributed only 3% of the world's manufacturing exports and 2% of commercial services.
- Smaller economies are more fragile to fluctuations in the market, and are less able to access capital and the other resources required to scale up their operations.
- Bigger economies can subsidise their own producers. In 2007 the United States subsidised its agricultural production by $31.6 billion, which far outweighed its total overseas development aid budget of $25.8 billion in 2008. This competition in the market can leave the poorest farmers unemployed. African farmers get hit hard as they cannot sell food products to overseas markets, and overproduction in wealthier countries is sold cheaply or dumped as 'aid', undermining local industries.

Trade agreements often fail to appreciate the possible consequences on health. Doctors or public health professionals are rarely asked to contribute to trade negotiations. Educating future health professionals in basic trade concepts is therefore crucial.

The trading of goods, services and intellectual property is governed by the treaties and standards of the World Trade Organization (WTO).

- *Goods* cross borders daily. These include anything physical (e.g., clothing, agricultural products, electronics, medicines and chemicals).

- *Services* include sectors such as health services, law, communications, construction, education, energy, finance and tourism.
- *Intellectual property* is a property that covers a variety of intangible assets. Examples of these include musical, literary, and artistic works, discoveries and inventions, phrases, words, symbols and designs. Intellectual property includes copyright, trademarks, patents and industrial design. The most important intellectual property right when one is dealing with public health and international trade is patents. Securities and financial instruments are also tradable but are not part of today's WTO system.

A patent is a grant of a property right given by the sovereign state to the inventor 'to exclude others from making, using or selling the invention' for a limited period. In the case of today's WTO members, a patent is granted for 20 years. Patents are particularly important when considering pharmaceutical products. A pharmaceutical company will apply for a new drug patent which will grant a 20-year monopoly to exclusively produce and sell the drug at a price of its choice.

International organisations

The end of World War II marked the beginning of a new era for the world economy. Policymakers increasingly recognised that international trade was essential for economic growth, moving away from the isolationist policies of the war period. Efforts to create an international structure, namely the International Trade Organization, failed, and instead an international agreement was created—the General Agreement on Tariffs and Trade (GATT). Its purpose was the 'substantial reduction of tariffs and other trade barriers and the elimination of preferences, on a reciprocal and mutually advantageous basis.' It was signed by 23 countries in 1947, took effect in 1948 and served as the only multilateral mechanism to handle international trade relations until 1995, when it was incorporated together with other trade-related frameworks, introducing the WTO.

The WTO recognised that trade rules needed to be formalised and institutionalised. It provides the basic legal framework for international trade, establishing and upholding the basic guidelines for engagement between member states. These served to harmonise rules and create standard approaches to trading. Today, they include more than 20 agreements, of which five are critical to public health:

- GATT
- General Agreement on Trade of Services (GATS)
- Agreement on Trade-Related Aspects of Intellectual Property Rights (TRIPS)
- Agreement on Technical Barriers to Trade (TBT)
- Agreement on the Application of Sanitary and Phytosanitary Measures (SPM)

Today, the WTO comprises 160 members, serving as a forum where governments can negotiate on international trade. All member states must comply with WTO's international standard requirements. The WTO structure includes three main components: ministerial conferences, the General Council and the Secretariat.

Trade is essential for economic growth and poverty mitigation. WTO supporters argue that international trade rules increase global economic outputs and, thereby, living standards. Others criticise the WTO decision-making process as it can favour the interests of economically developed countries. Commercial interests may conflict with the interests of health, safety, human rights, the environment and development.

The World Health Organization (WHO) undertakes to protect and promote the mental, physical and social well-being of the world's population. It has made efforts to identify links between trade and health, first described in a 2002 joint WHO–WTO report (*WTO Agreements*

& *Public Health*). The WHO undertakes trade-related activities under a number of its departments and programmes:

- immunisation, vaccines and biologicals
- medicines policy, essential drugs and traditional medicine
- ethics, equity, trade and human rights
- public health, innovation and intellectual property
- the Tobacco Free Initiative

The WHO holds ad hoc observer status at the WTO councils on the Agreement on TRIPs and GATS, and serves as member of the TBT and SPM committees.

Regulations and free trade agreements

'It hit me very early on that something was terribly wrong, that I would see silos full of food and supermarkets full of food, and kids starving …. In Fair Trade we see ourselves as this infinitesimal part of the world economy. But somebody's got to come with an alternative model that says children eating is Number 1.'

Medea Benjamin (former UN nutritionalist)

Trade agreements deal with the distribution of goods. Inequitable distribution can adversely affect access to health care. In contrast, free trade agreements aim to create open trading between two or more countries, thereby promoting economic growth. This growth comes about as a result of specialisation, division of labour and via comparative advantage. For example, Germany is efficient at producing cars and the Netherlands at producing light bulbs; the countries should therefore trade those goods instead of making them more inefficiently themselves.

Patent protection of drugs may have serious health consequences for the poor. This was highlighted by the AIDS crisis in Africa in the 1990s when the prohibitive cost of antiretroviral drugs contributed to many premature deaths. Responding to international concerns, the Doha Declaration (2001) stated that 'the TRIPS agreement does not and should not prevent members from taking measures to protect public health. Each member has the right to grant compulsory licenses and the freedom to determine the grounds on which licenses are granted.' The WHO recommended incorporation of these flexibilities into national patent laws. However, by 2011, only 57% of low-income countries had legal provisions for compulsory licensing.

The Indian Patents Act 1970

Eighty percent of the drugs used by Médecins Sans Frontières are manufactured in India. This was possible following the changes to patent legislation which encouraged generic drug production.

Before 1970, multinational companies dominated the Indian pharmaceutical market with a share of 85%, and local production was kept to a minimum. The Indian Patents Act 1970 removed production patents completely, and 'process patents' were reduced from a monopoly of 16 years down to 7 years to encourage innovation.

Local generic pharmaceutical companies took advantage of these new opportunities, and the price of medicines fell dramatically. The Indian Patents Act 1970 was in place until India joined the World Trade Organization, thereby accepting the rules and law under the Agreement on Trade-Related Aspects of Intellectual Property Rights.

Benjamin Ebeling (Denmark) and Jesper Nørgaard Kjær (Denmark)

Trade in health services

Trade in health services is becoming globalised in four main ways:

- *Increasing movement of health workers.* The movement of health workers around the globe has a huge impact on health systems. Some countries (e.g., the Philippines) produce an excess of health care workers, who then work overseas and remit money to their families.
- *Increasing movement of patients/consumers.* Health tourism enables affluent patients to access high-quality services anywhere in the world. For example, the low cost of medical treatment in India and Thailand encourages health tourism from rich as well as resource-poor nations.
- *Increasing cross-border service delivery.* Interactive technologies, such as telemedicine, enable the provision of diagnostic services and consultations regardless of geography. Electronic technologies enable the rapid delivery of services such as radiology and pathology.
- *Bilateral and multilateral trade agreements for health delivery.* These largely support health system development in resource-poor countries

Trade policy indirectly affects health through its impact on the social determinants of health. This is evident when, for instance, local incomes rise as a result of new trade agreements but the liberalisation of trade does not necessarily result in poverty reduction.

Work and health

The International Labour Organization has a set of international labour standards 'aimed at promoting opportunities for women and men to obtain decent and productive work, in conditions of freedom, equity, security and dignity.' These standards complement basic human rights.

Working conditions have a huge impact on health. Accidental injury contributes to the heavy burden of disease in many countries. The failure to appreciate the importance of health and safety regulations is a major cause of disability (e.g., operating unsafe machinery or working without appropriate protective equipment).

Forced labour is work obtained from a person under real or perceived threat. Labour exploitation is often an element of human trafficking. In the Palermo Protocol to Prevent, Suppress and Punish Trafficking in Persons, human trafficking is the combination of movement or harbouring of a person, use of deception or coercion, and placement into situations of exploitation. Trafficking of people, for all forms of exploitation, including labour exploitation, is an international criminal offence and is commonly referred to as *slavery*.

Forced labour can be identified when there is a lack of consent to work and an associated menace of a penalty (International Labour Organization, 2015). There may, for instance, be:

- threats or actual physical harm
- restriction of movement and confinement to the workplace or to a limited area
- debt-bondage
- withholding of wages or excessive wage reductions that violate previous agreements
- retention of passports and identity documents
- threat of telling authorities that the worker is of illegal status

Although the consequences of labour exploitation and health are not well documented, studies show huge health implications on the people involved. In a study investigating the health conditions of trafficked men and women for UK labour exploitation, 40% reported that they experienced physical violence while they were being trafficked, 81% reported one or more physical health symptoms and 57% reported one or more posttraumatic stress symptom (Turner-Moss, 2014).

Child labour exploitation and health

Labour exploitation is prevalent and neglected. More than 168 million children (5–17 years old) are working, and of these, 85 million are engaged in the 'worst forms of child labour' (International Labour Organization, 2015). These include trafficking, armed conflict, slavery, debt bondage, sexual exploitation and hazardous work.

Labour exploitation operates in, and sometimes throughout, supply chains. These supply chains are built to meet the demands of consumers. This allows a unique opportunity to question and insist on accountability for what is happening across the world. Labour exploitation has diverse impacts on health.

Working children are exposed to adult occupational risks, and are therefore especially vulnerable. Most receive no safety training and use no protective equipment, which, if available, is designed for adults. The lack of documented evidence on child injuries is often used as an excuse for inaction.

The sparse literature on the health of adults trafficked for labour exploitation reveals that these individuals also experience high burdens of mental and physical illness. A substantial proportion will have experienced violence and abuse. Those who are trafficked are often tightly controlled and have limited, if any, access to health services. If they do manage to present to health services, health professionals are often unprepared to recognise their situation and vulnerability or cater for their complex needs.

Eleanor Turner-Moss (UK)

Trade versus aid: the most effective route to health equity

The structural injustice of some trade negotiations and agreements is seen by many as a primary cause of continued poverty in many lower-income countries. It has been suggested that correcting any injustice is a more urgent and effective priority than increasing the amount of donated aid.

Emergency and developmental aid serve different roles. Aid often has political ties and purpose, particularly in bilateral agreements. Charitable construction projects, for instance, often undermine local authority and resources. Local farmers can be undercut or bankrupted by food aid. Local health services can be shattered as a skeletal health workforce is offered better paid roles in international aid organisations. Local governments often account for foreign aid and use it when prioritising their economy. Aid may indirectly end up financing military equipment by lowering local governments' spending on schools and hospitals. Other known outcomes of aid include harm to international competitive performance (decreasing exports) and damage to local governance as they avoid difficult decisions.

Nevertheless, aid can also build societies and have positive outcomes through structural and sustainable changes. Sustainable aid teaches and develops local capacity, does not displace local jobs and addresses deep-rooted challenges.

Neither aid nor trade policy offers a clear route to global health equity. Trade liberalisation can have unintended consequences by increasing income inequality, worsening psychosocial stress and introducing unhealthy lifestyle and diet (**Table 4.2.1**).

Improving trade

'A bite of Fair Trade chocolate means a lot to farmers in the South. It opens the doors to development and gives children access to healthcare, education and a decent standard of living.'

K. Ohemeng-Tinyase (Ghana)

TABLE 4.2.1 ■ **Trade versus aid**

Towards health equity	Pros	Cons
Trade	• Opening of markets that can bring in new technology and medicine • Increased international cooperation => steady and independent flow of cash and goods • Increased trade will focus attention on good governance, the benefits of a broadly stable currency and internal security in developing countries	• Increases income inequality • Increases competition => psychosocial stress • Some countries do not have the ability to trade because of low raw materials or lack of education • Cheap imports can impair local industries in developing countries
Aid	• Aid is linked to need and help those who cannot engage in trade • Even distribution of resources. In theory, no one in need should be overlooked • Can target specifically identified groups or areas on the basis of need • Can change structural barriers, e.g., corruption, education or infrastructure • Can provide expert advisors who can prepare the country for the challenges of globalisation	• Dependent upon economic situation of developed, donor countries • Indirect finance of weapons • Patronising concept • Manipulation by politicians from donor countries • Increasing bureaucracy and control

Data from < http://debatewise.org/debates/2795-trade-vs-aid/>.

There are many ways in which the globalisation of trade may benefit health. For example, an increase in cross-border delivery of health care systems often allows improved surveillance, helps serve underresourced areas and reaches vulnerable populations.

Strategies to ensure a just trading system with a fair approach to health include:

■ transparency with consumers
■ training health care professionals about the impacts of trade agreements
■ increasing the number of safeguards around public–private partnerships
■ creating high levels of standards in trading of health services
■ developing a database around global trading in health services

Methods such as these could have significant impacts by ensuring that health considerations are a component of relevant trade negotiations.

Conclusion

The conditions in which individuals work and the prices they can achieve for goods are subject to national and international agreements. These have a significant impact on their quality of life and health. Trade agreements can affect health issues directly by increasing the prices of medicines, or indirectly by increasing poverty and inequality. Health professionals should play a key role in protecting vulnerable populations from inequitable trade agreements

KEY POINTS

- Trade agreements can affect health issues directly or indirectly.
- The World Trade Organization formalises and institutionalises global trade.
- New trade agreements can affect health issues directly through patent protection
- The views of health care workers should be considered when trade agreements are being formulated.

Further reading

Easterly W: *Reinventing foreign aid*, Cambridge, 2008, MIT Press.

International Labour Organization: *Combating forced labour: a handbook for employers and business.* Geneva, 2015, ILO.

The Lancet series on trade and health, 2009. <http://www.thelancet.com/series/trade and health>.

Turner-Moss E, Zimmerman C, Howard LM, Oram SJ: Labour exploitation and health: a case series of men and women seeking post-trafficking services, *J Immigr Minor Health* 16(3):473–480, 2014.

World Health Organization, World Trade Organization: *WTO agreements & public health*, Geneva, 2002, WTO Secretariat.

4.3 Health and Industry

Johanne Iversen (Norway)　■　Anna Rasmussen (Denmark)

Introduction

'There are certain things that microbes don't do: microbes do not lobby politicians to allow them to continue to spread; they don't spend billions of dollars to convince people that it's cool to be infected; they don't fund scientists to say it's not so bad to get that infection or re-brand themselves as "light" bacteria that might be less harmful'.

Thomas R. Frieden, Director, Centers for Disease Control and Prevention (2011)

NCDs share common risk factors, including tobacco use, unhealthy diets, misuse of alcohol and lack of physical activity. The tobacco and food industries have, historically, been very effective lobbyists for their own commercial interests, and this has impeded the development of the effective health policies necessary to combat the adverse effects of NCDs.

Tobacco

'In the 1940s, cigarettes would be shown in classy situations, endorsed by celebrities - real A-list Hollywood stars in America - the ads would make claims about tobacco quality or manufacturing science and, bizarrely, some brands had what almost amounted to health claims.'

Peter York

Smoking contributes to 8.8% of all deaths worldwide and 4.1% of all disability-adjusted life years (DALYs) (WHO). The WHO's second-ever global convention, the Framework Convention on Tobacco Control, was passed against the wishes of pro-tobacco lobbyists. The tobacco industry's own internal documents, released by US litigation settlements in 1998, revealed a decades-long history of coordinated and extensive efforts to 'attack WHO' and to 'contain, neutralise and reorient' WHO's tobacco control activities. Countries acting to protect public health increasingly face legal assaults by multinational companies. For example, the Australian government faced lawsuits from Philip Morris, a multimillion dollar tobacco company, when it introduced the requirement for plain packaging on cigarettes in 2011.

The most effective policies to reduce smoking include higher taxation on tobacco products, the control of cigarette advertising (including plain packaging) and the prohibition of smoking in public areas. The WHO (2017) recommends that at least 70% of the price paid by the tobacco consumer should be excise tax as the global tobacco epidemic leads to the death of nearly 6 million people each year. Plain packaging targets the tobacco industry's use of branding by ensuring that all packets have the same neutral appearance. Australia and the United Kingdom have both introduced standardised packaging legislation on cigarettes. In the face of taxation and regulation in richer countries, the tobacco industry has focused on less economically developed countries, using unethical marketing strategies, including some directed at teenagers (**Fig. 4.3.1**) and poor people.

this patent time frame, no other company is allowed to produce a drug that infringes on the patent rights of the original. After the patent has expired, however, the market is, theoretically, open to competition from manufacturers of generic drugs.

A generic drug is a drug that is 'usually intended to be interchangeable with an innovator product' (Kaplan and Mathers, 2011). It is 'to be bioequivalent to a reference drug specified in the approval application' (Olson and Wendling, 2013). Generic drug treatments do not currently have to repeat the process of preclinical and clinical trials before being licensed provided that they demonstrate their bioequivalence.

The development and application of generic drugs may be delayed in a number of ways by pharmaceutical companies wishing to extend their patents. For example, minor modifications of the original patented drug may enable the pharmaceutical company to apply for a 'secondary patent', thus delaying the production of cheaper generic versions of the drug for many years.

In India and some other countries, patenting of both new uses of known substances and new forms of known substances that do not enhance 'efficacy' is illegal. The *World Medicines Report* (2011) notes that whilst there has been 'a modest decline (2%–3%) in the percentage of original and licensed brand usage since 2000' (i.e., an increase in generic drug use), there is a high degree of variability across countries. Branded products are more commonly used in high- and middle-income countries, whilst lower-income countries favour the use of generics.

Regulation and medication standards

Following successful clinical trials, regulatory bodies are responsible for granting licences for pharmaceutical products. Each country or union of countries has its own approval body, the most well known of which are the Food and Drug Administration and the European Medicines Agency. Indian regulation is controlled by the Central Drugs Standard Control Organization, and Chinese medications are controlled by China's food and drug administration.

The process used for approval by the European Medicines Agency lacks transparency, and its current regulations do not involve an assessment of drug efficacy. In contrast, until 1994, the Norwegian government required all medications to prove their additional efficacy, a process known as the *needs clause*. This ensured that new medications were both in line with the health priorities as a nation and that patients were not exposed to too many medications for similar purposes.

Following regulatory approval, there remains a need to ensure the quality and safety of all drugs available on the market. This is generally easier to achieve in high-income countries, but substandard medicines are widely marketed internationally, with an estimated US$35 billion to US$44 billion annual turnover. This means that an estimated 1% of drugs in the developed world to 10% of all medications in resource-poor countries are likely to be substandard. Substandard and falsified medical products were categorised into substandard, unregistered or unlicensed products, and falsified products (WHO, 2017). This distinguishes between authorised medical products that fail to meet the necessary quality standards/specifications and products which fraudulently misrepresent their identity, composition, or source. For a medication to be considered counterfeit, there must be deliberate or fraudulent mislabelling with respect to identity and/or source. Substandard medications cause potential harm to patients and they also promote a loss in confidence in the national health care system.

Pharmaceutical marketing, advertising and involvement in medical education

'Conflicts created by a range of common interactions with industry for medicine generally, and for academic medicine in particular ... have a corrosive effect on three core principles of medical professionalism: autonomy, objectivity, and altruism.'

The Association of American Medical Colleges (2008)

The pharmaceutical industry markets its products through advertising, delivery of meetings to professional health care workers and direct contact with patients. The lobby group Pharmaceutical Research and Manufacturers of America estimates that between $US27.7 billion and US$57.5 billion was spent on drug marketing in the United States in 2004. This marketing activity inappropriately influenced the prescribing habits of physicians. Pharmaceutical advertising directly to consumers may help them to be more informed about health issues, but can also promote spending on pharmaceutical products which may not be helpful or may even actively harm patients.

Pharmaceutical companies also market their products through their participation in the provision of continuing medical education. An analysis of Italian continuing medical education found that pharmaceutical companies make up to 60% of the budget for these sessions. Companies may thereby exert undue influence on aspects of health care training in pursuit of their commercial aims.

Reducing bias in marketing and medical education

A major systematic review of 538 studies on prescriber's perceptions and practices showed that most people failed to appreciate the influence of free lunches and gifts on their prescribing habits. Health care students have tried to raise awareness of this issue through a range of different advocacy initiatives, including Prescriber Promise and the American Medical Student Association's Scorecard.

Prescriber Promise is a UK initiative, launched in 2014, and strongly supported by PharmAware (a group of UK students promoting awareness of the risks of interactions with the pharmaceutical industry). It states that 'practising medicine based on good quality evidence allows health professionals to provide care in the best interests of their patients. However, evidence can become distorted and biased if it is influenced by ulterior motives. Pharmaceutical companies are often accused of distorting evidence for their own benefit as their financial interests often conflict with the interests of my patients.' The promise is an online pledge which publicly acknowledges that individuals will not accept any type of hospitality or free education which may create a conflict of interest with their relationship with their patients. (<http://www.pharmaware.co.uk/prescriber-promise.html>)

In 2007 the American Medical Student Association released its first Scorecard, which graded universities according to whether there was a policy regulating interactions between students and pharmaceutical and device companies. It was expanded in 2008 to assess these policies more rigorously and included details of the policies such as policies on attending conferences, receiving gifts and gaining free meals (<http://www.amsascorecard.org>).

Emily Ward (UK)

The industry response

The pharmaceutical industry has demonstrated some commitment to addressing concerns about its policies. In March 2009 GlaxoSmithKline announced a Pool for Open Innovation for Neglected Tropical Diseases, looking at 16 different diseases. The company made public information about its ongoing molecular research, including its preliminary test results, and agreed not to charge royalties for this information in low-income countries.

Other initiatives are based on greater collaboration to improve efficiency. Scientists from multiple pharmaceutical companies have looked at knowledge sharing in the 'precompetitive' industry. Alongside regulatory authorities, they recommend an increase in public–private partnerships as an alternative drug development model.

The regulatory authorities can also contribute by reintroducing ideas such as the needs clause which pushes pharmaceutical companies to rigorously trial their products against those of competitors in order to be accepted.

Conclusion

'Research today is immersed in a struggle for control of resources. Science is governed by guidelines set by the elites, pharmaceutical industry or political knowledge. We need dialogue to understand the ethical problems that we face and the implications of our actions as researchers or health workers.'

Escobar Emanuel (Argentina)

The pharmaceutical industry is a key component of health care systems. Researchers, as well as health care workers, need to be aware of potential conflicts of interest when interacting with these large organisations. An understanding of the processes which lead to drug development and marketing is an essential component of continuing medical education.

> **KEY POINTS**
>
> - The pharmaceutical industry has great power and influence in global health.
> - The phases and costs of drug development are complex, and there is potential for research bias.
> - Generic and branded medications are different.
> - Medical education can be compromised by inappropriate advertising by the pharmaceutical industry.

Further reading

Angell M: *The truth about drug companies*, New York, 2005, Random House Trade.

Davidoff F, de Angelis CD, Drazen JM, et al: Sponsorship, authorship and accountability, *CMAJ* 165(6):786–788, 2001.

Goldacre B: *Bad pharma*, London, 2013, Harper Collins.

Kaplan WM, Mathers C: *The world medicines situation 2011*, ed 3, Geneva, 2011, World Health Organization.

Law J: *Big pharma: how the world's biggest drug companies control illness*, London, 2006, Constable & Robinson.

Olson LW, Wendling BW: *The effect of generic drug competition on generic drug prices during the Hatch-Waxman 180-day exclusivity period*, Washington, 2013, Bureau of Economics, United States Federal Trade Commission.

Turner JR: *New drug development: an introduction to clinical trials*, ed 2, New York, 2010, Springer-Verlag.

CHAPTER 4.5

4.5 Health Policy and Research

Eleanor Turner-Moss (UK)

Introduction

Health policy is defined by the WHO as 'decisions, plans, and actions that are undertaken to achieve specific health care goals within a society.' *Policy* defines a shared vision and strategic plan, outlining priorities and the expected roles of different stakeholders. *Research* is the systematic investigation of hypotheses. It is important to establish facts and best practice so as to inform policy and practice, but this pragmatic evidence is not always available.

Health policy

Public health policies have a profound effect on health. The 10 greatest public health achievements of the 20th century in the United States involved strong health policies. These included control of infectious diseases, fluoridisation of drinking water, and safer roads and workplaces (Centers for Disease Control and Prevention, 1999). *Health policy* can refer to legally binding legislation and regulations, as well as to more informal (nonbinding) rules and guidelines. This term may also be used to describe the overall goals of an organisation. Health policies are potentially compromised when, for instance, they have been agreed at an international level without detail of the practical steps required for their implementation.

The formulation and effective implementation of health policy depends on many political, cultural and socioeconomic forces in addition to its quality and practicality.

The process (approach), content (quality of information) and outcome (monitoring/auditing processes) are all important aspects of policy development. **Fig. 4.5.1** provides a model of the steps involved in delivering public health policy and research which the US Centers for Disease Control and Prevention call the '10 essential public health services'.

Challenges in health policy

Public health is an underfunded and low-priority field of health care despite its importance and the huge potential for cost-effective interventions especially in areas of preventative medicine. Policies in areas other than health care, for instance in education and transport, influence health care outcomes through their effects on the social determinants of health. A lack of relevant research data means that policy decisions may be based on flawed assumptions and adversely influenced by political dogma.

As with research, funding is crucial for the development of effective health policy. The WHO depends on funding from both member states and charitable organisations. Nevertheless, its core activities such as vaccinations, integrated health services and action against NCDs are chronically underfunded as some states fail to honour their funding pledges. The focus on specific diseases by some charitable organisations may result in a conflict between national health care policy and the interests of philanthropic donors.

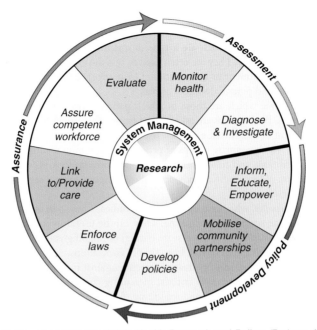

Figure 4.5.1   Designing and Delivering Public Health Research and Policy. *(Redrawn from Centers for Disease Control and Prevention: The public health system and the 10 essential public health services, 2014. <https://www.cdc.gov/nphpsp/essentialservices.html>.)*

TABLE 4.5.1 ■ **The advantages and disadvantages of different types of study design**

	Advantages	**Disadvantages**
Randomised controlled trials	Large studies Confounding factors and other sources of bias are carefully controlled	Selected population (usually in richer countries) Limited generalisability
Case–control studies	Relatively cheap Focus on causal factors	Requires recall of past events Controls not truly equivalent
Cohort studies	Prospective, can establish causal sequence and estimate incidence	Time-consuming and costly Risk of attrition of cohort
Cross-sectional studies	Inexpensive Snapshot of a population Outreach regardless of whether a population is accessing services Can assess multiple outcomes Good for opinions/local priority	Relies on self-report, resulting in potential inaccuracies and bias Out of date quickly Cannot establish causal sequence Not good for rare diseases

Research

> *'Ultimately, clinical research means patients get access to new treatments, interventions and medicines, and investment in research means better, more cost-effective patient care.'*
>
> **National Institute for Health Research Clinical Research Network**

The two main categories of research are qualitative and quantitative research (**Table 4.5.1**). Qualitative research aims to understand human behaviour and practice through word data.

Quantitative research is more concerned with numerical and statistical methods. Examples of trials include:

- *Randomised control trials,* which are a type of quantitative research regarded as the gold standard in clinical trials. They are often used to test the efficacy and efficiency of different types of medical treatment or intervention. Great efforts are made to control for all confounding factors and potential sources of bias.
- *Case–control studies,* which are those in which patients with a disease are compared with healthy controls. Both groups are asked about factors that might have caused or influenced the development of their disease.
- *Cohort studies,* which compare groups of people with common identified risk factors, experiences or conditions and follow them up through time to look at what diseases develop. They are a form of longitudinal study, and follow patients up for a set period, or sometimes throughout their lives.
- *Cross-sectional studies,* which are observational studies. They look at what is going on in a population at one specific point in time. They can be useful in collecting data on the efficacy of a particular intervention, disease burden or ongoing issues, but they often cannot differentiate different causal factors from simple associations.

Audit is a more formal means of evaluating practice against intended policy. The audit cycle has five stages: selecting standards and criteria, measuring current practice, comparing practice with standards, making improvements and reauditing. Auditing identifies practices which require improvement as well as compliance with established guidelines.

Challenges with research

The research agenda is often politically driven. Research content is controlled by academics, funders, journals and publishers; all may be affected by vested interests. Research development is also subject to bias and funding availability. Research should be conducted within health care environments to ensure that best practice is adopted.

In 1999 the Global Forum for Health Research analysed expenditure in health research throughout the world. It used the term *10/90 gap* to summarise the paradoxical spending patterns—the least amount of money spent on health issues that affect the largest number of people, who are also the poorest. Twelve countries provide 80% of research spending. Today, the 10/90 concept is less relevant, difficult to measure and can no longer be addressed simply by advocating high-income countries should spend more. The disease burdens in previously low-income countries are becoming increasingly complex as a new 'middle class' develops similar NCDs more familiar to wealthier nations. Inequity remains more striking in countries where neglected diseases of extreme poverty sit alongside those of overindulgence, sedentary lifestyles and increasing longevity.

The funding of medical research is, increasingly, dependent on the private sector (**Fig. 4.5.2**). In the United States, more than 60% of pharmaceutical research and more than 70% of clinical trials are financed by the pharmaceutical industry. These often focus on redesigning or optimising therapies for well-understood diseases in pursuit of profit. Paradoxically, these are often for NCDs which we know are preventable but for which the research into effective public health practice remains poor.

Access to research publications should be available to all. This can be a problem for those who are not members of an institution or who are working in low-income settings where publishers' fees are unaffordable. There have been several recent efforts to enable access to research, innovation and knowledge. These include open-access resources such as the Public Library of Science, BioMed Central, *The Lancet Global Health* and HINARI.

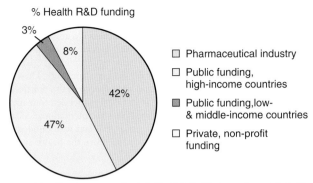

% Health R&D funding

3%

8%

42%

47%

☐ Pharmaceutical industry

☐ Public funding, high-income countries

■ Public funding, low- & middle-income countries

☐ Private, non-profit funding

Figure 4.5.2 Sources of funding for research globally (2004). *(Redrawn from data in The World Medicines Situation. WHO, 2004.)*

Getting involved in global health research

As a student, global health activities can be a rewarding way to influence both local and international health issues. Global health research also offers a very valuable skill set and a means of having lasting impact at both a health level and a policy level.

During 6 weeks studying global health in my fourth year of medical school, we decided to conduct a survey on the current provision of geriatric education in sub-Saharan Africa. We assessed how the challenges faced by a rapidly ageing population might be addressed. Questionnaires were sent to institutions across the region, to review the existing state of education in geriatrics and potential barriers to education. This research was published in a peer-reviewed journal, and we were able to raise awareness of the need for an improvement in geriatric education both in local approaches and in national policy.

Miriam Orcutt (UK)

Evidence-based policy and practice

Evidence-based medicine is the 'process of systematically reviewing, appraising and using clinical research findings to aid the delivery of optimum clinical care to patients' (Rosenberg and Donald, 1995). It challenges the traditional model of 'medicine by authority', encouraging a more discriminating scientific approach and application to clinical practice.

The acceptance and emphasis placed on evidence-based medicine and health policy is relatively new. The term *evidence-based policymaking* has been used in political currency in the United Kingdom to signify the entry of a government with a modern commitment to informed rational decision making.

High-quality research is crucial for guiding improvement of global health policy as well as health system design and service planning. Policy based on systematic evidence is seen to produce better outcomes. The increased involvement of researchers and doctors in policymaking is essential to ensure correct interpretation of data and translation into meaningful policy.

Implementation

After a health policy has been produced, it must be accepted and disseminated, implemented and evaluated. Implementation of research and health policy is challenging, and involves the practical application of principles and rules that may not match the priorities of the local politicians, health workers and public. It may require that funding is diverted from other priorities.

The World Health Organization's strategies on health policy and research

Health policy and systems research is an emerging field that seeks to understand and improve how societies achieve shared health goals, how different actors interact in the policy, and the necessary processes for effective policy implementation. It is interdisciplinary; a blend of economics, sociology, anthropology, political science, public health and epidemiology. These together draw a comprehensive picture of how health systems respond and adapt to health policies, and how health policies can shape, and be shaped by, health systems and the broader determinants of health.

The Alliance for Health Policy and Systems Research is an international collaboration of 350 partners globally. It is led by the World Health Organization and was founded in 1999. It promotes health policy and systems research as a means to improve the health systems of low- and middle-income countries.

It has three main objectives:
- to stimulate the generation and synthesis of policy-relevant health systems knowledge,
- to promote the dissemination and use of health policy and systems knowledge;
- to strengthen the capacity for the generation, dissemination and use of health policy and systems research knowledge amongst researchers, policymakers and other stakeholders.

The WHO strategy on research for health (2012) is as follows (**Fig. 4.5.3**):
- *capacity:* building capacity to strengthen health research systems;
- *priorities:* supporting the setting of research priorities that meet health needs particularly in low- and middle-income countries;

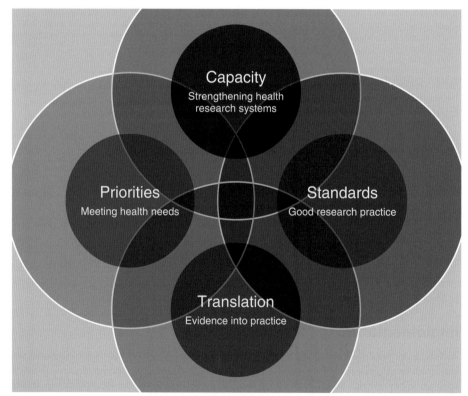

Figure 4.5.3 **WHO strategy on research for health.** *(Redrawn from WHO Strategy on Research for Health. Geneva, 2012, WHO.)*

- *standards:* creating an environment to create good research practice and enable the greater sharing of research evidence, tools and materials;
- *translation:* ensuring quality evidence is turned into products and policy;
- *organisation:* action to strengthen the research culture within the WHO and improve the management and coordination of WHO research activities.

Conclusion

Both health care research and health policy development are underfunded. They exist in a complicated web of political, corporate and other vested interests. Research, policy and practice are poorly aligned and poorly implemented. Effective health care policy must take account of the interconnected social determinants of health.

KEY POINTS

- Health policy and research are essential for improvement in global health.
- The greatest global health crises can be the most neglected.
- Research questions can be tainted by personal, political or profit-driven vested interests, and rarely address the issues of the poorest.
- Health policy is rarely truly evidence based.
- Implementation of health policy is variable, and is influenced by its quality, applicability, funding and public acceptance.

Further reading

Brownson RC, Chriqui JF, Stamatakis KA: Understanding evidence-based public health policy, *Am J Public Health* 99:9, 2009.

Centers for Disease Control and Prevention: Ten great public health achievements—United States, 1900–1999, *MMWR Morb Mortal Wkly Rep* 48:241–243, 1999.

Forum 2012 Beyond Aid: Research and innovation as key drivers for health, equity and development.

Overseas Development Institute: How can the analysis of power and process in policy-making improve health outcomes? *Moving the agenda forward Briefing paper* (online), 2007. https://www.odi.org/sites/odi.org.uk/files/odi-assets/publications-opinion-files/478.pdf.

Rosenberg W, Donald A: Evidence based medicine: an approach to clinical problem-solving, *BMJ* 310: 1122–1126, 1995.

Whitty C: What makes an academic paper useful for health policy? *BMC Med* 13:301, 2015. https://bmcmedicine.biomedcentral.com/articles/10.1186/s12916-015-0544-8.

4.6 Education and Health

Stijntje Dijk (Netherlands)   Aliye Runyan (USA)
Margot Weggemans (Netherlands)

Introduction

The relationship between health and education is complex and crucial. Education is one of the strongest social determinants of health, enabling informed decision making which affects health directly or indirectly. Education affects our understanding and interpretation of risk, our opportunities, our social status and our access to services.

Health care professionals play a key role in determining the health literacy of their patients and local communities. The extent to which health care providers understand and can adapt to the literacy level of their individual patients and population influences the success of health prevention programmes and the effectiveness of treatment.

Health professional education requires reform of existing curricula. These need to address the specific needs of health systems, the promotion of interprofessional and transprofessional education and the development of flexible competencies. The global shortage of health care professionals as well as the maldistribution of educational institutions requires urgent attention.

The need for education

Education ranks as a key determinant of health, along with income distribution, employment, working conditions and the social environment. Fifty-five percent of children who do not attend school are girls. Few health care professionals realise that educating a woman to secondary school level is a stronger predictor that her child will survive until the age of 5 years than other factors, such as the number of community health care workers. The children of mothers with secondary education or higher are twice as likely to survive beyond the age of 5 years compared with those whose mothers have no education (UNESCO, 2011).

This is thought to be due to what is known as a *multiplier effect*. Girls who have been educated marry later and have fewer children. They are also better paid in the workplace and more able to engage in political, social and economic decision-making processes. Their children are not only more likely to survive but are also better nourished and educated.

There are a number of direct and indirect benefits to being at school during the day. School offers children a safe environment where they are less likely to injure themselves, are safer from abuse, and are protected from forced child labour, child marriage, drugs, cigarettes and alcohol. It provides a place where children can be supported, can be supervised, can learn to build relationships, and can fit into society. Schools are also locations for the easy delivery of health interventions such as vaccinations, deworming and nutrient supplementation.

For this reason, several aspects of the MDGs and SDGs focus on the complex interrelationship between education and health. For example, a subsection of MDG 3 was to 'eliminate gender disparity in primary and secondary education, preferably by 2005, and in all levels of education by no later than 2015.' SDG 4 focuses on the provision of 'inclusive equitable quality education', whilst SDG 5 seeks to 'achieve gender equality and empower all women and girls' (see Chapter 6.6). Free primary school for all children has also been identified as a human right under the 1989 Convention of the Rights of the Child. Despite these policies, many children do not have access to education. They are particularly at risk when their families are in vulnerable groups such as indigenous or low socioeconomic groups.

Functional adult literacy: an essential tool in overcoming abject poverty

Uganda has one of the lowest literacy rates in the world, particularly amongst women. The inability to read and write restricts women's access to information and services; they cannot vote without support, read medical instructions for themselves or understand if they are being cheated. Literacy skills can empower women to engage with issues that affect their lives. Rose Ekitwi has been running community-based functional adult literacy groups in Uganda since 2005 to tackle this problem.

Rose's father was murdered when she was just 7 years old. Her aunt refused to send her to school, so she grew up unable to read or write. She married a pastor, and finally learnt to read and write at theological college. Her husband was tragically murdered shortly afterwards. Despite these adversities, Rose has been determined to tackle adult illiteracy in her local community. She now runs more than 80 literacy groups across Uganda with support from a UK charity.

The functional adult literacy programme (**Fig. 4.6.1**) focuses on providing literacy and life skills to help women move their families out of abject poverty. It enhances women's self-esteem, and enables them to understand their rights, take part in community decision making and begin income-generating activities so they can provide for their families. The programme is run by training 20 group leaders in an area who then go on in pairs to run a group of up to 20 other adults in their local area, each from a different family. This enables approximately 400 families at a time to gain education and training.

The programme is extremely practical, covering topics as diverse as keeping livestock, basic hygiene issues such as handwashing and childcare and managing small budgets. Clara, an English student visitor to the programme reported: 'I discovered that the women's literacy groups were learning how to keep chickens, not recite the alphabet.' The groups have been a tremendous success and have enabled thousands of adults to read across five districts of Uganda.

Rose Ekitwi (Uganda)

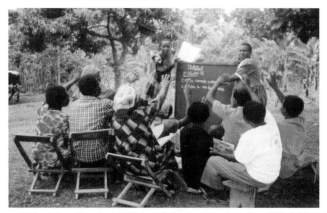

Figure 4.6.1 A functional adult literacy lesson. *(Copyright Rose Ekitwi, Uganda.)*

Health literacy

'Health literacy is the degree to which individuals have the capacity to obtain, process and understand basic health information and services needed to make appropriate health decisions.'

Institute of Medicine

There are an estimated 758 million illiterate adults in the world, 63% of whom are women (UNESCO Institute for Statistics, 2016). More than 121 million children, 57.8 million of primary school age (**Fig. 4.6.2**), are not enrolled in school, and of those who are, many do not get an education that will prepare them for life in rapidly changing societies. This problem does not lie only within the developing world: even in the developed world, around 100 million people are functionally illiterate.

Individuals with low health literacy are often less likely to use preventative services and are more likely to visit emergency departments. Higher levels of illiteracy contribute significantly to the disease burden of poor communities and countries, and reinforce health and economic inequalities.

Health literacy and skills-based health education is key in the prevention and treatment of conditions in which knowledge, behaviours, attitudes and skills are important. Examples of these diseases include vector-borne infections such as malaria and diseases related to water and sanitation such as diarrhoeal diseases, trachoma and schistosomiasis.

The ability of the care provider to communicate effectively is an important factor in enabling patients to access necessary health information. Components of health literacy, such as access to

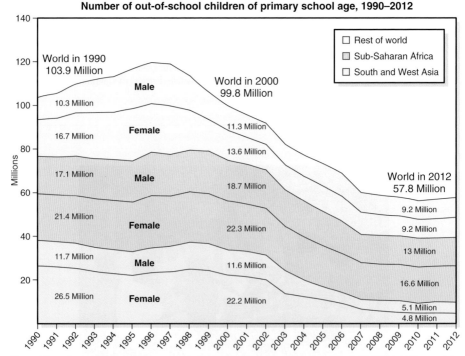

Figure 4.6.2 Out-of-school children of primary school age. *(Redrawn from Fig. 9, UNICEF: 25 Years of the Convention on the Rights of the Child, 2014, UNICEF. https://www.data.unicef.org>.)*

information and knowledge, informed consent and negotiating skills, should constitute a part of the overall development effort. Inability to access information is a key challenge for vulnerable groups in particular, many of whom may be poorly educated.

Health education

'Health education is any combination of planned learning experiences using evidence based practices and/or sound theories that provide the opportunity to acquire knowledge, attitudes, and skills needed to adopt and maintain healthy behaviors.'

Report of 2011 Joint Committee on Health Education and Promotion Terminology

Health education aims to provide individuals and communities with the information they need to make decisions that affect their health and to help them live healthy lives. Health promotion programmes can aim to encourage or modify behaviours, values and attitudes to protect or enhance health, and are core components of most health care professionals' roles.

Health promotion involves the following supporting environmental features (**Fig. 4.6.3**):

- policies: set of guidelines for activities;
- regulations: ability to implement policies;

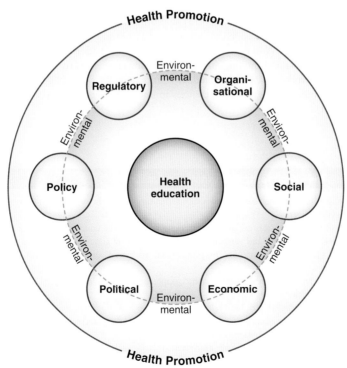

Figure 4.6.3 Health promotion. *(From Celletti F, Reynolds TA, Wright A, Stoertz A, Dayrit M (2011) Educating a New Generation of Doctors to Improve the Health of Populations in Low- and Middle-Income Countries. PLoS Med 8(10): e1001108. https://doi.org/10.1371/journal.pmed.1001108)*

- organisation: coordinating resources to implement a programme;
- financial: incentives for activities;
- social: people to do activities;
- political: legislative support for regulations/laws.

Health professionals need to be able to communicate properly and to be advocates for their patients' needs. They are ideally placed to educate both individual patients and the community at large. To do this effectively, they need diverse skills; for instance an ability to assess the level of understanding, communicate complex information at an appropriate level, and challenge inaccurate beliefs in a supportive and nonconfrontational manner. Physicians often overestimate the health literacy levels of their patients, and very few medical trainees feel confident about either their knowledge of health literacy or the use of skills for interacting with patients who have low health literacy.

Transforming health professional education: creating health professionals for the new century

'Transformative scaling up of health professional education and training is defined as the sustainable expansion and reform of health professional education and training to increase the quantity, quality and relevance of health professionals, and in so doing strengthen the country health systems and improve population health outcomes.'

Celletti et al (2011)

More than 1 billion people worldwide lack access to quality health services. *A Universal Truth: No Health Without a Workforce* (2013) reported an estimated global shortage of 7.2 million health workers, whilst 83 countries faced a health worker crisis. During the World Health Assembly in 2006, the Global Health Workforce Alliance was launched to address specific aspects such as health worker education and training, migration and financing. In particular, the need for more community health workers was highlighted. It is imperative that health professional education ensures the right mix of skills and competencies in line with ever-changing and evolving global needs (**Box 4.6.1**).

BOX 4.6.1 ■ The vision for transformative education

- Greater alignment is needed between educational institutions and the systems that are responsible for health service delivery
- Country ownership of priorities and programming related to the education of health professionals with political commitment and partnerships to facilitate reform at national, regional and local levels
- Promotion of social accountability in professional education and of close collaboration with communities
- Clinicians and public health workers who are competent and provide the highest quality of care for individuals and communities
- Global excellence coupled with local relevance in research and education
- Vibrant and sustainable education institutions with dynamic curricula and supportive learning environments, including good physical infrastructure
- Faculty of outstanding quality who are motivated and can be retained

---

Reproduced with permission from WHO: Transforming and scaling up health professionals' education and training. WHO Guidelines, 2013. Adapted from Celletti et al (2011).

Changes throughout the centuries

During the last century, the most significant change in education has been the move from curricula focusing on individual subjects or disciplines towards programmes where teaching and learning are integrated. The current educational structure aims to improve the performance of health systems by adapting core professional competencies to specific local needs. All health professionals should thereby engage in evidence-based and ethical practice as members of locally responsive and globally connected teams.

The training of health professionals needs to be aligned to 'society's priority health needs'. This requires a good understanding of the social determinants of health and the health care needs of people who are vulnerable and marginalised. Transformative learning, as proposed in the report 'Health professionals for a new century: transforming education to strengthen health systems in an interdependent world' (Frenk et al., 2010), aims to produce change by enabling future health care professionals to address local priorities. This includes the development of effective teamwork and the ability to base decisions on a robust analysis of available data.

Integrated teaching brings together different disciplines enabling different professions to learn with, from, and about each other.

Learning frameworks and medical electives

There is an increasing recognition of the need to train a range of health workers, including local community workers and volunteers, in addition to doctors. A number of competency frameworks have been developed but a framework of particular interest is the CanMEDS competency framework, which is now being used on all five continents (**Fig. 4.6.4**). The Royal College of Physicians and Surgeons of Canada developed a framework built around seven roles, making up the explicit abilities that a skilled health professional should have. The described roles are:

1. *medical expert*: applying knowledge skills and attitudes to patient care;
2. *communicator*: communicating effectively with patients, families, colleagues and other professionals;
3. *collaborator*: working effectively within a health care team;
4. *health advocate*: advancing the health and well-being of patients and populations;
5. *manager:* participating effectively in the organisation of the health care system;
6. *scholar*: committing to reflective learning as well as to the creation, dissemination and application of medical knowledge;
7. *professional:* committing to ethical practice and high personal standard of behaviour.

These CanMEDS roles are interconnected. Increased emphasis is placed on the team behaviours of health care professionals. Excellence in health professional education should ensure that graduates possess and use all desirable competencies to improve the health of individual citizens and society. The WHO includes issues of quality, equity, relevance and effectiveness when discussing health care and human rights. In 2010 the Global Consensus for Social Accountability of Medical Schools urged schools to improve their response to current and future health-related needs and challenges in society.

The term *global health* is used to stress the global commonality of health issues which transcend class, race, ethnicity, income and culture, as well as national borders whilst emphasising the importance of the social determinants of health. An understanding of the relevance of all these issues is essential for all health care professionals, not just those working overseas, and should be an objective in all educational programmes.

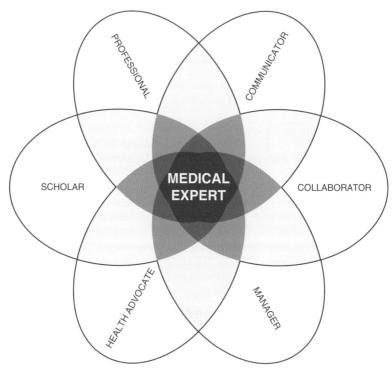

Figure 4.6.4   The CanMEDS framework. *(Reproduced with permission from the Royal College of Physicians and Surgeons of Canada, from Kelly K, Fung K, Maclean L: Canadian Otolaryngology – Head and Neck Surgery clerkship curricula: evolving toward tomorrow's learners. J Otolaryngol Head Neck Surg. 42(1):33, 2013.)*

'In the past, desperate conditions on another continent might cynically be written out of one's memory. The process of globalization has made such an option impossible. The separation between domestic and international health problems is no longer useful.'

Margaret Chan, former WHO Director General

There is significant variation in the approaches taken to include global health education within health care curricula. A competency model includes seven domains:

- capacity strengthening
- collaborating and partnering
- ethical reasoning and professional practice
- health equity and social science
- programme management
- sociocultural and political awareness and strategic analysis

In the absence of formal learning opportunities, students often pursue their own programmes and electives in global health. Nonformal learning opportunities include student-led or online courses and participation in projects and activities or international exchanges.

Professional exchanges through the International Federation of Medical Students' Associations

The International Federation of Medical Students' Associations (IFMSA) runs one of the largest student-run exchange programmes in the world. Currently, more than 1.5 million medical students from approximately 98 countries participate. The programme provides predeparture and postdeparture training and support cover for health, safety and ethical issues. It aims to promote cultural understanding and cooperation amongst medical students and all health professionals. Omar shares his personal experience of working in a different country and how that led him to take on a role directing the IFMSA programme.

In 2011, as a fourth-year medical student from Morocco, I undertook a life-changing elective in Toulouse, France. During the elective, I developed my practical skills and personal medical knowledge. I also became a more holistic doctor, and improved my personal understanding of global health and cultural issues.

I gained an understanding of the epidemiology of my host country, which was very different from my own. I cared for patients with some diseases I would not have encountered at home and also had the chance to diagnose one case of tuberculosis, a condition common in Morocco but rare in France. This experience helped me to understand the challenges faced by the two different health systems and taught me that disease does not respect country boundaries.

I was impressed by the opportunities offered by the IFMSA and so returned to Morocco and worked on founding an association to represent Moroccan medical students. One year later, IFMSA-Morocco started a professional exchange programme. In 3 years more than 350 medical students from Morocco have been able to go for an exchange to more than 25 countries, and vice versa. Those who have travelled have learnt about new health systems and cultures and enhanced their intercultural understanding.

Omar Cherkaoui (Morocco)

Experiencing health care in a different geographical and cultural setting is one of the commonest types of medical elective. Overseas placements facilitate exposure to different clinical diseases, pathology and diagnostic procedures. Students can broaden their clinical skills and practical experience, undertake placements in international public health or participate in research. These placements must, however, be arranged with agreed educational objectives and in an ethical manner so that neither patients nor host institutions are compromised.

Reforming and expanding health professional education

The Declaration of Alma-Ata on primary health care talked about putting people at the centre of health care. However, many countries do not accommodate this aspiration. Stronger links between education, communities and health service delivery need to be established. Health educational reforms therefore must be developed and implemented in line with these aims. Many actors are involved in educational reform (**Fig. 4.6.5**) but students should also have an active role in curricula development.

Conclusion

> *'Today, because of rapid economic and social change, (medical) schools have to prepare students for jobs that have not yet been created, technologies that have not yet been invented and problems that we don't yet know will arise.'*

> **Andreas Schleicher, OECD Education Directorate, 2010**

The education of health care workers should incorporate an interdisciplinary-based, patient-centred and competency-based approach, in which the community assumes a significant role. It is increasingly

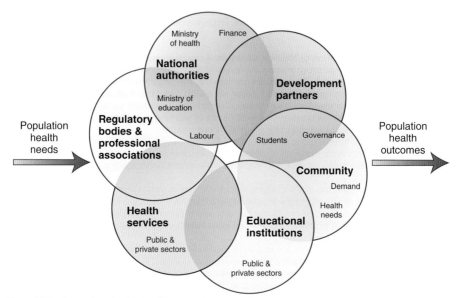

Figure 4.6.5   Actors involved in health care education. *(Redrawn from Fig. 5 in World Health Organization: Transformative scale up of health professional education, Geneva, 2011, World Health Organization. Available from http://whqlibdoc.who.int/hq/2011/WHO_HSS_HRH_HEP2011.01_eng.pdf?ua=1>).*

important that health care professionals can work across boundaries and are equipped to work effectively and ethically throughout the world.

Students and health care professionals have a duty to advocate education for health, both for their patients and local communities and within their own curricula. This will ensure that the global population becomes more health literate and is cared for by an appropriately skilled and competent global health workforce.

KEY POINTS

- Literacy and education are key factors in determining community and patient health.
- Health care professionals need the skills to communicate with, be advocates for, and empower their patients to provide better health outcomes.
- Health professionals' education needs redesigning to enable them to meet the needs of society.
- Students play key roles in advocating change and are valued contributors to educational reform.

Further reading

Celletti F, Reynolds TA, Wright A, et al: Educating a new generation of doctors to improve the health of populations in low and middle income countries, *PLOS Med* 8(10):e1001108, 2011.

Fletcher A: *Meaningful student involvement: guide to students as partners in school change,* ed 2, Olympia, 2005, CommonAction Consulting.

Frenk J, Chen L, Bhutta ZA, et al: Health professionals for a new century: transforming education to strengthen health systems in an interdependent world, *Lancet* 376:1923–1958, 2010.

UNESCO: *Education Counts,* Paris, 2011, UNESCO.

UNESCO Institute for Statistics: *UIS Fact Sheet no. 38,* Montreal, 2016, UIS.

World Health Organization: *Transformative scale up of health professional education,* Geneva, 2011, World Health Organization. Available from: http://whqlibdoc.who.int/hq/2011/WHO_HSS_HRH_HEP2011.01_eng.pdf?ua=1.

Law, Ethics and Human Rights

Junior Editor: Anya Gopfert (UK)

Introduction

A basic premise of the World Health Organization (WHO) is that health is a human right. Many people are denied access to health care or fail to seek such care on account of ethnic or religious practices. As a result, health outcomes for different populations differ significantly. Addressing some of these complex and challenging issues in global health requires multidisciplinary teamwork. This section introduces some of the key legislation, ethical and social theories, and the human rights frameworks which underpin work in this field.

5.1 Human Rights and Health

Josephine de Costa (Australia)   ■   Meggie Mwoka (Kenya)

'The essence of global health equity is the idea that something so precious as health might be viewed as a right.'
Paul Farmer, United States

Introduction

The concept of *human rights* derives from Western political theory regarding the interaction between the state and the individual. Human rights are the basic freedoms and protections to which people are entitled simply because they are human beings. They recognise that every person has a right to the fundamental things necessary for an adequate standard of living—ranging from freedom from arbitrary detention to freedom of expression. Three important definitions surround the human rights framework:

- *Inalienable*: Not able to be violated in any circumstance.
- *Positive obligation*: An obligation on a person or government to *actively* act in a certain way (e.g., to provide a functioning legal system).
- *Negative obligation*: An obligation on a person or government *not* to do a particular act (e.g., to refrain from the arbitrary imprisonment of people).

The history of human rights

What we consider *inalienable* in human rights today (**Fig. 5.1.1**) is very different from that generally recognised hundreds of years ago. Some of the original documents relevant to human rights were religious documents (e.g., the Hindu Vedas, the Babylonian Code of Hammurabi, the Bible, the Koran and the Analects of Confucius). The rights and responsibilities listed in these documents were often limited to a single group of people, usually those who were adherents of a particular religion.

Subsequently, various national legal frameworks were developed, including Magna Carta (1215), the English Bill of Rights (1689), the French Declaration on the Rights of Man and of the Citizen (1789) and the US Constitution and Bill of Rights (1791). These rights were significant as they placed a *positive obligation* on the state to protect the rights of the individual. This contrasted with religious texts, which generally put the responsibilities for human rights on individuals and communities (as opposed to governments).

The human rights abuses of the Holocaust during the Second World War led to the creation of the United Nations in 1945. This was to be a body for global governance with a major focus on peacekeeping. The protection of human rights was a fundamental purpose of this institution. A principal objective of the United Nations was 'to promote social progress and better standards of life in larger freedom'. This led to the adoption of the Universal Declaration of Human Rights (UDHR) by the UN General Assembly in 1948; it listed the fundamental rights that should be

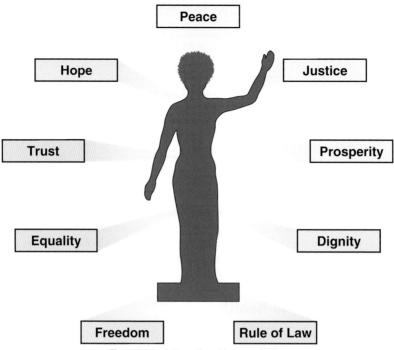

Figure 5.1.1 International human rights.

available for all people. Whilst the creation of the UDHR was an important milestone in the setting out of which rights *should* be respected, it was not a legally binding document.

> *'Peace can only last where human rights are respected, where the people are fed, and where individuals and nations are free.'*
>
> **Dalai Lama**

The implementation of the UDHR was challenging as people and cultures have different notions about what is moral or 'right' behaviour (moral relativism). It is inappropriate to pass judgement on the cultural norms in other communities just because they are incongruent with norms elsewhere.

Human rights agreements

Current concepts of *human rights* developed from Western political ideas in three stages:
- *civil and political rights* (rights in the public sphere)
- *economic, social and cultural rights*
- *group or people's rights* (rights in the private sphere)

Two key binding treaties place legal obligations on states to protect the human rights of their citizens. These legal frameworks are the International Covenant on Civil and Political Rights (ICCPR) and the International Covenant on Economic, Social and Cultural Rights (ICESCR).

International Covenant on Civil and Political Rights, 1966

The ICCPR obliges governments to respect and ensure that all individuals subject to its jurisdiction have access to the rights prescribed in the ICCPR. These include the right to life, freedom of religion, self-determination, freedom of speech, freedom of assembly, electoral rights and rights to due process and a fair trial. In addition to the main body of the ICCPR, there are two addenda (optional protocols). The first of these creates the Human Rights Committee, a court-like body that provides individuals with the opportunity to make complaints about violations of the ICCPR. The second protocol provides for the abolishment of the death penalty. As of 2017, 169 countries had ratified the ICCPR.

International Covenant on Economic, Social and Cultural Rights, 1966

The ICESCR requires signatories to work towards the realisation of their civilians' full economic, social and cultural rights. These include labour rights, the right to an adequate standard of living, the right to health and the right to education. The ICESCR specifically recognises that some states may take longer than others to achieve full protection of certain rights. As of 2017, 166 countries were party to the ICESCR (2017 data).

The human right to health

The human right to health should be understood as the 'right to the highest attainable standard of physical and mental health'. It is enshrined in Article 12 of the ICESCR, and encompasses both freedom and entitlements. The right to health is understood as including the right to control one's health and body, to be free from external interference and to have access to a health care system in pursuit of the highest attainable level of health. Authorities are obliged to ensure that adequate health services are available, along with healthy and safe working conditions, adequate housing and nutritious food. The right to health does not imply a right to be *healthy*, as the latter is subject to individual variation.

> *'Human rights that do not apply to everyone are not human rights at all.'*
>
> **Volker Beck**

Human rights are fundamentally interconnected. Their realisation is dependent on a variety of economic and social factors. These include gender, education, social status, freedom of religion and access to food and housing. Such factors are underpinned by other rights; for example, the right to equality before the law (ICCPR Article 26), the right to education (ICESCR Article 13), the right to freedom of religion (ICCPR Article 18) and the right to a safe workplace (ICESCR Article 7[b]).

Health should be considered within a human rights framework as it is affected by sociocultural as well as physical considerations (**Fig. 5.1.2**).

> *'Violence against women is perhaps the most shameful human rights violation. And it is perhaps the most pervasive. It knows no boundaries of geography, culture or wealth. As long as it continues, we cannot claim to be making real progress towards equality, development and peace.'*
>
> **Kofi Annan, former Secretary-General of the United Nations**

One strategy whereby health can be developed within a human rights framework is the *health in all policies* (HiAP) approach. HiAP is 'a type of large-scale inter-sectoral action which improves

Examples of the links between **Health** and **Human Rights**

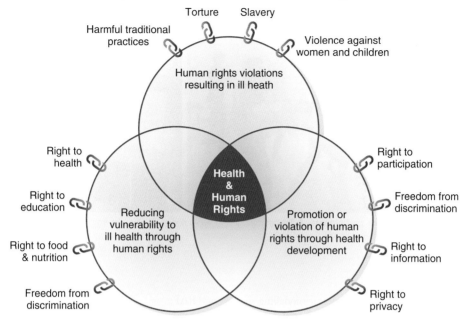

Figure 5.1.2 **Links between health and human rights.** *(Redrawn from Columbia Center for New Media Teaching and Learning: Human rights and health, <healthandrights.ccnmtl.columbia.edu/human_rights/ human_rights_and_health.html>.)*

Daphne: stop violence against women!

Physical and sexual violence against women is a global problem. This is often perpetrated by a woman's intimate partner or a family member. Eighty percent of victims stay with their abuser, with only 12% of all abusers ever coming to the notice of the justice system.

Violence carries both short-term and long-term consequences affecting physical and psychological well-being. The high prevalence of violence against women brings them into regular contact with doctors. As many as one in five women seen in emergency departments have suffered abuse which doctors may fail to recognise.

A Daphne programme (**Fig. 5.1.3**) was created in 2010 by a group of students to address the human rights violation of violence against women. Workshops for medical students (in cooperation with local universities), community services for victims, peer education in high schools and social campaigns were developed. As the project evolved, women learned how to react, where to find help and how to protect their families. International courses have now been established in Slovakia, Italy and northern Africa. There is nothing more satisfactory than to hear from a course participant 'I'm not scared anymore; now I know what to do.'

Anna Szczegielniak (Poland)

health through attention to the full range of determinants'. As a result, various policies, each relating to a different human right, are effectively integrated and contribute to improved public health.

However, the implementation of HiAP at a national and international level faces numerous obstacles:

- difficulties in reaching agreement between government departments or sovereign governments to implement such policies;

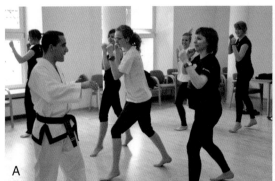
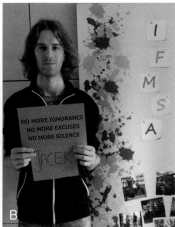

Figure 5.1.3   Daphne participants. A Training women in self-defence. **B** Support from IFMSA for Daphne programme. *(© IFMSA-Poland.)*

- lack of effective economic modelling supporting HiAP;
- the time frame of most elected governments being significantly shorter than the time required to deliver successful HiAP projects.

The unfortunate outcome of these obstacles is that HiAP is rarely implemented as fully as it could be. Despite these difficulties, HiAP, where implemented, facilitates the management of health issues within a human rights framework.

Conflicts in prioritising different human rights

All rights apply to all human beings equally, regardless of 'race, colour, sex, language, religion, political or other opinion, national or social origin, property, birth or other status' (ICCPR Article 26). This is known as the *principle of nondiscrimination* in all rights; no person's right can be placed before the same right of any other person.

Academics have debated whether or not there is a hierarchy of human rights—should one right be regarded preferentially as compared with any other right? Whilst this hierarchical view has been surpassed by the view that all human rights are equal, two issues remain.

- Firstly, states may be able to *derogate* from (i.e., breach) their international human rights obligations. For example, under the ICCPR, in times of 'public emergency' such as war, a country is allowed to breach the human rights of its citizens (ICCPR Article 4[1]). Such derogations are strictly defined. However, governments may *not* derogate from the right to life, freedom from torture, slavery and arbitrary imprisonment, the right to equality before the law and freedom of thought, conscience and religion (ICCPR Article 4[2]). These rights are *nonderogable* and therefore are enforceable in extreme situations, such as war. The impact of legal frameworks in emergency situations may differ, as do the ethical challenges of conflict situations (Oraa, 1999).
- Secondly, health professionals may encounter situations where the rights of an individual (or that individual's parent or guardian) conflict. These may encompass cultural, religious, ethnic and other issues. The following case (p. 135) illustrates the difficulties which occur in accommodating potentially conflicting rights (e.g., health, life and religion).

TABLE 5.1.1 ■ Comparison of the charity, needs and rights-based approaches

Charity approach	Needs approach	Rights-based approach
Focuses on input not outcome	Focuses on input not outcome	Focuses on process and outcome
Emphasises increasing charity	Emphasises meeting needs	Emphasises realising rights
Recognises moral responsibility of rich towards poor	Recognises needs as valid claims	Recognises individual and group rights as claims towards legal and moral duty bearers
Individuals are seen as victims	Individuals are objects of development interventions	Individuals and groups are empowered to claim their rights
Individuals deserve assistance	Individuals deserve assistance	Individuals are entitled to assistance
Focuses on manifestations of problems	Focuses on immediate causes of problems	Focuses on structural causes and their manifestations

In all situations, it is recommended that health care organisations have a strategy to deal with competing human rights interests; for example, the Ontario Human Rights Commission's policy on competing human rights (<http://www.ohrc.on.ca/en/policy-competing-human-rights>).

Rabbi versus doctor: a conflict of rights

Haemophilus influenzae causes frequent and often life-threatening meningitis in infants. In 1994 the Israeli Ministry of Health added the Hib conjugate vaccine to the regular infant immunisation programme that is provided free of charge. In 2 years the incidence of invasive *H. influenzae* dropped from 34 per 100,000 to less than 5 per 100,000, and the programme was thought to have essentially eliminated the disease.

A 14-month-old boy presented in a hospital in Israel with signs of meningitis. He had not been vaccinated because of the religious beliefs of his parents, who also refused any procedures, including a lumbar puncture. Treatment for suspected *H. influenza* meningitis was started. The day after his hospitalisation, the parents discharged the child from hospital against medical recommendations on the advice of their rabbi. As the child's illness was severe, the hospital obtained a court order requiring that the boy be returned to hospital. The family took him to an ultraorthodox hospital, where the hospital rabbi was able to convince the parents to accept an alteration in therapy. The child recovered, and appropriate prophylaxis was given to his family. However, his parents still refused to vaccinate the child and his siblings. It is not uncommon to encounter behaviours that conflict with current medical knowledge. This boy had a preventable illness, and the case shows the importance of engaging with faith leaders who also have medical knowledge: the hospital rabbi played a critical role in this child's survival.

Jae Hyoung Lee (Korea)

Human rights-based approach and development

The human rights-based approach (HRBA) recognises the need for development activities to respect, protect and fulfil human rights in accordance with the international human rights legal framework. In this respect, human rights act as a guideline as to how activities should be conducted, at the level of design, planning or implementation. Those being supported are seen as citizens rather than as beneficiaries. A comparison of this approach with alternative approaches is shown in **Table 5.1.1**.

Health policy

The running and management of all health systems is guided by health policies.

According to the WHO, *health policy* refers to decisions, plans and actions that are undertaken to achieve specific health care goals within a society, for the short or medium term. On various aspects of health (e.g., health budgets, criteria to be a certified health practitioner), support for HRBA in health policies has increased. In 1997 the UN Secretary General, Kofi Annan, adopted the HRBA for the entire UN system, incorporating it into policies and programmes in various sectors. When these human rights-based health policies are being created, core human rights principles must be applied at all stages of design, implementation, evaluation and monitoring. These principles include:

1. universality and inalienability
2. indivisibility
3. interdependence and interrelatedness
4. equality and nondiscrimination
5. participation and inclusion
6. accountability and rule of law

The term *human rights* within HRBA can be confusing as it is widely used in a number of ways. Failure to distinguish between various rights means that many people assume, inappropriately, that all rights are *legal* rights. A rights approach, inappropriately formulated, may lead to an unrealistic list of demands to 'duty bearers', usually governments, causing opposition to this policy. HRBA, when implemented appropriately, should promote collaboration between all stakeholders.

A human rights-based approach to dementia

Scotland's National Dementia Strategy (2010) is founded in human rights. Key to this approach has been the involvement of people with dementia as well as their carers. The strategy is based on the PANEL approach, which the Scottish Human Rights Commission has promoted and which is endorsed by the United Nations.

The PANEL approach emphasises the following rights for everyone:

- participation in decisions which affect their human rights;
- accountability of those responsible for the respect, protection and fulfilment of human rights;
- nondiscrimination and equality;
- empowerment to know their rights and how to claim them;
- legality in all decisions through an explicit link with human rights legal standards in all processes and outcome measurements.

From Health and Social Care Alliance Scotland: Being human: a human rights based approach to health and social care in Scotland, Glasgow, 2017, Health and Social Care Alliance Scotland.

Conclusion

Key international agreements underpin our current understanding of human rights. The concept of using an HRBA is valuable for planning services in global health, and, when applied correctly, encourages an empowering and enabling approach to problem solving.

KEY POINTS

- The human right to health was established by the International Covenant on Economic, Social and Cultural Rights.
- The international human rights framework sets out certain fundamental rights and freedoms which apply to all people without discrimination on the basis of ethnicity, religion, gender, socioeconomic status or various other factors.

- Human rights are interconnected and interdependent. The realisation of one human right is often dependent on other related rights.
- The interconnected nature of human rights and the associated impact on health is encompassed by a 'human rights-based approach' to health policy being taken.

Further reading

Amnesty International: *What are human rights?* <https://www.amnesty.org.uk/what-are-human-rights>, 2015.

Farer T: The hierarchy of human rights, *Am Univ Int Law Rev* 8(1):115–119, 1992.

Greaves LJ, Bialystok LR: Health in all policies - all talk and little action?, *Can J Public Health* 102(6):407–409, 2011.

Hunt P, Backman G: Health systems and the right to the highest attainable standard of health, *Health Hum Rights* 10:81–92, 2008.

Hunt P, Backman G, Bueno de Mesquita J, et al: The right to the highest attainable standard of health. In Detels R, Gulliford M, Karim QA, Tan CC, editors: *Oxford textbook of global public health*, ed 6, Oxford, 2015, Oxford University Press.

Oraa J: The protection of human rights in emergency situations under customary international law. In Goodwin-Gill G, Talmon S, editors: *The reality of international law*, Oxford, 1999, Oxford University Press.

5.2 Law and Health

Josephine de Costa (Australia)

Introduction

The international legal framework and issues concerning global governance have developed over the last 50 years but compliance with this framework is essentially voluntary. 'Soft laws' (including nonbinding resolutions of international organisations) are not binding but are usually adopted with an expectation that they will become 'hard laws' over time. International conventions regarding public health (e.g., the Framework Convention on Tobacco Control) and the rules of major organisations (e.g., the WHO's International Health Regulations) have increased in importance. Areas of international law relevant to health include international criminal law, trade law, humanitarian law, environmental law and human rights law. All peoples should now have access to a set of legal structures that avoid the violation of their inherent rights.

Legal instruments

Local, national and international legal agreements, as well as interventions such as deregulation and methods of taxation, make a huge impact on public health. The social and economic environment also has a significant health impact. Laws affect other domains, including trade, border security and travel restrictions related to outbreaks of infectious diseases.

An *agreement* is a decision made between nation states. A *treaty* is an international agreement that is entered into by two or more nations. A treaty can be likened to a contract between countries in the sense that both parties willingly assume obligations. A *convention* describes a formal statement of principles that are agreed upon by nation states.

When a country agrees to the contents of an agreement, there are different mechanisms by which it can agree to be bound. Nation states may become *signatories* to an agreement. Depending on the international agreement, this may require either a 'simple signature' or a 'definitive signature'. The definitive signature is an express consent from the state to be bound by the terms of the agreement and does not require ratification. A simple signature applies to most multilateral treaties, and is subject to ratification. It represents the agreement of the nation state in good faith not to act in a way that would defeat the object and purpose of the agreement. When a country *ratifies* an agreement, it expressly agrees to be bound by the terms dictated within the agreement. This requires that consent/approval is granted by the local national parliament. This step is significant as it is at this time that a nation state may implement the content of the treaties into its domestic law.

Global governance

This is a process of consensus forming which involves a range of international actors and states. This process aims to generate guidelines and better relationships between domestic and international stakeholders. A key actor or organisation (e.g., the World Trade Organization) may be given a nominal lead role on an issue. There are concerns that the increased role of these large international

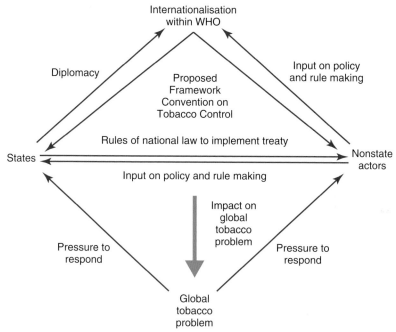

Figure 5.2.1 **The Global health governance dynamic: tobacco.** *WHO*, World Health Organization. *(Redrawn from Fidler D: Global health governance. Overview of the role of international law in protecting and promoting global public health, 2002. Available from <http://cgch.lshtm.ac.uk/ghg3.pdf>.)*

organisations has reduced the role of national governments and their leadership over their own country, thereby compromising their sovereignty.

One of the key issues in international governance is the lack of translation of international agreements to domestic situations. Three gaps are often recognised in this process:

- *The jurisdictional gap.* This describes the problems which result from the absence of an international authoritative body with the power to promote effective global governance.
- *The incentive gap.* This is the gap which results from a lack of national motivation leading to a breakdown in international collaboration.
- *The participation gap.* This is the concept that international cooperation is largely organised and operated by states with few civil society stakeholders.

Public health issues and legal challenges illustrating jurisdictional and incentive tensions posed by the tobacco industry are shown in **Fig. 5.2.1**.

A further example of the jurisdictional and incentive disconnect is illustrated in the following case study (p. 140).

Human rights law

Human rights law promotes and protects human rights at an international, domestic and regional level. The two most important international treaties on fundamental human rights are the ICCPR and the ICESCR. There is a complex relationship between international human rights law and domestic law. Each state decides how it incorporates international obligations (under the ICCPR or ICESCR) into its domestic law. The extent to which these obligations are incorporated into domestic law can have a significant impact on their efficacy, and on the ability of citizens to rely on such laws for protection.

Modern day slavery: a right to freedom?

The issue of slavery has been of international concern for many years. Increasing numbers of legal instruments have been agreed, by both human rights and legislative bodies. However, slavery continues because of significant jurisdictional and incentive gaps.

A 32-year-old single mother of two children spent her life savings to work abroad in a new job to earn money so as to feed her two children. On arrival, her passport was confiscated by her new employer. Her new job included assisting a physically challenged child as well as household chores. She was badly treated and abused by her employer but then found that she was unable to leave the country without her passport and grew increasingly desperate. She finally escaped to her country's embassy, which helped her to return home. On returning home, she was reunited with her children and found work as a tailor. Sadly, she required prolonged regular psychiatric counselling following the trauma of her abuse.

Thirty million people are victims of modern-day slavery, a US$150 billion global industry, fuelled by poverty and marred by ill health and distress. The global health care community is morally obliged to facilitate health care and health care services to serve the victims of slavery. As more people are freed, so more services are required. Resource-poor countries are the most affected by modern-day slavery, and a holistic approach is necessary to close jurisdictional and incentive gaps in tackling this global issue.

Abilash Sathyanarayanan (India)

For example, the American Bill of Rights (the name given to the first 10 amendments to the American Constitution) protects various fundamental human rights, including freedom of speech, freedom of religion, and the right to keep and bear arms. As these rights are enshrined within the constitution, they have the highest available legal protection. Thus the US Government may not make laws that contradict the protection of these rights or the ability to exercise them freely. As a result, the limited checks required for firearm ownership result in a level of injury which is similar to that associated with road traffic accidents.

Few states have incorporated their human rights obligations into their domestic constitutions. They either incorporate individual rights into preexisting domestic statutes or create a separate statute, or charter, of human rights. The Australian state of Victoria has adopted such a separate charter, the Charter of Human Rights and Responsibilities Act (2006), which should respect human rights. In practice, the charter has had little impact, and is more of a normative or aspirational document rather than one with binding legal obligations.

Discrimination against lesbian, gay, bisexual and transgender patients: the legal basis

Discrimination against lesbian, gay, bisexual and transgender (LGBT) populations can have a negative impact on health outcomes. There are scant data on the health and well-being of the LGBT population. This issue was missed in Article 26 of the International Covenant on Civil and Political Rights. There are significant differences between countries in the legal status of sexual acts between adults of the same sex.

As of 2014 81 jurisdictions had criminalised consensual sexual conduct between adults of the same sex. Thirty-eight of these were in Africa. Offenders could be punished by incarceration in prison for up to 14 years. Homosexuality is a capital offence in five countries. This illegal status impacts on patient disclosure of sexuality, resulting in inadequate provision of care, potentially endangering the patient's own health and that of others.

Several international agencies have drawn attention to the negative effect of criminalisation on health but progress in this area has been slow. There is a widespread need to condemn discrimination on the grounds of gender or sexual identity. Health care workers must engage with governments to review any discriminatory laws and policies.

The LGBT population faces many obstacles when accessing health care. Documented barriers include:

- Availability of treatment for LGBT-specific conditions.
- Denial of treatment.
- Inadequate or substandard care. LGBT individuals often experience verbal abuse, disrespectful behaviour or inadequate attention from health care professionals.
- Inappropriate linking of sexuality or gender identity to diagnoses.
- Avoidance of interaction with LGBT patients.

Changing of perceptions is difficult, especially in more conservative regions. In May 2014 the African Commission on Human and Peoples' Rights adopted a landmark resolution protecting the rights of LGBT people.

Meggie Mwoka (Kenya) and Jessica Dean (Australia)

Trade law

The General Agreement on Trade and Tariffs was signed by 23 countries in 1947. It aimed to try to reduce tariffs and trade barriers and to foster international trade. It was superseded in 1995 by the World Trade Organization. There are currently 164 member states (2017).

Trade law impacts on health care in a number of different ways. Notable examples include:

- The impact of trade laws on the pharmaceutical industry.
- International instruments relating to noncommunicable diseases (WHO Framework Convention on Tobacco Control; the WHO Global Strategy on Diet, Physical Activity and Health; and the WHO Global Strategy to Reduce the Harmful Use of Alcohol). The extent to which these international agreements are translated into domestic law differs greatly; marketing restrictions, product regulation and focused taxation have been introduced by many countries. Legal restrictions, for example labelling of drugs or food, also have a big impact in this field.
- Work-related injuries are still a major cause of death and disability. National laws for health and safety make a significant difference to the number and severity of work-related injuries. The International Labour Organization has brokered many international agreements; nevertheless, the number of workplace-related injuries has increased significantly, particularly with industrialisation. Only 10% of workers in low-income countries are protected by occupational health and safety legislation. This contributes significantly to the correlation between low economic status and high risk of workplace-related injury.

Criminal law

International criminal law can be applied for crimes against humanity, including torture and abuse. National criminal law applies in cases when people are harmed as a result of incompetence in health care delivery by individuals or corporations. To stand trial in a local, national, or international court, an accused individual must be considered to be mentally competent as this affects the legal process. Health care workers may be required to give their professional opinion in court.

Other examples of the intersection between criminal law and health include:

- Policies which criminalise activities posing a high risk for health (e.g., same-sex or paid sex activities). These policies may be counterproductive by driving practices underground, worsening the health problem.
- Law relating to intentional gender-related violence such as rape and homicide. Increased levels of criminal regulation, heavy sentencing and strict law enforcement help to reduce this form of violent crime.
- Narcotic drug control. Domestic laws differ considerably between countries. For example, cannabis is used legally for medicinal use in some countries.

Environmental law

International treaties are the major source of environmental law, and principles such as sustainable development were enshrined in the Rio Declaration at the United Nations Conference on Environment and Development (1992).

Interactions between environmental law and health include:

- Public health harms (e.g., environmental damage through air or water pollution). This can be rectified through litigation by citizens or public bodies.
- Travel-related injuries have been reduced by domestic legal restrictions around traffic speed, driving licenses and road design.
- Pesticide poisoning in lower middle-income country (LMIC) seriously harms health in the absence of effective national legal and regulatory mechanisms. The Rotterdam Convention on the Prior Informed Consent Procedure for Certain Hazardous Chemicals and Pesticides in International Trade (2004) regulates international trade in these chemicals.
- The Vienna Convention for the Protection of the Ozone Layer (2008) aims to protect human health and the environment.

Although legal instruments impact on both individual and population health, the application of such agreements may be challenging in complex situations.

Law, conflict situations and health

Millions of people suffer the effects of war and conflict. Public health and human rights are inevitably compromised. The human rights law framework (international criminal law, international humanitarian law, international human rights law) is a means whereby conflict situations can be reviewed and evaluated. Three elements should be considered separately from any relevant domestic laws.

- *International criminal law* covers many different legal issues, such as drugs and human trafficking. Through the International Criminal Court, based in The Hague, individuals can be charged with crimes including genocide and crimes against humanity. Whilst these may seem to overlap with international human rights law under the ICCPR, different legal requirements may apply. A person found guilty by the International Criminal Court can be imprisoned. A government found guilty of breaching a citizen's human rights can only be issued with a direction to reform its actions.
- *International humanitarian law*, through the Geneva Conventions (1949), regulates the behaviour of people involved in armed conflicts. It does not set out whether they can engage in the conflict but guides how they must treat each other while the conflict is ongoing. International humanitarian law regulates the types of weapons that can be used and the treatment of prisoners of war, and protects civilians, health care workers and religious personnel. It is triggered only when armed conflict is widespread.
- *International human rights law*. This area of international law is designed to promote human rights at several levels (regional, social and domestic).

Human trafficking

The Palermo Protocols (2003) are three UN protocols to:

- prevent, suppress and punish trafficking in persons, especially women and children
- prevent smuggling of migrants by land, sea and air
- prevent the illicit manufacturing of and trafficking in firearms

These protocols provide a common definition and set international standards around trafficking. They were developed within a *criminal justice framework* but do not include binding provisions to protect the human rights of trafficked persons. They have several limitations:

- The core of the crimes defined within the protocols are abuse, violence and exploitation. Some argue that the trafficking of people across national borders should be seen as a crime in itself.
- There is a level of ambiguity within the definition of trafficking. For example, some consider prostitution itself to constitute trafficking, whilst others consider prostitution as work labour.
- They do not adequately protect vulnerable workers (e.g., by preventing binding arrangements and guaranteeing the right to join workers' unions).
- They fail to address situations when states are complicit in trafficking.

Human trafficking

At 15 years of age, Sahiba was sold by sex traffickers for profit to be a child bride. She was raped and beaten every night. The problem of sex trafficking remains rife worldwide. As Sahiba's story shows, state institutions such as hospitals and the police often fail to acknowledge or support such individuals. There are also huge physical (e.g., STIs, pregnancy) and emotional (e.g., depression, posttraumatic stress disorder) health impacts.

Sahiba's mother died giving birth to her. Ill-treated by her sister-in-law, who took over the household, Sahiba decided to run away from home to eke out a living. Aged 15 years, she asked a trusted neighbour where she could get a job, and was introduced to a woman who sent her to a town for a 'good job'. As this provided an opportunity for financial independence, Sahiba agreed to take the job, but on the journey was raped by an older man and was subsequently locked up in a house and repeatedly abused. To escape this ordeal, she agreed to marry. Her husband and other men continued to abuse her.

Sahiba had managed to keep her SIM card although her phone had been confiscated. She eventually managed to call her brother, who immediately went to the police. The police officer refused to register a report. In despair, her brother contacted a charitable agency, and Sahiba was finally rescued. She then required counselling to overcome posttraumatic stress disorder. These experiences will remain with her for the rest of her life.

Erliani Abdul Rahman (Singapore)

Conclusion

Health can be affected by many legal frameworks. Human rights law, humanitarian law, trade law, environmental law and criminal law can impact on health. The international human rights law framework is probably the most important of these as human rights violations impact on health in many ways. Health care professionals therefore require a good understanding of this framework, and can be powerful advocates for enforcement of these instruments.

KEY POINTS

- Two key international human rights law documents are the International Covenant on Civil and Political Rights and the International Covenant on Economic, Social and Cultural Rights.
- Various international legal bodies impact on health. Particular areas of relevance include human rights law, humanitarian law, trade law, environmental law and criminal law.
- In complex situations, different bodies of law may apply or even appear to contradict one another.
- In conflict situations, international criminal law, humanitarian law and human rights law may all apply.
- Key challenges in global health governance include the jurisdictional, incentive and participation gaps.

Further reading

Gostin LO, Sridhar D: Global health and the law, *N Engl J Med* 370:1732–1740, 2014. <http://www.nejm.org/doi/full/10.1056/NEJMra1314094>.

Gostin L: Law and the public's health, Chapter 3.4. In Detels R, Gulliford M, Karim QA, Tan CC, editors: *Oxford textbook of global public health*, ed 6, Oxford, 2015, Oxford University Press, p 293–302.

United Nations: *International law and justice.* <http://www.un.org/en/sections/issues-depth/international-law-and-justice/index.html>.

5.3 Access to Health Care for Vulnerable Groups

Joseph Cherabie (Lebanon)   Fadi Halabi (Lebanon)
Wajiha Jurdi Kheir (Lebanon)   Storm Parker (UK)

> *'The enjoyment of the highest attainable standard of health is one of the fundamental rights of every human being without distinction of race, religion, political belief, economic or social condition.'*
> Constitution of The World Health Organization, 1946

Introduction

Universal health coverage requires physical access to nondiscriminatory, affordable health care services, as well as to comprehensive health-related information. Women, children, people with disabilities, people with HIV/AIDS, migrants, the elderly, people with a diagnosis of a mental health illness, and lesbian, gay, bisexual and transgender (LGBT) people are groups vulnerable to human rights violations. Although most of these at-risk groups have been assured equal rights, these are often not delivered without appropriate legal enforcement. The right to health and health care access is universal. This 'right' is determined by socioeconomic, cultural and environmental factors (i.e., the social determinants of health).

The determinants of health which can lead to health disparities

Disparities in health, whether between individuals, populations or groups of differing societal status, result in social disadvantage. Factors impacting on an individual's health are shown in **Fig. 5.3.1**. These include an adequate standard of living, good nutrition, housing and clothing, water sanitation, safe drinking water, good working conditions, education and gender equality, all of which ultimately contribute to a healthy life. Not only are these determinants required for good health, good health in itself allows achievement of many other elements, such as education and employment.

Social inequities, for example those resulting from the persecution of minority groups, are unjust but can be addressed through changes in societal attitudes and policy. They can also result in the differences in health seen between different socioeconomic groups within a population.

Nondiscriminatory health care

Discrimination affects individuals' lives on many levels. It affects personal behaviour and access to employment and health. As a result, marginalised groups may be unable to receive appropriate health care.

Mental health conditions are known to be underdiagnosed, in part due to the social stigma associated with mental health illnesses. Frameworks such as the Principles for the Protection of Persons with Mental Illness and the Improvement of Mental Health Care (United Nations, 1991) outline standards for mental health care and the rights of people with mental health conditions.

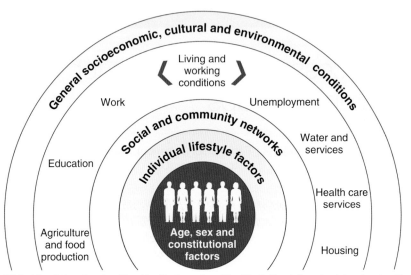

Figure 5.3.1   The determinants of health. *(Redrawn from The King's Fund: Broader determinants of health, 2015. http://www.kingsfund.org.uk/time-to-think-differently/trends/broader-determinants-health.)*

These standards are often unmet. Some patients, including some with mental illness, do not present to medical services because they fear the label of a stigmatising diagnosis and discrimination by health care staff.

The International Guidelines on HIV/AIDS and Human Rights provide guidance for governmental and other organisations providing care for people with HIV and AIDS. It is the responsibility of the state to make laws to protect this group from discrimination, and to make efforts to change societal attitudes. Despite this, people with HIV and AIDS continue to experience debilitating social stigma and discriminatory behaviour by health care workers. These attitudes negatively impact on the quality of care, and may discourage individuals from seeking appropriate and timely treatment. This potentially limits their life expectancy and reduces their quality of life.

LGBT individuals include people with various sexual, cultural, ethnic and social identities. They all experience discrimination in their communities, and are denied some of the most basic human rights. In some countries, it is illegal to engage in same-sex sexual relations. Cultural insensitivity may result in poor care by health care staff who are homophobic. LGBT individuals may not disclose their sexuality to health care professionals for fear of discrimination. These factors contribute towards a poor doctor–patient relationship and poorer health outcomes.

The impact of health discrimination and denial of rights to the transgender population in India

India's transgender population has a long history. Stigmatisation and discrimination against this population over the years has compromised their rights and alienated them from society.

Knowledge of the availability of services among members of the transgender community is good, but many barriers, stemming directly from their gender identity, prevent access to appropriate services. This leads to social isolation and amplifies the impact on the social determinants of health, such as poverty and poor education. It also results in inappropriate health care treatment, particularly in the area of sexual health. There is a need for greater awareness of the detrimental effects of discrimination and denial of rights on health.

Ellen Adams (UK)

Physical accessibility

Physical access to health care facilities, resources and services can be difficult for indigenous populations, ethnic minorities, women, children, adolescents, the elderly, the disabled and those with HIV/AIDS. This access also requires disabled-friendly roads and health care services within a safe distance, especially in rural areas. Other essential requirements include safe drinking water, sanitation facilities and local access to nutritious foods. The average local income of a geographical area determines the number of health care facilities and practitioners. Inevitably, this means that there is poor provision for people of low socioeconomic status, who have greater health care needs.

People with disabilities often encounter physical inaccessibility through a lack of disabled-friendly settings, particularly in rural areas and slums. It is not the individuals' disability that puts these people at risk of increased morbidity and death, but the social barriers that they face. They can be seen as a burden on society, and are therefore marginalised. Impingement on their human rights affects both their psychological and physical well-being. The Standard Rules on the Equalization of Opportunities for Persons with Disabilities states that countries should remove all obstacles that hinder disabled peoples' interaction with the physical environment.

Taking action for people with disabilities in Uganda

Disabled people, especially females, may be stigmatised. They may face violence and can be denied basics such as food, clothing and shelter.

Anne Kobusingye contracted polio at the age of 7 years, leaving her disabled. She persevered to overcome her disability and set up a grassroots organisation to tackle stigma and improve the quality of life for those with disabilities. She created employment opportunities for people with disabilities along with improved access to basic education, health information and vocational training (**Fig. 5.3.2**). 'The disabled have no voice to speak out; they are in a prison of self-pity, poverty, hatred, stigma and all sorts of oppression just because of disability. In Uganda, there are national programmes to help people with disabilities but they don't reach people. I therefore resolved to reach Ugandans with disabilities in my district.'

Anne Kobusingye (Uganda)

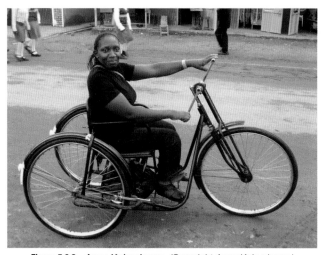

Figure 5.3.2   Anne Kobusingye. *(Copyright Anne Kobusingye.)*

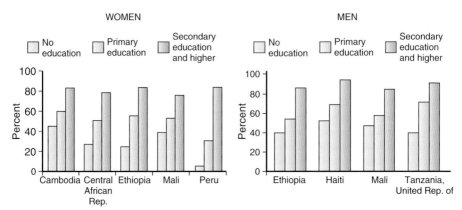

Figure 5.3.3 Young people aged 15–24 years who know a healthy-looking person can transmit HIV. *(Data from UNICEF: Girls, HIV/AIDS and education, New York, 2004, UNICEF.)*

Another vulnerable group with regard to poor physical access is the elderly. They may be unable to easily reach health care facilities because of their own frailty, the physical access to buildings and the distances they need to travel. This may contribute to their poor health outcomes and high morbidity.

Access to information

Information access 'includes the right to seek, receive and impart information and ideas concerning health issues.' This right should not impair the right of the individual to confidentiality. People with physical and psychosocial disabilities are often excluded from decisions regarding their treatment when health care professionals make assumptions about their ability to give informed consent. They are seen as objects rather than as individuals, and this is degrading, unethical and an impingement on their human rights.

Access to information can prevent harm. The fight against HIV/AIDS includes prevention through education about safe-sex practices. Healthy adolescents should be made aware of the risks of HIV transmission; many are unaware of these risks because of a lack of education and information as a result of inadequate resources (**Fig. 5.3.3**).

Economic accessibility

Health care services, facilities and resources should be affordable for all individuals, in particular for socially vulnerable groups. The ICESCR states that 'equity demands that poorer households should not be disproportionately burdened with health expenses as compared to richer households.' Homeless people have higher morbidity and mortality rates than the rest of the population. They are a vulnerable group with many physical and mental health needs as a result of substance and alcohol misuse, unhygienic living conditions, risky sexual behaviour, physical and sexual abuse, and smoking. They frequently face barriers to health care access, because of stigma, lack of continuity of care, lack of primary care access, and unaffordable health insurance or treatment. The poor therefore delay seeking necessary health care and spend their income on food and shelter.

Refugees (a term used here to cover refugees and asylum seekers) are underprivileged and experience extreme discrimination. Despite the efforts of international and local agencies to

The most prominent humanitarian account comes from Peter Singer of Princeton University. His arguments rely on utilitarian ethics (i.e., maximising interests and preferences for all involved). According to Singer, if it is in our power to prevent something bad from happening, without thereby sacrificing anything of comparable moral importance, we ought, morally, to do it. His humanitarian approach has clear implications for the daily activities of individuals, institutions and multinationals. It makes the 'duty to assist others' an intrinsic part of our obligations.

Singer's fundamental arguments are that:

- *Distance between people is not a criterion that justifies lack of action.* For example, we cannot say that an individual starving in another country is not morally important to us just because that person is in another country.
- *The same moral obligations impact on each individual regardless of the circumstances or actions of others.* For example, it may be tempting to think that duties can be less strict if others do not follow them. However, the lack of action by others is not an adequate reason to excuse our own obligations.
- *If it is in our power to prevent resource scarcity, then it is an individual moral duty to address the problem.* He suggests any solution is morally essential as long as it does not translate into a personal sacrifice of comparable or higher moral importance. For example, if we find ourselves passing by a shallow pond where a child is drowning, it is our moral responsibility to help that child despite the likelihood that it might result in a minor inconvenience such as delayed time or messed clothing.

Singer's arguments have significant implications for charitable giving as part of the global health agenda, and apply equally to personal, institutional and even national finances. It is important to channel these efforts into effective charities that have evidence of positive impact. There are numerous associated ethical issues in attempting to apply Singer's theory.

Cosmopolitanism and blamefulness (Pogge)

If we consider the issue of responsibility, 'who is to blame' for global health problems, the ethical perceptions shift. According to Thomas Pogge, the identification of blame defines the response and subsequent action. 'Blameworthiness' implies an obligation to rectify the harm caused. Thus those who caused the inequity have a stronger moral responsibility than those who had no control over the cause. It requires detailed clarity regarding the causes of inequities as they may be influenced by many variables, thereby affecting the apportionment of blame. This point of view requires a thorough insight into evidence pertaining to global development.

The social, political and economic determinants of health are major causes of structural inequity. This inequity is exacerbated by the coercive behaviours of some global institutions which result in major consequences for global health. Unfortunately, declarations such as the ICESCR (1966) and the Framework Convention on Tobacco Control (2009) have failed to resolve many relevant health challenges. Financial considerations and power determine many global health outcomes.

Pogge's cosmopolitanist arguments suggest that those who are materially involved in institutions perpetuating an unethical state of affairs have the responsibility to change priorities within these organisations. He emphasises the moral obligation for them to campaign to remove underlying structural violence and rectify any harm caused.

Ethical procurement of supplies in the National Health Service

In accordance with cosmopolitanism theory, health care systems have a moral duty to ensure that goods and services are supplied ethically. In failing to do so, we, ourselves are acting unethically. This obligation also extends to manufacturers as well as to consumers.

The National Health Service (NHS) spends in excess of £30 billion each year on the procurement of goods and services. Manufacturers of these goods may employ:

- unsafe working conditions with associated health and safety hazards
- low wages with payment significantly below the living wage
- child labour
- excessive and unsafe working hours
- poor labour contracts
- restrictions on rights of assembly

This demonstrates an uncomfortable paradox—improving the health of the UK population but adversely affecting health globally. The conditions described are examples of the wider social determinants of health.

Ethical Procurement for Health aims to ensure that workers producing goods used by the NHS meet fundamental labour standards. NHS purchasers stipulate that these workers' rights must conform to the ethical standards of the International Labour Organization .

The voice of doctors and other health care professionals has the potential to be very powerful in decisions regarding procurement by the NHS. Cosmopolitanism theory suggests that health care professionals *everywhere* should engage in ethical trading practices to take steps to improve the conditions and welfare of people involved in the supply of goods and services.

Martha Martin, Amelia Martin, Felicia Yeung, Sam Gnanapragasam and Akanksha Mimi Malhotra (UK)

Noncosmopolitanism

The concept of noncosmopolitanism regards the state as the most important actor in rectifying equity. Justice, therefore is secured only within established institutions following political debate. Noncosmopolitanism theory states that the social contract between the individual and the community acts as the foundation for ethics (**Fig. 5.4.2**).

Noncosmopolitans recognise that, despite the principle of equal moral standing for all, variations occur in the treatment of individuals. Some ethicists such as Rawls and David Miller suggest that the obligations (see **Fig. 5.4.2**) are built and channelled through political institutions. An alternative viewpoint, *social egalitarianism* (see later), focuses on social values.

Rawls's difference principle: 'Social and economic inequalities, for example inequalities of wealth and authority, are just only if they result in compensating benefits for everyone, and in particular for the least advantaged members of society.'

John Rawls, A Theory of Justice, 1971

Individual	Community
Obligations: • Pay taxes • Register for selective service • Vote • Attend K–12 education (mandatory since 1938) • Obey the laws • Participate in public debates • Preserve property rights	**Obligations:** • Provides protection fire & police; national level military • Establish courts & a system of justice; resolve disputes • Hold elections • Legislate the laws • Establish property rights & protect businesses • Build & maintain the roads

Figure 5.4.2   The social contract (Walzer). This is an agreement between an individual and the state/place of residence (community). *K–12 refers to educational grades between kindergarten and college in North America and some other countries. (Redrawn from Bowser, Diane (Ph.D.) Lectures on John Rawls. Ethics Course at The Art Institute of Pittsburgh, 2001–2011.)*

Rawls's global duties in *The Law of Peoples* (1999) helps us to understand the political implications for national and global health. The main target for assistance at a global level is the establishment of a 'well-ordered' or functional political infrastructure. Emphasis is placed on the worst-off individuals, leading to equalising opportunities for all.

At a global level, no state should intervene in national affairs except to establish an appropriate political culture. Any intervention is limited to providing mere advice or support. With this theory, a process of global fair distribution of resources is not required, and is even seen as undesirable, as justice should naturally stem from fair societies.

An alternative approach is *social egalitarianism*. This argues that individuals' opportunities depend on their social standing, which is, in itself, shaped by the way society is organised. The underlying structures of the society must be addressed to provide greater opportunities, equity and justice for all. The focus of this approach is on the people and civil society, whilst institutions are the mechanism whereby society delivers its obligations.

The ethics of international aid

International aid has been subject of ethical debate for many reasons. It is a key topic to which these theories have been applied within the global development field. Some of the reasons for controversy include:

- The exponential increase in the allocation of aid going into emergency projects (earthquakes or floods) versus developmental projects (sanitation or health care infrastructure). This is seen to highlight the focus of global health actors on short-term approaches.
- The effectiveness of donation is difficult to measure given the various factors influencing results. These include the lack of accountability and transparency of donors (self-interests) and receptors (corruption and autocracy), and the multiplicity of donors, leading to disorganised governance.
- The large amount of aid which is spent in the donor rather than recipient countries.
- The stringent conditions often attached to aid, which may limit national sovereignty and lead to an unequal power relationship.

Crossing culturing differences

Different ethical codes are encountered when one is travelling for tourism, education or aid provision. Tourism is often regarded as a positive economic activity as it promotes employment, redistributes income and alleviates poverty. However, it can have adverse environmental impacts (e.g., carbon dioxide generated by air travel) and can lead to degradation of local cultural and environmental features. This has led to the development of the theory of *sustainable tourism*. This tourism makes a positive impact on the local environment and society.

The Green Tourist Association in Toronto developed the concept of urban green tourism as part of its sustainable city plan. This approach (**Fig. 5.4.3**) encourages cities to build in hosting visitors as part of its day-to-day business, and encourages businesses and those visiting to think carefully about the impacts of their travel.

Challenges of travel and ethical health care practice

International travel provides excellent opportunities for health care professionals. It widens their horizons, promotes professional and personal development, and provides an insight into the needs of multicultural societies.

'They ignored me because I was a girl, and they said to my (male) clinical partner. "You have to do this procedure now, or the patient will suffer. He has no money so he cannot pay for a proper dentist

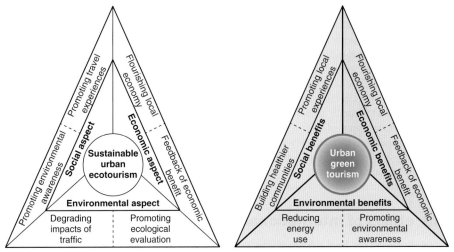

Figure 5.4.3 Three-dimensional targeting model of sustainable urban ecotourism, and a proposed model for urban green tourism. *Left:* Aspects of sustainable ecotourism (social, economic and environmental factors) with two targets for each. *Right:* Modification of these targets to clarify the benefits of urban green tourism in line with the recommendations of the Urban Green Tourism Association. *(Left: Redrawn from Wu Y, Wang H, Ho Y (2010) Urban ecotourism: defining and assessing dimensions using fuzzy number construction. Tourism Management 31 (6) 739–743. Right: redrawn from Dunlop I (2013) The making of a guidebook to the City of Hamilton as a practical exercise in context-sensitive place marketing and community economic development. University of Waterloo 2013.)*

to do it. It is you or nobody." My partner looked at me and I knew he was thinking that we hadn't been trained to do that yet and we didn't have the language to explain this to the patient or to ask for his consent. I thought to myself that nothing had prepared us for this.'

Dentistry student

Many practical and ethical challenges arise during which students may find it difficult to cope with different cultures, languages and practices of medicine. Students often report feeling uncertain about the best way to help host communities, given their limited experience. Additionally, students may struggle with the application of their own professional standards in a different cultural environment. When encountering a different culture, students may undergo a challenge with ethical relativism, perhaps believing that their ethical approach is superior. Few institutions equip students for the challenging situations they may face overseas.

Peer-led ethical teaching for global health electives

Ethical challenges are frequently encountered by students undertaking overseas medical elective attachments. A student–faculty group designed, implemented and evaluated peer-led workshops for 57 students preparing to visit overseas. The workshop included the sharing of personal stories, introduction to relevant ethical frameworks and the opportunity to work through some real-life ethical scenarios. Students gained confidence and reported feeling much better prepared following the workshop.

Peer teaching enables role-modelling, sharing of personal experiences and frank and open conversations on difficult topics. These attributes are relevant for students navigating complex ethical and professionalism issues, such as those arising when they are working overseas. Our team systematically reviewed the literature regarding ethical challenges experienced by students overseas. We collected personal accounts from students at our institution and internationally, and categorised them by ethical theme.

Key recurrent issues included:

* when to question clinical practice
* whether to adapt to different professional cultures
* responding to patients who cannot afford vital care
* being asked to perform tasks outside their competency
* power and privilege
* being a burden

We developed a framework for real case studies following informal consultations with students and by reviewing existing programmes of the International Federation of Medical Students' Associations. The following questions were relevant:

1. What are the ethical issues/themes here?
2. What is my role in this situation?
3. What factors should I consider?
4. What resources or forms of support are available to help me think about/manage this?
5. What should I do next?

Students commented positively on the structure and methodology, and were better able to identify ethical issues and apply learning from the workshop to specific written scenarios.

Thomas Hindmarch, Felicity Knights, Vita Sinclair and Anika Rahim, with the support of Molly Fyfe and Paula Baraitser (UK)

> **BOX 5.4.1** ■ **Principlism: ethical decision making in health care**
>
> How can we make ethical decisions?
> *Principles of Biomedical Ethics* (Tom Beauchamp and James Childress) proposes four principles:
> ■ Non-maleficence – do no harm
> ■ Beneficence – do good, act in the best interests of others
> ■ Autonomy – maximise freedom for individual or community
> ■ Justice – treat equal cases equally and unequal cases differently
>
> *Reproduced with permission from Beauchamp TL, Childress JF: Principles of biomedical ethics, ed 5, Oxford, 2001, Oxford University Press.*

The ethical issues encountered by health care students are similar to those encountered by fully trained professionals. Many health care professionals in European and Western countries have been taught medical ethics according to principlism (**Box 5.4.1**).

This theory arose from Western cultures and, arguably, does not reflect global moral perspectives. It focuses on individual physician and patient interactions, and fails to incorporate issues such as context, culture and community. This is inevitable because of differing beliefs about the duties, rights and roles of individuals in various cultures. For example, confidentiality would be breached by Western standards in countries where treatment decisions are determined by the family/friends without the explicit consent of the patient. In Western societies, when these principles come into conflict, the principle of autonomy tends to be seen as the overriding principle in an informed adult with mental capacity. In contrast, many other societies would hold issues such as beneficence and nonmaleficence (i.e., not doing any harm to others in an individual's family or society) to be more important. This is a classic reason that some cultures and societies struggle with the concept of human rights, based around the importance of autonomy.

Pinto et al. (2009) propose four alternative pillars for global engagement:

■ *Humility:* Appreciating our limitations (e.g., medical training in one context does not mean competence everywhere) and appreciating the expertise of local practitioners and communities. This approach suggests that we must challenge 'medical tourism', which undermines existing health care, and also challenge neocolonialism.

■ *Introspection:* Understanding your own motives, perspectives, burden and experiences. Considering the sustainability of one's actions.

■ *Solidarity:* Aligning ourselves and working in partnership, developing an understanding of the experiences of others and establishing ongoing relationships. This arises from a global village perspective: 'My health is intricately connected to your health.'

■ *Social justice:* Diminishing the net inequity in the world. Looking beyond the patient to the health system, communities, societies and the environment they live in and reflecting on how these affect health. Sharing this learning and reacting against our learned helplessness.

There are many circumstances in which international global health volunteers place themselves in unethical situations, or even volunteer with unethical organisations.

This hands-on experience, in the absence of legal repercussions, is one of global health's weakest links. A sense of social responsibility motivates volunteers to invest personal time and resources to help others, and a lack of resources may lead the host country to accept them. However, altruistic intentions are often insufficient and may produce more harm than good, whilst not meeting the needs of the community. An ethical and sustainable model is needed, and collaboration between international/foreign organisations and local health sectors is always essential.

The dark side of international medical volunteering

International surgical missions provide treatment to patients in need. Diagnosis and early treatment are important, but follow-up and longer-term support therapies are often required. A lack of sustainable support and regulation of these endeavours can mean that such missions result in harm.

Diego, a 32-year-old man, presented to the hospital emergency department with chronic left leg pain, swelling and several bouts of fever. Three months previously, he had fractured his leg in a motor vehicle accident and had an internal fixation and short leg cast. About 2 months before, he was treated by foreign medical volunteers during an orthopaedic surgical mission when external fixation of the distal part of his left tibia was performed. Diego was given antibiotics for 15 days, and although he was already developing fevers and a swollen leg during that period, he did not know who to inform—there was no one to conduct follow-up. Two weeks later, Diego presented to another hospital with a deformed, hot, erythematous left leg with exudate oozing out of the pins of the external fixator. An X-ray showed extensive osteomyelitis with soft tissue ulceration and cellulitis. He subsequently required amputation of his leg. International medical-surgical missions are one of global health's greatest triumphs. However, as shown in this case, comprehensive care with appropriate follow-up is absolutely essential. Humanitarian missions must be based on ethical principles of nonmaleficence and beneficence.

Helena Chapman (Dominican Republic)

Conclusion

Good ethical practice is an integral part of all global health activities. It requires an understanding of local environmental and cultural issues. Detailed planning as well as appropriate support is essential when new projects are being developed.

KEY POINTS

• There are two main schools of thought within equity-focused global health ethics: cosmopolitanism and noncosmopolitanism.
• Cosmopolitanism focuses on health responsibilities with a global context.
• Noncosmopolitanism (or political theory) focuses on health duties within national boundaries.
• Health care professionals should prepare themselves to address challenging ethical issues when working abroad.

Further reading

Benatar S, Brock G, editors: *Global health and global health ethics*, Cambridge, 2011, Cambridge University Press.

Brock G: *Global justice: a cosmopolitan account*, Oxford, 2009, Oxford University Press.

Frenk J, Moon S: Governance challenges in global health, *N Engl J Med* 368(10):936–942, 2013.

Pinto AD, Upshur REG: *An introduction to global health*, Abingdon, 2013, Routledge.

Sudhir A, Peter F, Sen A, editors: *Public health, ethics, and equity*, Oxford, 2006, Oxford University Press.

5.5 Social Theories and Health

Amanda Craig (UK)　　Charlotte Thomassen-Kinsey (Denmark/UK)

Introduction

Social scientists evaluate interactions between health care programmes and local society structures. They are also able to explore the perspectives of individuals and their health beliefs in the local setting. As the study of health and medicine can be considered to be as social as it is scientific, three main social theories have been used to explain the interaction between individuals in society, the medical profession and illness: functionalism, Marxism, and symbolic interactionism.

Functionalism suggests that medicine has a functional place in society in maintaining social cohesion. *Marxism* explains how medicine maintains individual health, keeping workers at work, and ensuring that society is able to prosper economically. Both of these social theories take a top-down approach to exploring and explaining society. *Symbolic interaction* takes a bottom-up approach by looking at the interaction between the individual, and health and medicine. In this model, individuals control their health and treatment options.

Functionalism, Parsons and the sick role

Functionalism is a social theory which takes a top-down approach to societal institutions. It argues that institutions interact positively and cohesively with individuals. Talcott Parsons (1952) formulated an 'organic analogy' which suggests that society functions very much like the human body: if one organ stops working, the body becomes ill and malfunctions. Likewise, if either a person falls ill or an institution fails, society will become dysfunctional. Society therefore requires healthy workers and well-run institutions. A functionalist perspective regards illness as a form of social 'deviance' within society. This is seen in Asian and African societies, where the good of society is regarded as being relatively more important than that of the individual. In many of these cultures, the individual's key purpose is seen to be as a contributor to society. This has significant impact on the values of the society and culture in decision making.

Parsons developed the notion of the sick role, whereby a sick individual may adopt certain patterns of behaviour so as to minimise the disruption caused by the illness. The sick role is learnt through socialisation—as children, we are taught how to behave when ill. A 'sick' individual disrupts society's cohesive balance as that person is unable to perform his or her regular societal duties and responsibilities.

Parsons suggests that when an individual falls ill, the sick role is played out as follows:

- If illness is not through the individual's own fault, the individual is not perceived by society to be responsible for being sick.
- As the individual is not responsible for being sick, he/she is exempt from some of his/her normal roles within society. However, the sick individual should regain his/her health as the sick role is temporary.
- If recovery does not occur, the sick individual must consult a health care professional who is able to legitimise the illness. The sick individual has now become a patient. There is

---

Exploring the organic analogy: the impact of the sick role on the family and society

Aisha is a 15-year-old African girl who dreams of being a vet. When her father became ill, it affected the whole of her family and community.

Aisha's parents have three children and work long hours to afford the cost of sending her to school. They have high aspirations for her. She only has a couple of years left in school, and studies hard to pass her university entrance exams.

Unfortunately, Aisha's father falls ill and she has to take time off school to look after him. He becomes unable to work and loses his job. As a result, Aisha fails her exams and cannot return to school as her parents cannot afford the fees.

Aisha's story links into Parsons' organic analogy (every part of society has to work for it to function cohesively), and the notion of the sick role.

---

agreement between the sick individual and those around him/her that he/she is trying to regain his/her health. If the sick individual does not follow the advice of the health care professional, he/she is seen to be jeopardising his/her health.

This approach places a responsibility on the individual to maintain his or her health for the good of society. In many societies, doctors play a key gatekeeper role as they have to assess whether an individual is fit to work. Their decision can legitimise an individual's 'right' to be ill, and thus his or her access to the sick role, as well as additional resources such as social payments. This interaction has implications for both society and the individual.

Freidson (1970) identified a further three versions of the sick role, depending on the severity of the illness:

- *The conditional sick role:* a temporary illness which gives access to the sick role (e.g., the common cold).
- *The unconditional legitimate sick role:* a chronic illness with potential long-term access to the sick role (e.g., Parkinson disease).
- *The illegitimate sick role:* illnesses in which the individual is deemed to have personal responsibility for the development of that illness (e.g., obesity). This notion does not allow for factors such as the social determinants of health and may contribute to stigma by society.

The sick role has been influential in showing how the ill person plays a role within society and how that society functions if a person is ill. However, it may not capture the patient's experience of the illness, especially in situations where there is disagreement between the doctor and the patient on the diagnosis.

The sick role is mainly relevant to an understanding of acute illness. In chronic illness, patients usually have to adjust their life to their condition rather than necessarily relinquishing their societal role. Within many societies, individuals are seen as having the dominant responsibility for their own lifestyle and well-being. Social and cultural factors may deny an individual being granted the sick role (e.g., because of class, gender or ethnicity). Overall, the sick role and functionalism can provide only a partial understanding of the way sick individuals have a role within the cohesive function of a productive society.

Marxism, health and medicine

> *'The bourgeoisie has stripped of its halo every occupation hitherto honored and looked up to with reverent awe. It has converted the physician, the lawyer, the priest, the poet, the man of science, into its paid wage laborers.'*

Karl Marx, The Communist Manifesto

Marxism takes a top-down view of society. From a Marxist viewpoint, capitalism fosters inequality between workers and the 'ruling classes' and is detrimental to both individual and population health. This perspective has implications when applied to specific health care problems. Smoking is a socially constructed habit, with a huge global negative health care impact. Marxists point out that smoking enables capitalism to prosper, as taxes and revenue from cigarette sales far exceed the cost of smoking to the health care system. The medical industry remains in business as smoking provides new patients. From a traditionally Marxist perspective, much of ill health can be explained by class and linked to poor working conditions, and low-income workers may be directly affected by industrial diseases, injuries and stress through their day-to-day work. The Marxist approach argues that health problems should be addressed, recognising the inequalities in society and the importance of the social determinants of health in the generation of these inequalities.

Critics suggest that Marxists should focus their attention on the dynamics of the medical process, the experience of the illness and the state of being a patient. Hart (1985) also argues that as capitalism has provided health care gains and medical advances that have prolonged life expectancy, it should not be viewed in an entirely negative manner.

Capitalism and China's baby milk scandal (2008)

China relies on imported milk formulas to feed babies and infants. The baby milk powder industry is one of many industries that make significant profits from health care provision. A Marxist perspective enables us to understand the scandal of 2008 as well as methods to prevent similar disasters.

In 2008 more 300,000 babies were affected by the contaminated milk formula widely bought and used in China. The formula was found to contain an industrial chemical (melamine) more commonly found in plastics. With the addition of this chemical, the milk, when tested, appeared to contain more protein. This enabled the milk producers to water down their product so it could go further. Six babies died as a result of this contaminated milk, causing a national and international scandal.

The Marxist approach shows how companies prioritised corporate interests and profitability over the safety of babies. This perspective is relevant when one is considering ways to mitigate against similar disasters. It suggests that capitalist industries focus excessively on profit, to the potential detriment of patients. There is therefore a need for regulation of industry by a cross-section of society. Extension of this philosophy also questions the validity of partnerships between the commercial and not-for-profit sectors.

Charlotte Thomassen-Kinsey

Symbolic interactionism

Within the sociology of health and illness, _symbolic interactionism_ focuses on the decision of the individual to seek professional medical help. In contrast to functionalism and Marxism, symbolic interactionism rejects the idea that illness is inevitably the direct result of a disease. One of the key factors in determining whether a patient self-labels as unwell, chooses to access care and chooses to comply with medical recommendations is _stigma_.

Exploring stigma

> 'Before you become unwell, you are exposed to stigma in society and the negative attitudes that people hold towards people who have mental health problems. When you do become unwell yourself, you know that these views exist and expect that they will be attached to you. This fuels self-stigma.'
>
> **Anonymous research volunteer, Scottish Recovery Network**

Stigma occurs when an individual is socially excluded and not fully accepted in society. It may be based on stereotypes and prejudice that may not always be correct. It can also be a way of exhibiting social control over the group. Health care professionals have a key role to play in educating society about diagnoses, and can be key in perpetuating or tackling stigma.

Stigma in society helps to generate and perpetuate self-stigma in which an individual starts to apply society's negative associations about a group to themselves. These negative associations may be accepted over time by the individual as self-evident 'truths' that influence the individual's beliefs and attitudes. Compassionate consultations with health care professionals, especially around the time of diagnosis, can be key in helping individuals to maintain hope and avoid shame.

Individuals who are concerned about stigma or being labelled with a diagnosis they do not want to receive may avoid accessing health care until forced to by an emergency situation. At this point, patients may be very unwell, and their recovery may be seriously compromised. This is a real challenge for public health interventions, and is frequently relevant to diagnoses perceived as terminal (e.g., cancer) and in mental health issues.

Stigma at the end of life

Stigma is culturally and socially constructed, and therefore differs significantly around the world. This case study describes the stigma around a dying patient in India with violation of her human rights. It describes how the health care team is attempting to educate the local population, modelling an alternative path for patient care to tackle this stigma.

'Did you just feed her?' The bite in her tone was obvious. We looked at her, confused. Subhadrabai lay motionless on her woven cot, covered in flies, watching silently as her daughter-in-law moved menacingly towards us.

'You're the ones that fed her. Now you clean the excrement tomorrow.'

She swept out of the backyard, and we looked at each other in stunned silence. Subhadrabai gazed at us, too weak to move, eyes filled with a pain too deep to fathom.

I work in a rural hospital providing community care. Subhadrabai, a 75-year-old woman with hemiplegia, was one of our patients. Perhaps her folly stood in transferring her assets to her son before her demise. Subhadrabai's family wanted her dead. She was a pain, with her constant ailments and then her paralysis. Who had the time to care for someone who was so obviously outliving a reasonable lifespan? Subhadrabai could not understand what she had done to deserve the scorn of those she loved, and she had often wished she was dead. She looked forward to our weekly visits with a childlike simplicity, and would often ask us to bring her favourite foods.

We now make it a point to remind our local society that the dying are still human beings. Our health care team make it clear that ill-treating or discriminating against these patients, for example by refusing to feed them, is a violation of human rights. We speak to each family we visit about the sacrifice parents make for their children. We also make it clear that it is our responsibility to care for them at the end of their lives, as a disease does not diminish their inherent value. We teach by example, through love and care for those who have nothing to give us in return.

When Subhadrabai died, her last rites were performed with pomp. Relatives went on a pilgrimage to the Ganges to immerse her ashes. It is with great shame and sorrow we realise that in a culture that prides itself in the honour and respect of elders, it is easier to pray for the soul of the deceased than to care for the body of one who is still alive.

Ishita T. Johal (India)

Conclusion

Three key social science theories affect thinking about health, medicine and illness. *Functionalism* looks at the way in which institutions, such as health care, relate to society. *Marxism* provides an alternative perspective to capitalism, positioning economic prosperity at the heart of health care. *Symbolic interactionism* considers the way in which the individual patient interacts with the health care system to legitimise the illness. Stigma is a key factor in the patient experience, and health care professionals have a significant role to play in tackling inaccurate stereotypes and delivering nonjudgemental care.

KEY POINTS

- Social theories that can be applied to global health include functionalism, Marxism and symbolic interactionism.
- Parsons' notion of the sick role explores how society perceives different forms of illness, and the responsibilities of individuals as they recover their health.
- Marxism views health care institutions as part of capitalism. They perpetuate economic inequality.
- Stigma is a significant challenge for patients, particularly those with illnesses which cannot be readily cured. It may affect access to care and treatment.
- Symbolic interactionism and the health belief model help to explain the factors influencing an individual's decision to seek and adhere to medical care.

Further reading

Bradby H: *Medicine, health and society*, Thousand Oaks, 2012, Sage Publications.
Gernsbacher MA: Stigma from psychological science: group differences, not deficits—introduction to stigma, *Perspect Psychol Sci* 5:687–713, 2015.
Scambler G, editor: *Sociology as applied to medicine*, ed 6, Oxford, 2008, Elsevier.

5.6 Culture, Religion, Ethnicity and Health

Fiona Headley (UK)

'Diversity in the world is a basic characteristic of human society, and also the key condition for a lively and dynamic world as we see today.'
Jinato Hu

Introduction

Culture refers to the shared ideas, customs and social behaviour of a particular group of people. *Religion* is defined as a particular system of faith or worship. An individual's religious beliefs may be either part of or separate from their culture. *Ethnicity* defines a social group that has common national or cultural traditions. This is distinct from *race*, which categorises individuals using physical characteristics. These terms are often used to classify individuals into groups. However, it is vital to appreciate the differences within, as well as between, these groups, and to avoid stereotyping.

Impact of culture, religion and ethnicity on health

Culture, religion and ethnicity may impact on health via the social determinants of health. For example, the Koran's prohibition of alcohol may protect Muslims from the health risks of excess consumption, but the modesty of women's dress (**Fig. 5.6.1**) may hinder their ability to partake in certain physical activities. Furthermore, health disparities are frequently observed between the dominant ethnic group and ethnic minorities. This may be the result of behavioural factors due to cultural differences, discriminatory factors such as social exclusion and lower socioeconomic background.

Health beliefs and use of health care

Two individuals may have the same disease, but their experiences of this as an illness may be very different. An individual's health beliefs are influenced by culture, ethnicity and religion. For example, there are cultural and religious differences in the medicalisation of depressive symptoms. Some Buddhists regard symptoms of depression as a natural part of life, not as a form of mental illness, whereas depression in Chinese people may be dominated by somatic symptoms. An individual's health beliefs can have profound effects on health care outcomes. They impact on health-related behaviours, including the decision to seek health care, the expression of illness management decisions and adherence.

The use of health care services is significantly affected by financial considerations, geographical access to health care and social beliefs. For example, the cultural practice of male guardianship in some Islamic countries may limit a woman's access to health care at times when her guardian

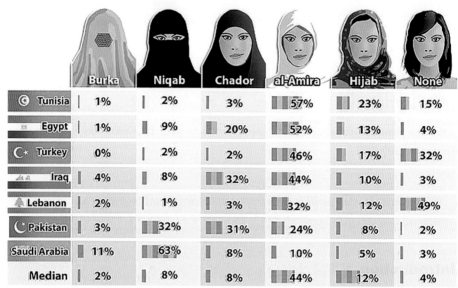

	Burka	Niqab	Chador	al-Amira	Hijab	None
Tunisia	1%	2%	3%	57%	23%	15%
Egypt	1%	9%	20%	52%	13%	4%
Turkey	0%	2%	2%	46%	17%	32%
Iraq	4%	8%	32%	44%	10%	3%
Lebanon	2%	1%	3%	32%	12%	49%
Pakistan	3%	32%	31%	24%	8%	2%
Saudi Arabia	11%	63%	8%	10%	5%	3%
Median	2%	8%	8%	44%	12%	4%

Figure 5.6.1   The differing beliefs on appropriate dress for Islamic women. *(Courtesy of Daily Mail / Solo Syndication.)*

is not present, or will not consent. Ethnic minorities are also commonly disadvantaged because of cultural and linguistic differences. However, many faith-based organisations provide access to health care for all, regardless of religious beliefs.

Individual preferences may determine management options. For example, a Jehovah Witness may refuse lifesaving blood transfusions. Furthermore, some individuals may wish to incorporate traditional medicines, faith healing or alternative medicines into their management plan. It is necessary to enquire about an individual's use of such practices, and to ensure that the patient's wishes are respected.

Communicating and working with colleagues and patients from different backgrounds

'No culture can live if it attempts to be exclusive.'

Mahatma Gandhi

Cultural competence refers to behaviours, attitudes and policies that enable health professionals to work effectively within the context of the cultural needs of the individual. Several models have been created to help people develop cultural competence. An example is Campinha-Bacote's model, which breaks down cultural competence into an ongoing process of cultural awareness, cultural knowledge, cultural skill, cultural encounters and cultural desire (**Fig. 5.6.2**). A limitation of this model is the lack of reference to intracultural differences in beliefs as highlighted by Kleinman and Bensen.

Cultural competency can aid in health outcomes, by attempting to understand and adapt to cultural differences in health beliefs. This is a necessary skill for health professionals wherever they work. An understanding of the impact of cultural and religious factors on patients' experiences and health care needs is critical, particularly for patients facing serious or terminal diagnoses. Beliefs in key issues which define a patient's experience of their illness, such as the soul after

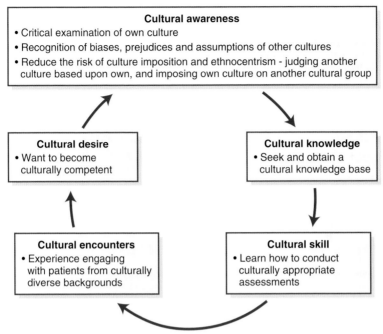

Figure 5.6.2 **Model of cultural competency.** *(Redrawn from Campinha-Bacote J: The process of cultural competence in the delivery of healthcare services: a model of care, J Transcult Nurs 13(3):181–184, 2002.)*

death or a belief in miracles, differ substantially by gender, education and ethnicity. Both patients and family caregivers frequently rely on spirituality and religion to help them deal with serious illness.

Avoiding discrimination and achieving equity

Discrimination is the unjust treatment of a group of people, for example those of a particular culture, ethnicity or religious group. Awareness of the existence and effects of such discrimination is important so as to act to prevent or limit this behaviour. The following examples illustrate some of the challenges encountered in achieving equity in health care:

- *Psychiatry.* In psychiatry, the perspective of the health care professional is not entirely objective. As health and illness are subjective entities, evaluation of these requires moral judgement. However, 'cultural relativism' suggests that morality differs between societies and that no single concept of morality is universally valid. Consequently, Western biomedical definitions of health and illness may be invalid from a cross-cultural perspective. An example is the overdiagnosis of schizophrenia, and underdiagnosis of mood disorders in African Americans. Cultural specificity is further demonstrated by the presence of culturally bound syndromes. These are psychiatric syndromes that are recognisable only within a specific culture. For example, taijin-kyofusho is a Japanese culturally bound phobia based on social fear and anxiety. Individuals avoid social interaction as they have a fear of offending others. In contrast, Western individuals are more egocentric, and prioritise their personal concerns above those of others.
- *Life and death.* Individual views on life and death are strongly influenced by cultural attitudes and religious beliefs. Difficult ethical issues such as brain death, euthanasia,

abortion and stem cell research are highly emotive and trigger strong views. Western views are commonly more individualistic than those from other cultures.

■ *Sexual behaviour and norms.* Sexual behaviour and norms differ across the world. For example, abstinence from premarital sexual relationships is required by some religions and cultures. The cultural practice of female genital mutilation has been condemned by the United Nations but continues to be widely practised.

Female genital mutilation

Female genital mutilation (FGM) is 'partial or total removal of the female external genital organs for nonmedical reasons'. It is an ancient cultural practice that is still prevalent in many African countries. The practice of FGM illustrates a tension between cultural relativism and rights, and the upholding of human rights.

The use of the term *female genital mutilation* (instead of *female circumcision*) has been criticised by some individuals from cultures in which FGM is practised, as it casts a moral judgement; it lacks cultural relativity. Conversely, human rights activists argue that morality is *universal*. The practice of FGM is associated with many complications, including death, and is often undertaken without adequate consent. Human rights activists argue that FGM violates human rights, and so should be discouraged or prohibited.

Is it possible to discern individual choices from those based on social and cultural obligations established over a life course? Such questions highlight the complexity of issues involving culture, ethnicity, religion and morality.

Fiona Headley (UK)

Conclusion

Culture, ethnicity and religion impact on an individual's perception of health and illness. They influence health-seeking behaviour, the ability to access appropriate health care services, and the management of illness. Examples of the impact of culture, ethnicity and religion on health are evident when addressing life and death issues, sexual health and psychiatric illness. Health professionals should aim to develop cultural awareness and accommodate individual beliefs and wishes.

KEY POINTS

- Health is a concept which is socially, culturally and religiously determined.
- Culture, religion and ethnicity have a significant impact on determinants of health, health beliefs, health-seeking behaviour and the doctor–patient relationship.
- Service design should consider the cultural, religious and ethnic backgrounds of patients and colleagues.
- Health care professionals and providers should aim to be culturally competent.

Further reading

Fadiman A: *The spirit catches you and you fall down: a Hmong child, her American doctors, and the collision of two cultures*, New York, 1997, Farrar, Straus and Giroux.

Helman CG: *Culture, health and illness*, ed 5, London, 2007, Hodder Arnold Publication.

Kleinman AA, Benson P: Anthropology in the clinic, the problem with cultural competency and how to fix it, *PLoS Med* 3(10):e294, 2006.

Pool R, Geisser W: *Medical anthropology*, Oxford, 2005, Oxford University Press.

Scambler G: Ethnicity and health. In Scambler G, editor: *Sociology as applied to medicine*, ed 6, Oxford, 2008, Elsevier.

Specific Global Health Challenges

Junior Editors: Laura Bertani (USA)　　Elizabeth Wiley (USA)

Introduction

The highest burden of health challenges is faced by low-income countries (LIC) and middle-income countries. People with a lower socioeconomic status are particularly affected. The importance of a multifactorial approach in addressing global health challenges is illustrated by the following case study.

A family's global health challenges

This report describes the problems experienced by three generations of a family in the slums of Asunción, Paraguay. Multiple coexistent medical problems are compounded by the lack of access to resources and finance.

Rogelio, the father of two children, worked as a mechanic. Four months ago he lost his right leg in a traffic accident. He cannot afford a prosthesis or therapy, and uses crutches to get around. The town's roads and public transport are not suitable for wheelchairs. He is unable to provide for his family as he cannot work. His frustration led him to take an overdose of painkillers. He has been referred to a psychiatrist, and is still on the waiting list to be seen.

Rogelio's mother, Lorena, had a stroke 2 years ago. She had a long history of high blood pressure and high cholesterol level but was unable to take appropriate medication because of its expense. She is now unable to help with childcare.

Lorena's husband, Juan, has contracted dengue fever and has been in hospital for weeks. The family can barely afford his hospitalisation, and frequently have to make trips to the pharmacy to bring supplies and medications. Rogelio's wife, Juana, is 8 months pregnant She works selling sweets and fizzy drinks in the street, and brings her two young children to assist. As a result, the children cannot attend school. Her first child died of malaria aged 3 years.

Whilst one may conceive of various ways to help this family, the lack of access to services pushes them further into a cycle of poverty and dependence, causing a 'double burden' on individuals, families and communities.

Elizabeth Wiley and Laura Bertani (USA)

6.1 Communicable Diseases

Daniel Tobón-García (Colombia)

Introduction

Communicable diseases can be defined as diseases transmitted from an animal to another animal, from animal to human, from human to human or from human to animal. They may be caused by viruses, bacteria, parasites or fungi. These diseases particularly affect high-risk populations such as children, pregnant women, the elderly and the immunocompromised.

Communicable diseases are an enormous threat to human health, and disproportionately affect the world's poorest and most vulnerable populations. The growing challenge of antimicrobial resistance makes their spread more difficult to control. For the terminology used in evaluation of communicable diseases, see **Table 6.1.1**.

Diseases can be transmitted and spread in a variety of ways:

- food-borne (e.g., salmonella, *Escherichia coli* infection)
- waterborne (e.g., cholera, rotavirus infection)
- sexual transmission or blood-borne (e.g., hepatitis B, hepatitis C, HIV infection)
- vectors (e.g., malaria, Chagas disease, dengue, Zika virus disease)
- airborne (tuberculosis, meningitis, influenza)
- traumatic contact (dog bites; e.g., rabies)
- direct contact (e.g., Ebola virus disease)

Communicable diseases affect the health status of populations, and also have significant economic consequences as they cause disability and reduce productivity. Additionally, health care costs can impoverish families. They disproportionately affect the poorest countries, and the global distribution of specific diseases is highly varied (**Fig. 6.1.1**).

Since 2000, with the implementation of the Millennium Development Goals (MDGs), international organisations have especially targeted the control of malaria, HIV/AIDS and tuberculosis (TB) but other globally important infectious diseases include hepatitis, influenza and diarrhoeal diseases. Other less prevalent infectious diseases are grouped together under the title of the *neglected tropical diseases* (NTDs).

Much of the burden of communicable disease can be controlled with existing interventions such as sanitation, clean water and vaccines. With access to essential medicines, these measures are effective and affordable. **Table 6.1.2** illustrates the way in which communicable diseases impact on individual MDGs.

Malaria

Malaria is a potentially life-threatening vector-borne disease caused by infection transmitted by the female *Anopheles* mosquito. In 2013 97 countries reported cases of malaria. Malaria commonly occurs in the tropics, although it can also occur in nonendemic areas. For 2015 the World Health Organization (WHO) estimated that 214 million new cases of malaria and 438,000 malaria-related

TABLE 6.1.1 ■ Communicable disease terminology

Prevalence	Proportion of a population found to have a disease or a risk factor
Incidence	Number of new disease cases in a given time divided by the number of people who were at risk
Morbidity	Proportion of sickness in a specific territory
Mortality	Number of deaths in a population per unit of time
Vector	Organism that transmits an infectious agent from a reservoir to a host
Case	Individual with a particular disease
Case fatality rate	Proportion of persons with a particular disease (case) who die of that condition
Elimination of a disease	Reach zero incidence of a disease
Eradication of a disease	Complete elimination of the disease and its causative agent
Reemerging infectious disease	An existing disease that has increased in incidence or has taken new forms
Antibiotic/antimicrobial	Product that kills or inhibits the growth of a microorganism
Antimicrobial resistance	Ability of some microorganisms to survive antimicrobial agents
Epidemic	Occurrence of disease cases that exceeds what is expected in a given region

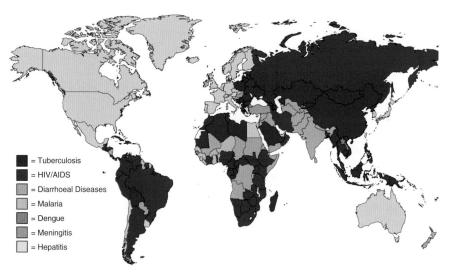

= Tuberculosis
= HIV/AIDS
= Diarrhoeal Diseases
= Malaria
= Dengue
= Meningitis
= Hepatitis

Figure 6.1.1 The deadliest infections around the world. *(Redrawn from Kholsa S: The planet's deadliest infectious diseases, by country, 2014. <http://www.salon.com/2014/11/01/the_planets_deadliest_infectious_diseases_by_country_partner/>)*

deaths occurred worldwide. Further, 306,000 children younger than 5 years died. This equates to almost one child dying every minute. Approximately 90% of malaria-related deaths occurred in sub-Saharan Africa. Infection can be prevented with basic measures such as insecticide-treated mosquito nets, indoor residual spraying and antimalarial drugs. Forty percent of malaria-related deaths occur in two countries: Nigeria and the Democratic Republic of the Congo.

TABLE 6.1.2 ■ **Correlation between the Millennium Development Goals and communicable diseases**

Goal 1: Eradicate extreme hunger and poverty. Both hunger and poverty contribute to the burden and perpetuation of communicable disease. Communicable diseases can have a negative impact on the poverty cycle, reducing ability to work and reducing income. Poverty also severely limits individuals' ability to cover health care expenses

Goal 2: Achieve universal primary education. The education of children can be adversely affected when mothers fail to address the need for basic hygiene

Goal 3: Promote gender equality and empower women. Improved maternal education should lead to better hygiene practice within families and reduced transmission of communicable diseases

Goal 4: Reduce child mortality. Communicable diseases such as respiratory infections, diarrhoeal diseases and malaria contribute significantly to child mortality

Goal 5: Improve maternal health. HIV infection and malaria are particularly relevant to maternal outcomes

Goal 6: Combat HIV/AIDS, malaria and other diseases. This goal directly focuses on communicable diseases

Goal 7: Ensure environmental sustainability. Open defaecation, slum dwelling and poor access to safe drinking water all significantly increase the risk of communicable disease transmission

Goal 8: Develop a global partnership for development. To appropriately address the threats posed by communicable diseases, public–private partnerships and multilateral collaborative work is needed. Examples include the Global Fund to fight AIDS, Tuberculosis and Malaria, Roll Back Malaria and Gavi, the Vaccine Alliance

From United Nations Millennium Development Goals. http://un.org/millenniumgoals/goal © United Nations. Reprinted with the permission of the United Nations.

Following the development of funding programmes for malaria control, major reductions in mortality and morbidity have been achieved. These programmes have also significantly contributed to a reduction in childhood mortality (MDG 4).

HIV/AIDS

'We live in a completely interdependent world, which simply means we cannot escape each other. How we respond to AIDS depends, in part, on whether we understand this interdependence. It is not someone else's problem. This is everybody's problem.'

Bill Clinton

(From Vultaggio M: *National Youth HIV, AIDS Awareness Day quotes: 10 inspirational sayings*, 2015. Available from <http://www.ibtimes.com/national-youth-hiv-aids-awareness-day-quotes-10-inspirational-sayings-1876760>.)

HIV, a blood-borne retrovirus, is transmitted via sexual contact, blood transfusions and intravenous drug use; mother-to-child transmission has also been reported. HIV causes AIDS, a progressive failure of the immune system leading to increased susceptibility to opportunistic infections, some cancers and, if inadequately treated, death.

Since the discovery of HIV in the early 1980s, more than 39 million lives have been lost because of HIV. In 2017 HIV/AIDS remains a significant global public health challenge. In 2015 an estimated 1.1 million people died of AIDS-related causes worldwide. Approximately 36.7 million people had HIV (2.1 million newly infected) at the end of 2015. Antiretroviral (ARV) drugs have significantly improved the prognosis for individuals with HIV. They reduce viral load, increase immune cell count, delay symptom onset, reduce contagion risk and increase life expectancy.

Circumcision and HIV prevention

Male circumcision provides a substantial degree of protection against HIV/AIDS.

Three randomised controlled trials found that circumcision reduced the risk of males acquiring HIV by 48%–60%. As a result, African countries are increasingly implementing circumcision into their health programmes. However, ethical, social and cultural concerns affect the practicality of instituting this practice in communities with a high risk of HIV infection.

Gabriel Tse (Canada)

The spread of HIV has been reduced through use of ARVs and other prophylactic measures but progress has not been evenly distributed. Almost one-third of all new infections occur among young people (15–24 years). Access to ARVs remains a challenge for some groups, and in 2015 only 46% of people with HIV were receiving treatment. Coverage amongst children was significantly lower than in adults.

Youth action against HIV/AIDS

Two different youth movements tackling the HIV/AIDS epidemic are described.

Pact is a coalition of youth organisations working together to coordinate the response to HIV to ensure the health, well-being and human rights of all young people. They promote the availability of HIV treatment in sexual and reproductive health services and policies, increase access to evidence-informed prevention and treatment. They advocate for the removal of laws that prevent young people from accessing services and for the allocation of resources on the basis of need and evidence, thus ensuring that HIV remains a priority in the post-2015 development agenda.

Africaid Zvandiri is another youth-led HIV/AIDS initiative, based in Zimbabwe. It started in 2004 as a group of children with HIV who decided to create a support group. It has since grown into a 'community-based program which provides prevention, treatment, care and support services for children and adolescents with HIV, integrated within the clinical care provided by government and private clinics.' HIV-positive young people are empowered in designing, implementing and monitoring all the projects and programmes of the organisation.

Daniel Tobón-García (Colombia)

HIV/AIDS in the history of global health

HIV/AIDS has played a unique role in the history of global health. This case study describes the development of an activist movement in support of treatment for patients with HIV/AIDS.

In the 1980s across the United States, many of those who had been infected with HIV mobilised to demand investment in treatment for themselves and their loved ones. As the disease had emerged in the 'gay' community in San Francisco and many did not believe it was a worthy recipient of medical resources, the gay community mobilised to demand treatment for people with HIV/AIDS.

In the 1990s antiretrovirals started to become available in developed countries at a cost of US$15,000 per year. The HIV/AIDS epidemic was devastating entire countries in Africa and pushing them close to social and economic collapse. The pharmaceutical industry was unwilling to reduce its prices despite an increasing death toll. A coalition of patients, faith leaders, politicians, activists and others worked together to highlight this gross injustice. Generic drugs were manufactured cheaply, and treatment was administered in these lower middle-income countries. HIV infection highlighted social and economic inequalities and sparked a global movement to tackle AIDS. By 2013 the average price for a first-line antiretroviral was just US$115 per year. This movement has been a model for further health campaign groups.

Mike Kalmus Eliasz (UK)

Tuberculosis

TB is caused by *Mycobacterium tuberculosis,* and is both preventable and curable. It is the second leading cause of death worldwide from a single infectious agent (after HIV). About one-third of the world's population has latent TB; only 10% of these will develop active TB. Immunocompromised patients, for example those with AIDS, have a greater chance of developing active TB.

The global distribution of TB is unequal, with most new TB cases occurring in Asia. In 2015 there were an estimated 10.4 million new cases worldwide, of which 11% occurred in patients with AIDS. There were approximately 1.4 million TB deaths and an additional 0.4 million deaths from TB amongst people with HIV. There has also been an epidemic of new cases of multidrug-resistant TB, with 480,000 new cases in 2015.

The rising incidence of drug resistance to anti-TB drugs restricts the availability of effective treatments, especially in lower middle-income countries (LMIC) and LIC. India, China and the Russian Federation accounted for 45% of the multidrug-resistant TB plus rifampicin-resistant TB cases. There remains an urgent need to:

- increase detection and treatment of individuals with TB
- address multidrug-resistant TB as a public health crisis
- enhance response to HIV/TB coinfection
- increase financing for TB initiatives
- ensure affordability and rapid adoption of TB innovations

The WHO's End TB Strategy (2017) is an ethical initiative, aligned with the framework of the Sustainable Development Goals (SDGs).

Hepatitis

Hepatitis is caused by a number of viruses, and hepatitis B and hepatitis C can lead to chronic liver disease. As a result, about 1.3 million people die and 390 million develop chronic infections per year. Many of these are caused by vertical (mother–child) transmission. Limited access to timely and effective diagnosis and treatment for viral hepatitis on account of health system weakness and costs poses a significant obstacle to the implementation of effective treatments.

Influenza

Influenza is a viral infection affecting the respiratory system. It can cause severe pneumonia, and even death, in the elderly, the very young or those with serious medical comorbidities. It is of special public health importance as populations may not possess effective resistance to infection because of the ability of the virus to mutate into new strains. A pandemic can arise when a type or subtype of an influenza virus emerges that is significantly different from previously circulating strains. A notable pandemic was the Spanish flu in 1918, which caused between 20 million and 50 million deaths worldwide.

Diarrhoeal diseases

'It is still just unbelievable to us that diarrhoea is one of the leading causes of child deaths in the world.'

Melinda Gates

(From <http://www.azquotes.com/quote/598583?ref=diarrhea>.)

Diarrhoea can be defined as the passage of three or more loose stools per day. In LMIC and LIC, it is generally caused by bacterial, viral or parasitic infection. Risk factors include contaminated food or drinking water and poor interpersonal hygiene. Simple public health measures such as health education regarding infection control, exclusive breastfeeding until the age of 6 months, and vaccination against rotavirus are effective preventative measures. Nearly 1.7 billion cases of diarrhoeal illness occur per year. Dehydration is the most dangerous consequence as significant amounts of water and electrolytes are lost during a diarrhoeal episode. This results in significant mortality, as well as long-term malnutrition, particularly in young children.

Management and control of communicable diseases

Increased urbanisation, population growth and indiscriminate use of natural resources, along with climate change, have contributed to an increase in the number and severity of natural disasters (e.g., floods, hurricanes and cyclones). This has major implications for the way diseases emerge, re-emerge and spread. Changing weather and settlement patterns affect the transmission and viability of certain infectious agents and vectors, which, in turn, shape the patterns of infectious disease spread. For example, a study in Venezuela over an 8-year period showed a 14% decrease in dengue fever cases during the El Niño season, in contrast to a 9% increase in cases during the La Niña season.

The spread of communicable diseases has been facilitated by mass tourism, and poses a global risk. For example, the severe acute respiratory syndrome (SARS) pandemic was first recorded in China in 2002, and its rapid spread was accelerated by air travel. There were 8000 cases and 774 deaths before control of SARS was ultimately achieved.

Since 2007 international health regulations have been a binding instrument of international law. They are based on an agreement among 194 of the WHO's member states to 'prevent, protect against, control and provide a public health response to the international spread of disease in ways that are commensurate with and restricted to public health risks, and which avoid unnecessary interference with international traffic and trade.'

Communicable diseases demand a complex response from nations and global health agencies. The WHO, as the leading agency in global health, has always played a leading technical and political role in prevention, management and control. The Millennium Declaration, with the inclusion of several health-related MDGs, led to increased funding for communicable diseases, specifically for HIV/AIDS, TB and malaria (SDG 3). Communicable diseases have historically attracted a great deal of vertical funding (i.e., funding earmarked for control of a specific disease or a specific intervention) from organisations such as the Bill & Melinda Gates Foundation and the Global Fund to Fight AIDS, Tuberculosis and Malaria. More recently, global health funding has focused on horizontal interventions which strengthen health systems as a whole. Nevertheless, there remains a strong argument for ongoing vertical interventions, alongside work to invest in health systems.

Medical students tackling antimicrobial resistance

The growing threat of antimicrobial resistance (AMR) poses a greater challenge than any other current public health issue. The consequences of AMR lead to increases in health care costs, which impact across business, politics and trade. They cause a reduction in gross domestic product and set back years of advancement in modern medicine.

With these threats in mind, medical students from Jamaica, Mexico, Canada, Chile, Brazil and Peru drafted a policy statement entitled 'Antibiotic Abuse'. This was submitted to become official policy of the International Federation of Medical Students' Associations. The policy statement highlighted the current state of antibiotic resistance. It emphasised the negative effects of AMR and suggested ways to mitigate its consequences. It also urged chief policymakers such as the World Health Organization, local government officials and medical schools to implement measures to offset the effects of AMR. This policy statement was the first of its kind, and represented the start of a student advocacy campaign.

Kevouy Reid (Jamaica)

Vaccines are economically and clinically effective in fighting communicable diseases, and have contributed to a decrease in the occurrence of infectious diseases. Smallpox was declared eradicated by the WHO in 1980, and the occurrence of polio and measles infections has been dramatically reduced.

Conclusion

Communicable diseases pose an ongoing global health challenge. Health system strengthening and vertical funding initiatives, together with enhanced international cooperation and political commitment, are essential in combating this challenge.

KEY POINTS

- Communicable diseases spread from one person to another or from an animal to a person.
- Communicable diseases can spread by contact, insect bites or air.
- HIV/AIDS, tuberculosis and malaria have attracted major funding, but diarrhoeal diseases are still a major source of morbidity and death.
- Antimicrobial resistance (AMR) is a major threat to good health.

Further reading

Joint United Nations Programme on HIV/AIDS: *Global AIDS response progress reporting 2015*, Geneva, 2015, World Health Organization. Available from: <http://www.unaids.org/sites/default/files/media_asset/JC2702_GARPR2015guidelines_en.pdf>.

World Health Organization: *Global tuberculosis report 2016*, 2017 <http://www.who.int/tb/publications/global_report/en/>.

World Health Organization: *World malaria report 2014*, 2017. <http://www.who.int/malaria/publications/world_malaria_report_2014/en/>.

World Health Organization: *Ethics guidance for the implementation of the End TB Strategy*, Geneva, 2017, World Health Organization.

6.2 Neglected Tropical Diseases

Anand Bhopal (UK)　　Sadie Regmi (UK)

> *'A civilization is judged by the treatment of its minorities.'*
> **Mahatma Gandhi**
> (From Stern EJ: Forgotten people, forgotten diseases: the neglected tropical diseases and their impact on global health and development. 2d ed, *Clin Infect Dis* 57:15:1793–1794, 2013. Available from <http://cid.oxfordjournals.org/content/early/2013/10/23/cid.cit631.full>.)

Introduction

One in seven people worldwide have an NTD. This term is used to describe a very varied group of diseases which primarily occur in those populations living in poverty, not simply in the tropics (**Fig. 6.2.1**). They cannot be defined by geography or pathophysiology. The WHO lists 17 diseases (**Table 6.2.1**) which it describes as 'a group of communicable diseases which thrive in impoverished settings and blight the lives of around one billion people worldwide, while threatening the health of millions more' (WHO, 2010).

NTDs highlight the inadequacies of health systems in LIC, and are at the heart of inequities in global health. On account of their high morbidity and relatively low mortality, they disable individuals, exacerbate poverty and impede community, national and international development (see **Table 6.2.1**). NTDs can usually be managed with current techniques and therapies. A rapid impact interventional package (Hotez et al., 2006) showed that the seven major NTDs in Africa could be treated with only four drugs costing about $0.40 per person.

NTDs have witnessed a surge in political, economic and scientific interest as they cause a burden of disease on a par with that associated with TB, malaria and HIV/AIDS.

Fever in a returning traveller

The following case of fever in a returning traveller is relevant to the clinical practice of health care professionals anywhere in the world.

A 13-year-old boy arrived in the emergency department with a 3-day history of malaise, severe muscle soreness, fever, chills and retro-ocular pain. Physical examination showed a petechial rash in the lower extremities, tachycardia, bilateral basal crackles and low blood pressure (90/70 mm Hg). Four days previously, he had returned from a 2-week-long trip to the Dominican Republic. Blood test findings were unremarkable, but a chest X-ray showed bilateral pleural effusions. He received a diagnosis of dengue fever.

A recent trip to the Caribbean region with a clinical presentation similar to the one described earlier is highly suggestive of a tropical infectious disease. Dengue is endemic in more than 100 countries, with estimates of 50 million cases of the disease occurring each year. The Dominican Republic has one of the highest numbers of cases in the Caribbean. There is no prophylaxis for dengue, and supportive measures were therefore implemented in this case, with full subsequent recovery.

Maria Espanol and Manuel Hache-Marliere (Dominican Republic)

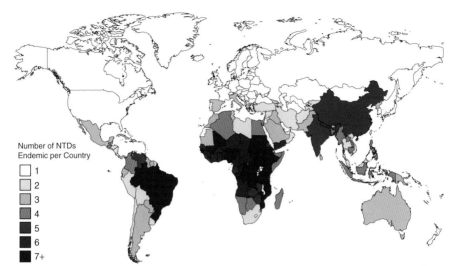

Figure 6.2.1 Global burden of neglected tropical diseases *(NTDs)* **map.** *(Redrawn from Uniting to Combat Neglected Tropical Diseases: <http://unitingtocombatntds.org/resources/burden-map-neglected-tropical-diseases/>, 2009–2010 data.)*

TABLE 6.2.1 ▪ The 17 neglected tropical diseases

Viruses	Kinetoplastids (protozoa)	Helminths	Bacteria
Dengue/severe dengue	Chagas disease	Cysticercosis/taeniasis	Buruli ulcer
Rabies	Human African trypanosomiasis (sleeping sickness)	Dracunculiasis (guinea worm disease)	Leprosy
		Echinococcosis	Trachoma
	Leishmaniasis	Food-borne trematodiasis	Yaws
		Lymphatic filariasis	
		Onchocerciasis (river blindness)	
		Schistosomiasis	
		Soil-transmitted helminthiases	

Modified from World Health Organization: Working to overcome the global impact of neglected tropical diseases: first WHO report on neglected tropical diseases, Geneva 2010, World Health Organization.

History of neglected tropical diseases

Since the inception of the WHO, individual diseases within the NTD grouping have had control strategies coordinated centrally by the organisation. During the 1950s, WHO General Assembly resolutions targeted leprosy, rabies, trachoma and helminthiases. In the following decades, onchocerciasis, dracunculiasis, human African trypanosomiasis, dengue and other human and zoonotic diseases were similarly targeted. In 1999 Médecins Sans Frontières launched an NTD programme, and the Bill & Melinda Gates Foundation provided significant funding a year later.

The term *neglected tropical disease* was formally adopted in 2005, and a clear vision and framework for tackling the diseases was established. Subsequently, the Global Network for Neglected Tropical Diseases was launched (2007), and a WHO NTD department was set up in 2008. Disease control efforts relied largely on individual drug donation programmes. Individual disease advocacy groups had a major influence on funding policy although this was not always aligned with the needs of patients.

TABLE 6.2.2 ■ **Summary of diseases targeted in the London Declaration**

Control	Eradication/elimination
Schistosomiasis	Lymphatic filariasis
Soil-transmitted helminthiases	Guinea worm disease
Visceral leishmaniasis	Blinding trachoma
Onchocerciasis	Human African trypanosomiasis
Chagas disease	Leprosy

The *WHO's Accelerating Work to Overcome the Global Impact of Neglected Tropical Diseases: A Roadmap for Implementation* (2012) inspired the collaboration of all major stakeholders in NTD control through the London Declaration on Neglected Tropical Diseases. This show of collective will, encompassing international organisations, nongovernmental organisations (NGOs), drug companies and research outfits, has made significant progress in NTD eradication. The WHO 2020 road map, strengthened by the commitment of the signatories of the London Declaration of 2012 (**Table 6.2.2**), guarantees that the 10 'core' NTDs will receive attention for the rest of the decade.

Research and development regarding neglected tropical diseases

Although cheap treatment is available for many NTDs, others, including Chagas disease, leishmaniasis and human African trypanosomiasis, still require innovative solutions. Available drugs have significant side effects which limit adherence to treatment. The problems of drug resistance coupled with inadequacies in local health systems as well as the lack of effective vaccines means that health care for patients with these NTDs remains inadequate. Research and development investments are often more aligned with purchasing power than with health needs. Between 1975 and 2009, only 15 of more than 1400 new chemical entities were specifically developed for NTDs. Conventional, profit-driven, drug development has failed diseases of poverty because those affected lack the ability to pay enough to stimulate pharmaceutical investment.

Although the so-called 10/90 gap, whereby only 10% of investment is spent on 90% of the world's disease burden, is thought by some to be changing, research and development (R & D) investments are still far from aligned with public health priorities. The WHO Consultative Expert Working Group on Research and Development: Financing and Coordination found that the global investment in R & D for neglected diseases continues to be much smaller than that required by the global burden of these diseases. Investment is minimal in the public sector. An analysis by the student global health organisation Universities Allied for Essential Medicines found that most of the 50 leading North American research universities devote less than 2% of their research budgets to neglected diseases.

Long-term control of neglected tropical diseases: the post-elimination strategy

The WHO (2012) acknowledges that 'at some point, external support and resources for NTDs will end.' Although efforts have been made to harmonise advocacy and to overcome technical challenges amongst disease initiatives, little emphasis has been placed on sustainability and national governance. Like many health problems, NTDs rely on a strong health care system for long-term control. In this regard, the historical examples of yaws and leprosy are educational.

Medical students in the fight against dengue fever in Brazil

Medical students used evaluation and information to demonstrate the impact of their programme to tackle vector-borne disease in Brazil.

In the 21st century Brazil became the country with the most reported cases of dengue fever. Brazilian medical students decided to tackle this issue.

They began to teach children aged 7 to 12 years about strategies to reduce vector reproduction in the home environment, recognising that the children would then educate other members of their families. They then conducted house-to-house visits in particularly high-risk areas to deliver further education on simple preventative measures.

They also compared the rate of dengue fever in the target population areas before and after their interventions. This project, which started at a local level, ultimately became a national initiative, 'Project Dengue Zero'. It demonstrated how students can act to change their communities and countries through the dissemination of appropriate information.

Arthur Mello and Ana Beatriz Lobato (Brazil)

Between 1956 and 1964 the United Nations Children's Fund (UNICEF), in conjunction with the WHO, undertook to control yaws. Their efforts achieved a 95% reduction in cases, at which point programmes were transferred to local primary health care. There were no attempts to strengthen already overstretched health systems. Cases of yaws increased rapidly, and 44 years later, the WHO had to launch a new elimination attempt.

> *'Village people started discriminating against me because of my ulcers. My friends withdrew from me and didn't want to be associated with me. I even had to stop going to school.*
> *People stopped coming to our house. They stopped speaking to me and my parents. They didn't involve any of us socially, and they avoided us. It was very upsetting for my parents as well. Community people stopped respecting them....*
> *After that, my parents stopped supporting me, and that was the worst point for me.'*
> **Sarita (leprosy patient)**

(From American Leprosy Missions: A blessing for Sarita. http://www.leprosy.org/patient-stories/sarita/.)

In the case of leprosy, control through drug treatment alone is not enough; education and rehabilitation must continue even when drug treatment is no longer needed. A World Health Assembly resolution was adopted in 1991 to eliminate leprosy by the year 2000—in this case, the target for elimination was reduction of burden to less than 1 in 10,000 in the population. On the accomplishment of these targets, the WHO declared global elimination had been achieved. However, because of the long incubation period of the disease and subsequent difficulties generating financial and political support for leprosy patients, the disease subsequently resurfaced.

These problems arose as a result of WHO's mislabelling of *elimination*. Some diseases were declared 'eliminated' when, in fact, they had merely been intensively controlled. 'Post-elimination' strategies were therefore not instituted effectively. As illustrated, leprosy and yaws are examples of diseases which have re-emerged with a vengeance in communities almost rid of these diseases. Whilst *elimination* certainly sounds more attractive than *intensified control*, misleading terminology has complicated and sometimes discouraged progress towards true elimination.

Conclusion

NTDs are a major global health burden. They can be treated with widely available cost-effective interventions. Long-term follow-up of patients is necessary for certain disease groups if re-emergence of disease is to be avoided. Ongoing pharmaceutical investment and research should address the needs of those with diseases of poverty.

- Neglected tropical diseases (NTDs) are diseases of poverty with high morbidity and low mortality.
- The disease burden of NTDs rivals that of tuberculosis, malaria and HIV/AIDS.
- Efforts have been made recently by all major stakeholders to tackle NTDs.
- Greater investment in NTD research and development is needed.
- Incentives for research must be aligned with public health priorities to address NTDs.
- Strong health care systems are critical to long-term control of NTDs.

Further reading

Hotez PJ, Molyneux DH, Fenwick A, et al: Incorporating a rapid–impact package for neglected tropical diseases with programs for HIV/AIDS, tuberculosis, and malaria, *PLoS Med* 3:e102, 2006.

Hotez PJ, Pecoul P: "Manifesto" for advancing the control and elimination of neglected tropical diseases, *PLoS Negl Trop Dis* 4(5):e718, 2010.

Uniting to Combat Neglected Tropical Diseases: *London Declaration on Neglected Tropical Diseases*. <https://www.gov.uk/government/uploads/system/uploads/attachment_data/file/67443/NTD_20Event_20-_20London_20Declaration_20on_20NTDs.pdf>.

World Health Organization: *Accelerating work to overcome the global impact of neglected tropical diseases: a roadmap for implementation*, Geneva, 2012, World Health Organization.

6.3 Noncommunicable Diseases

Shela Putri Sundawa (Indonesia)

Introduction

A noncommunicable disease (NCD) is a medical condition or disease that is noninfectious and nontransmissible amongst people. This definition is somewhat misleading as it fails to address the multifactorial nature of some of these illnesses. NCDs are often chronic in nature. The global NCD movement initially focused on four disease categories identified by the *Global Strategy for the Prevention and Control of Noncommunicable Diseases:* cardiovascular diseases, cancers, diabetes and chronic lung diseases. This focus has since broadened to include gastrointestinal, renal, and neurological and psychiatric disorders.

Epidemiology

'Four in five deaths from NCDs now occur in low- and middle-income countries. Without decisive action, the NCD burden threatens to undermine the benefits of improving standards of living, education and economic growth in many countries.'

Martin Silink, President, International Diabetes Federation
ECOSOC Annual Ministerial Review meeting on NCD, Doha (May 2009)
<https://ncdalliance.org/sites/default/files/resource_files/timetoact.pdf>

In 2012 38 million people died (68% of all global deaths) as a result of the sequelae of NCDs. Forty-two percent of those deaths were premature (i.e., before the age of 70 years). Despite the misperception that NCDs are more prevalent in the developed world, this burden, like most global health issues, disproportionately affects LIC and middle-income countries. In these countries, 74% of all deaths and 82% of premature deaths were attributable to NCDs (WHO, 2014).

In all WHO regions except Africa, NCD mortality has exceeded the mortality attributable to communicable, maternal, perinatal and nutritional conditions combined. The leading causes of NCD deaths in 2014 were cardiovascular diseases (17.5 million deaths), cancer (8.2 million deaths), respiratory diseases, including asthma and chronic obstructive pulmonary disease (4 million deaths), and diabetes (~1.5 million deaths) (WHO, 2014).

The WHO has identified six leading risk factors associated with NCDs: high blood pressure, tobacco use, high blood glucose levels, physical inactivity, obesity, and high cholesterol levels. Given that most of these risk factors are modifiable, many of the deaths and disabilities are preventable. Insufficient physical activity is a major contributor to deaths from NCDs as it contributes to obesity and its related comorbidities. Overall, physical inactivity causes 3.2 million deaths each year, and 69.3 million disability-adjusted life years (see Chapter 1.3).

Tobacco use is estimated to contribute to 6 million deaths each year, projected to increase to 8 million deaths by 2030. As the number of tobacco users worldwide is disproportionately increasing in the developing world, this increase in mortality is expected to predominantly affect LIC and middle-income countries. Antismoking measures such as plain cigarette packaging are strongly opposed by the tobacco industry.

Learning as a student about diabetes in Uganda

Christine Andreasen undertook an elective at a rural hospital in Busolwe, Uganda, in 2014 and experienced the difficulties of treating diabetes in a developing country setting.

'I decided to take my medical elective in a small community hospital in Busolwe in the summer of 2014 and experienced real poverty for the first time. We drove through rice fields and saw many people, including children and old women, working along the river. In the village, we could buy rice, soap, biscuits and locally grown vegetables, but not much else. Surprisingly, there was a small street shop every ten metres selling Coca-Cola. At the hospital, there were many patients with malaria, pneumonia and skin infections but I did not expect to see such large numbers of patients with diabetes and hypertension. The diseases that were the most challenging to treat were these 'Western lifestyle diseases'. According to the nurses, the numbers of diabetic patients had escalated in recent years and they were difficult to treat. Communication about the problems surrounding diabetes, including the need for lifelong treatment, was difficult in a foreign language. Similarly, it was difficult for patients to understand the dangers associated with input of sugary drinks.'

Christine Andreasen (Denmark)

Plain packaging in Australia

In 2011 Australia passed the Tobacco Plain Packaging Act and became the first country to require the removal of colour images and corporate logos from the packaging of all tobacco products. Cigarette packets now had to display the brand name in a mandated size and font alongside a health warning.

This new policy aimed to reduce the attractiveness of tobacco packaging as that was thought to encourage children or adolescents to smoke. As expected, the regulation outraged the tobacco industry. Philip Morris, a tobacco company, sought but failed to obtain compensation from the Australian government for the loss of trademarks. The American Legislative Exchange Council, a lobbying organisation, launched a worldwide campaign against plain packaging of cigarettes with the backing of tobacco companies and other corporate interests. It targeted governments that were planning to introduce bans on cigarette branding.

In 2014 a number of countries, led by the Ukraine, challenged Australia's anti-tobacco legislation through the World Trade Organization, stating that it violated World Trade Organization intellectual property agreement. This action was abandoned in May 2016, and many other countries have now implemented tobacco packaging laws similar to those in Australia.

Despite such fierce opposition from a very powerful and well-funded industry lobby, the success of Australia's bold move is clear. In the year from December 2013 to December 2014, tobacco consumption fell by 12.2%, and advocates claim that this was a direct result of the plain packaging legislation.

Shela Putri Sundawa (Indonesia)

Alcohol consumption contributes to approximately 3.3 million deaths annually. Heavy episodic drinking is most prevalent in the European and American WHO regions (WHO, 2014). In 2012 *hypertension* led to 9.4 million deaths and *diabetes mellitus* resulted in 1.5 million deaths. Although the current prevalence of diabetes is greater in upper middle-income countries, the global increase in the incidence of diabetes is accelerating more rapidly in LMIC.

Global impact of noncommunicable diseases

NCDs have pervasive and profound effects on the sustainable development agenda and SDGs. For example, the increasing prevalence of high blood pressure and gestational diabetes increases the risk of maternal morbidity. Exposure to second-hand tobacco smoke also increases the risks of childhood respiratory infections, sudden infant death and asthma. There is growing evidence that poor nutrition, particularly in childhood, contributes to NCD risk later in life.

'The possibility of influencing behaviour is very strong at the time when people tend to adopt these unhealthy behaviours. So we need to focus on the young because these diseases affect them and because the possibility of addressing the risk factors is a very great one at that age group.'

Sir George Alleyne, Director Emeritus, Pan American Health Organization

NCD risk factors have been steadily increasing in LIC and LMIC, and these increasingly contribute to the overall burden of disease in these countries. Risk factors are especially associated with poverty, and include the use of biomass fuels and coal for cooking and heating. Poor foetal and early childhood nutrition are also significant factors. Tobacco use, alcohol misuse, and consumption of foods high in saturated and *trans* fats, salt, sugar and sugar-sweetened beverages, as well as physical inactivity, have also increased. In contrast, many high-income countries have already made strides in curbing these risk factors.

Along with a higher burden of NCDs, patients in LMIC have difficulty in accessing timely diagnosis, care and treatment. Financial constraints, as well as political imperatives, have resulted in a lack of investment in cancer services in the public sector. Patients with cancer in high-income countries have up to twice the survival rate of those in middle-income countries.

The costs of treating NCDs, in terms of diminished or lost productivity and caregiver cost, can take a tremendous toll on families and communities, particularly those with already limited resources. On the basis of a World Bank qualitative survey of poor individuals in 60 countries, sickness and injury was the most frequent trigger for downward mobility. Like many global health issues, NCDs and poverty can propagate a cycle of impoverishment. Every year 100 million people fall below the poverty line because of out-of-pocket health costs.

Health system vulnerability can further exacerbate financial instability. The absence of universal health coverage and limited access to NCD medications on essential drug lists increases the burden of NCDs. Fewer LIC receive government funding to address NCDs (66% vs. 90% in middle- and high-income countries). In India, high out-of-pocket spending for health care has driven an estimated 1.4 million to 2 million Indians into poverty because of the cost of cardiovascular disease and cancer care. In one study of cardiovascular diseases in Bangladesh, Malawi, Nepal and Pakistan, only 7.5% of medicines were available in the public sector (WHO, 2011). LIC are also four times less likely to have NCD services covered by health insurance. Without this coverage, many families cannot afford adequate treatment, and the risks of poverty are increased.

The story of Suminah

Suminah ran a roadside food cart with her daughters in Indonesia. She was married when she was only 11-years-old, never went to school and gave birth to nine children. At the age of 61 years, she developed non-Hodgkin lymphoma. As she had no savings, her children paid her costs by dividing them amongst themselves, on the basis of their incomes, and drove her to the nearest city (4 hours away) for chemotherapy every week. She eventually gave up treatment as she was too weak to travel and undergo her chemotherapy. She died at the age of 63 years.

Suminah was my grandmother.

Shela Putri Sundawa (Indonesia)

Economically, NCDs are a threat to global well-being. A macroeconomic analysis showed that each 10% rise in the prevalence of NCDs is associated with a 0.5% decrease in annual economic growth. NCDs cost between 0.02% and 6.77% of gross domestic product (GDP) in LMIC, greater than the cost of malaria in the 1960s or AIDS in the 1990s.

Noncommunicable diseases in the post-2015 development agenda

In 2011 the United Nations held its first high-level meeting on NCDs. This was heralded as an opportunity to 'stimulate a coordinated global response to NCDs that is commensurate with their health and economic burdens'. More than 190 countries contributed to, and agreed on, a 'global action plan for the prevention and control of NCDs 2013-2020'. The plan challenged countries to target NCDs, including reductions in advertising for tobacco, expanded access to cervical cancer screening interventions and substitution of polyunsaturated fats for *trans* fats. The overarching goal of the action plan was to achieve '25 by 25', or a 25% reduction in NCD mortality, specifically cardiovascular diseases, cancer, diabetes or chronic respiratory diseases, by 2025 (WHO, 2013). Nine targets were included (**Fig. 6.3.1**).

These targets were adopted by the World Health Assembly in 2013 as part of the Global Action Plan for the Prevention and Control of Noncommunicable Diseases. The objectives are summarised in **Box 6.3.1**.

In 2011 Ban Ki-moon, the UN Secretary General, established a UN system task team to further the development of the post-2015 agenda. The team provided input on goals established in *The Future We Want*, the outcome document from the Rio+20 meeting in June 2012. They highlighted the importance of human rights, equality and sustainability in the new development goals, and noted that the MDGs failed to mention NCDs. A subsequent review in 2014 recognised that progress in NCD prevention remained highly uneven on account of a lack of essential resources. This review renewed the focus on cost-effective strategies to address NCDs and emphasised the importance of universal health coverage.

BOX 6.3.1 ■ The global action plan for the prevention and control of noncommunicable diseases

1. To raise the priority accorded to the prevention and control of noncommunicable diseases (NCDs) in global, regional and national agendas and internationally agreed development goals, through strengthened international cooperation and advocacy
2. To strengthen national capacity, leadership, governance, multisectoral action and partnerships to accelerate country response for the prevention and control of NCDs
3. To reduce modifiable risk factors for NCDs and underlying social determinants through creation of health-promoting environments
4. To strengthen and orient health systems to address the prevention and control of NCDs and the underlying social determinants through people-centred primary health care and universal health coverage
5. To promote and support national capacity for high-quality research and development for the prevention and control of NCDs
6. To monitor the trends and determinants of NCDs and evaluate progress in their prevention and control

A **25%** relative reduction in the overall mortality from cardiovascular diseases, cancer, diabetes, or chronic respiratory diseases

At least **10%** relative reduction in the harmful use of alcohol, as appropriate, within the national context

A **10%** relative reduction in prevalence of insufficient physical activity

A **30%** relative reduction in mean population intake of salt/sodium

A **30%** relative reduction in prevalence of current tobacco use

A **25%** relative reduction in the prevalence of raised blood pressure or contain the prevalence of raised blood pressure, according to national circumstances

Halt the rise in diabetes and obesity

At least **50%** of eligible people receive drug therapy and counseling (including glycaemic control) to prevent heart attacks and strokes

An **80%** availability of the affordable basic technologies and essential medicines, including generics, required to treat major noncommunicable diseases in both public and private facilities

Figure 6.3.1 **Global action plan for the prevention and control of noncommunicable diseases 2013–20.** *(Redrawn from World Health Organization: Global action plan for the prevention and control of noncommunicable diseases 2013-2020, Geneva, 2013 World Health Organization.)*

Conclusion

The global burden of NCD is immense. The poorest of the world's populations suffer from a double or even triple burden of diseases, when communicable diseases, NCDs and lifestyle diseases coexist. These require holistic interventions which deal with the underlying social determinants of health as well as the late sequelae of disease.

KEY POINTS

- Noncommunicable diseases (NCDs) generally have a long and slow progression.
- The four main types of NCD are cardiovascular disease, cancer, chronic respiratory disease and diabetes.
- NCDs are the leading cause of death worldwide, accounting for 63% of all deaths.
- Despite a historical burden of NCDs in high-income countries, the disease burden in low-income countries and lower middle-income countries is increasing.
- NCDs are largely preventable by modification of risk factors such as tobacco and alcohol consumption, sedentary lifestyle and poor diet.

Further reading

Daniels ME Jr, Donilon TE, Bollyky TJ, Tuttle CM: *The emerging global health crisis: non-communicable diseases in low- and middle-income countries*, New York, 2014, Council on Foreign Relations.

Hunter D, Reddy K: Noncommunicable diseases, *N Eng J Med* 369:1336–1343, 2013.

World Health Organization: *10 facts on noncommunicable diseases*, 2013. <http://www.who.int/features/factfiles/noncommunicable_diseases/en/>.

World Health Organization: *Global status report on noncommunicable diseases 2014*, Geneva, 2014, World Health Organization.

6.4 Ageing and Dying

Christian Kraef (Germany)

> '*Increasing longevity is one of humanity's greatest achievements. People live longer because of improved nutrition, sanitation, medical advances, health care, education and economic well-being.*'
>
> **Ageing in the 21st Century**

Introduction

The process of ageing is affected by numerous cultural, societal and psychological factors. National policies relating to pension provision and health care profoundly influence the experience of ageing and dying. Global demographic changes as well as cultural and political factors also impact on the individual's experience of ageing. There is a global need for a more holistic approach to the dying patient.

Demographic change

In most countries, the number of people older than 60 years is growing faster than that of any other age group. This presents a new array of societal challenges and opportunities. The global population has tripled in the past 65 years, and the world population has now exceeded 7.6 billion people. Between 2000 and 2050 the proportion of the population aged more than 65 years is predicted to double from 11% to 22%, with an associated change in the shape of the global population pyramid (**Fig. 6.4.1**). By 2050 80% of people aged more than 60 years are predicted to live in LIC and middle-income countries, and they will carry a higher burden of disease than their peers in wealthier countries.

Ageing of societies is occurring more rapidly than in the past. In France, doubling of the population older than 65 years took 114 years, whereas Brazil underwent this process in just 21 years. This phenomenon is called *compression of ageing* and is due to a combination of declining fertility and rising life expectancy. Improved global gender equity may have contributed to declining fertility in many parts of the world as women are increasingly able to determine their family priorities.

The consequences of the 'ageing society' affect many facets of life, and there is huge variation in the degree to which national governments have prepared themselves for this demographic shift.

Impacts of ageing populations

Ageing and dying are crosscutting policy issues involving every sector of society (e.g., housing, transportation, health, education, social security). The changing demographics of an ageing society put stress on social security systems. In 1950 there were 7.2 persons aged 20–64 years supporting one person older than 65 years in the Organisation for Economic Co-operation and Development (OECD) countries. This *support ratio* is currently about 4:1, and is predicted to fall to less

Dome truths and pillar talk
Global population, % of total

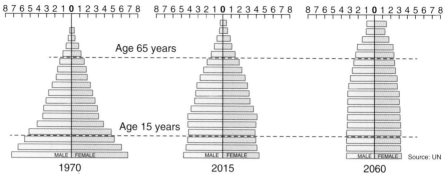

Figure 6.4.1   Changing population pyramids. Source = United Nations. *(Redrawn from <http://www. economist.com/news/21631911-end-population-pyramid-world-reshaped>, 13-Nov–14, Fig. 1.)*

than 2:1 in 2050. This poses a massive challenge to current retirement and pension systems. The so-called intergenerational contract in which young generations support older members of society has long been the frame for social policy in many wealthy countries. With the sharp fall in the support ratio, there are concerns that the current support arrangements for older people may be unsustainable.

Health systems are under increasing pressure because of increasing health comorbidities. Innovative models of patient care, aligned with the personal values and wishes of the patient, are required as new treatment options have become available. Debates about 'prioritisation and rationing' in health care, frequently directed at the problems of managing the ageing population, are current in many wealthier countries. Governments need to respond rapidly and effectively to projected demographic change so as to mitigate burgeoning pension and care costs and to utilise the skills and experience that many older people can offer (e.g., within the labour force or voluntary sector).

Pallium India is a community-based palliative care organisation providing an innovative care model which crosses disease boundaries

Pallium India is based in Kerala, the southernmost province of India. It has catalysed a network to offer locally funded care to approximately 15,000 patients with a wide range of chronic and life-limiting conditions. It provides most of its services through outpatient clinics held in public venues such as schools, and weekly home visits by multidisciplinary teams of clinical staff and local volunteers.

The organisation relies heavily on a network of more than 12,000 volunteers, and derives 90% of its funding from the local community. In the years since Pallium India's creation, the provision of home-based care in the state has increased from 2% to 70%.

Pallium India has a strong advocacy focus and has promoted palliative care education for undergraduate students. It campaigned for the amendment of the Indian Narcotics and Psychotropic Substances Act, which led to improved access to appropriate pain relief for the Indian population.

Pallium India is recognised as a leading model of palliative care provision in a resource-poor setting. Similar techniques are applicable in both developed and developing settings.

Felicity Knights and Daniel Knights (UK)
(Adapted from material originally presented at the Turning the World Upside Down event coordinated by Lord Nigel Crisp.)

Challenges for older people and those approaching the end of life

Older people should enjoy the same intrinsic rights as everyone else. However, age-based discrimination is prevalent worldwide. Discrimination includes the lack of representation of older individuals in scientific studies, restriction of resources for the elderly, elderly abuse and neglect.

The Commission on Dignity in Care for Older People report *Delivering Dignity* (NHS Confederation, Local Government Association and Age UK) described the neglect experienced by the elderly in health and social care. Recommendations to improve the quality of care and treatment that the elderly receive in a health care system included emphasis on needs assessment, building caring communities and listening to the elderly.

An often-underestimated aspect of ageing is the impact of dementia, one of the main causes of dependency and impairment of life quality in the elderly. According to the WHO, 47 million people worldwide have dementia, and each year over 9.9 million new cases are diagnosed. This is predicted to increase more rapidly in LIC and LMIC after 2020. Dementia places a high burden on the patient's family, as well as a heavy burden on the national economy. The WHO estimated the global societal costs of dementia were approximately US$604 billion in 2010. At the same time, many patients with dementia are vulnerable to neglect, mistreatment and inappropriate therapy. The number of cases of dementia are expected to double every 20 years, reaching 127 million in 2050. It is therefore essential that new societal strategies are developed and research in this field is accelerated.

Older people are known to experience a higher burden of troubling symptoms, including fatigue, depression and loneliness. The concept of *total pain* was introduced by the British pioneer of the palliative care movement Cicely Saunders. This concept describes pain as not only being physical but also containing psychological, social and spiritual dimensions. According to the concept of total pain, it is not sufficient to treat the physical pain (e.g., with analgesics) but it also necessary to understand and address the other dimensions from a multidisciplinary perspective. This facilitates effective end-of-life care.

Malia's experience of total pain

Malia is a 69-year-old woman with advanced breast cancer living in rural Uganda. The Mbararan mobile hospice team used the 'total pain' model to manage her care.

When the hospice team first met Malia, she was experiencing significant pain, constipation from using analgesics, anxiety about the future for herself and her family, in particular her 5-year-old grandchild, and concerns about the value of her life.

The nurse provided her with orally administered morphine solution, an antiemetic and a laxative, which resolved her pain. She was given a chicken to provide a regular source of income through egg production, a scholarship for her grandchild to ensure she would receive education after her death, and spiritual support from her local priest.

Addressing all four dimensions (physical, psychological, social and spiritual) of Malia's suffering was critical. The fact that the interventions were relatively cheap and simple to administer meant that this type of holistic care was entirely possible, even in resource-poor settings.

Felicity Knights and Dan Knights (UK)

Palliative care

'*Palliative care is an approach that improves the quality of life of patients and their families facing the problems associated with life-threatening illness, through the prevention and relief of suffering by means of early identification and impeccable assessment of pain and other problems, physical, psychosocial and spiritual.*'

WHO, 2002

Palliative care should begin from the point of diagnosis, with a gradual shift of emphasis from curative management to palliative management as the disease progresses. However, in practice, end-of-life care usually starts only when death is foreseeable and inevitable. The medical side of palliative care involves close assessment of the patient, proper pain relief and management of symptoms as well as an understanding of the patient's wishes. It requires a holistic assessment with involvement of all members of the care team.

> *'You matter because you are you, and you matter to the end of your life.'*
>
> **Dame Cicely Saunders**
>
> (From AZ Quotes: *Cicely Saunders quotes.* http://www.azquotes.com/author/20332-Cicely_Saunders.)

Good palliative care is an ethical obligation and is cost-effective. Appropriate training for health care workers and physicians working in this area is essential. However, palliative care is still hugely underrepresented around the world, and is not a part of many health care curricula. Many grassroots and advocacy initiatives aim to tackle this. An example is the Palliative Care Toolkit, a simple set of training sessions in basic palliative care that has been translated into many local languages and dialects.

In many LIC and LMIC, large parts of the population are unable to obtain appropriate pain medication. Palliative care remains particularly important in this context as it is frequently of low cost, and requires minimal resources. There remains an ethical need to address deficiencies in palliative care in countries with a large burden of terminally ill patients, especially when treatments such as chemotherapy or appropriate HIV therapy are unavailable.

Palliative care training for medical students

The German Medical Students' Association (Bundesvertretung der Medizinstudierenden in Deutschland) **formed a movement which successfully lobbied for palliative care training to become compulsory in all German medical schools.**

Recognising the importance of palliative care and its neglected status in the German medical curricula, the German Medical Students' Association founded a working group and subsequently a standing committee on palliative care in 2004. The aim was to lobby for the inclusion of palliative care as a mandatory subject in the German national medical curriculum. The directors of this standing committee partnered with professional associations in the field, formed policy recommendations and lobbied the German government for several years.

Increasing presence in the media, at congresses and at many consultative meetings led to a change in the national law to require integration of palliative care into the German medical curriculum as a mandatory subject in all 37 medical schools.

In March 2014 the success of this initiative was extended beyond Germany. The International Federation of Medical Students' Associations passed a policy statement on palliative care calling for better access to pain medication, palliative care and medical education in this field.

Christian Kraef (Germany)

Barriers to end-of-life care

There are three main obstacles to the implementation of palliative care in resource-poor countries: lack of government commitment, opioid availability and limited education. Family, community and cultural issues also play an important part in the access to palliative care.

The simplest indicator for the existence of palliative care and end-of-life care is the use of morphine. Although a vast oversimplification, a country's use of opioids may reflect its use of strategies for pain management and palliative care (**Fig. 6.4.2**). South Africa is the only sub-Saharan African country above the global mean per capita consumption of morphine. The use of morphine

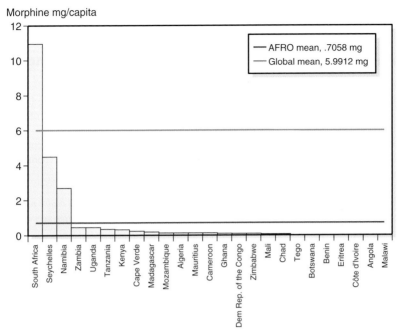

Figure 6.4.2 Morphine consumption in African countries. *AFRO,* WHO Africa region. International Narcotics Control Board: World Health Organization population data. *(Reproduced from Pain & Policy Studies Group, University of Wisconsin/WHO Collaborating Center, 2012.)*

as a cheap illicit recreational drug has compromised its use in palliative care as many countries prioritise drug control above health needs. The principle of 'balance' between these two imperatives is laid out in the 1961 UN Single Convention on Narcotic Drugs, and remains an ongoing policy and advocacy priority for global palliative care and pain management proponents.

Cultural and religious perspectives on ageing and dying

Cultural and religious beliefs can strongly influence an individual's approach and perspective to death, life after death and the appropriate management of death and dying. Recognition of these variables greatly improves the ability of policymakers and clinicians to offer good care, and to provide appropriate support to patients and their families at the end of life.

In most monotheistic religions, rituals and traditions mark the process of death and dying. In many religions it is important for relatives and friends to have access to the body after death so as to perform the burial process. This can be challenging when an autopsy is required, as many faiths require rapid burial after death. Incomplete appreciation of cultural beliefs can easily lead to insensitivity, and even offence, in the provision of palliative and hospice care.

The term *euthanasia* is used to describe intentional practices that end life prematurely so as to relieve pain and suffering. Views on euthanasia and legal approaches differ greatly across the world. In Belgium, the act of euthanasia is classified as homicide but is not prosecuted or punishable if the physician responsible meets certain legal criteria. Physician-assisted suicide is legal in some other countries (e.g., Switzerland) and some states in the United States (e.g., Oregon). In this case, the physician enables the patient to end his/her life by providing the medical means to do so. In some countries it is acceptable to provide pain relief medications to the point that they may hasten death, despite that not being the original purpose.

New approaches to policy around ageing and dying

Increasingly, national and international communities are developing policies to address the needs of their ageing populations. The Madrid International Plan of Action on Ageing (2002) was a landmark policy adopted by UN member states. It offered a comprehensive stance on the subject of ageing whilst formulating policy recommendations.

The declaration focused on three priority areas: older persons and development, advancing health and well-being in old age, and ensuring supportive environments. Key recommendations are summarised in **Box 6.4.1**.

> *'There is no "typical" older person. The resulting diversity in the capacities and health needs of older people is not random, but rooted in events throughout the life course that can often be modified, underscoring the importance of a life-course approach.'*
>
> **Margaret Chan, former WHO Director General**

In 2015 the WHO published its *World Report on Ageing and Health*, and in 2016 at the 69th World Health Assembly the *Draft Global Strategy and Plan of Action on Ageing and Health* was presented. These documents drew attention to ongoing deficiencies in health care for older people, highlighted the benefits of investing in older people and called for efforts to focus around 'maximis[ing] functional ability'. The draft strategy highlighted the relevance of ageing to 15 of the 17 SDGs, and proposed the following strategic objectives:

- commitment to action on health ageing in every country
- development of age-friendly environments
- alignment of health systems to the needs of older populations
- development of sustainable and equitable systems for long-term care
- Improvement of measurements, monitoring and research for health ageing

Another landmark resolution recognising palliative care as 'an ethical responsibility of health systems' was passed at the 67th World Health Assembly (2014). It called on countries to 'ensure adequate domestic funding … for palliative care initiatives, integrate relevant education and training and ensure access to controlled medicines.' This was also relevant to the more recent discussions around a coordinated global approach to the 'world drug problem' at a UN General Assembly Special Session in April 2016 and the 69th World Health Assembly in May 2016.

BOX 6.4.1 ■ Key summary points from the Madrid International Plan of Action on Ageing

- Focus on primary health care for older people
- Comprehensive inclusion of ageing, dying and end-of-life care in medical curricula
- Strengthen Social Security systems for demographic change
- Take ageing and demographic change into consideration in all sectors of policymaking
- Demographic change is a global challenge and needs to be addressed by governments, international organisations and nongovernmental organisations alike when framing development policy
- Consider ethnic, religious and cultural aspects of ageing and dying

---

Adapted from Ageing (Political Declaration and Madrid International Plan on Acting on Ageing, © (2002) United Nations. Reprinted with the permission of the United Nations.

Conclusion

The global population is ageing. The pace of change in response to the challenges posed by ageing differs significantly. Social and cultural norms, values and policies as well as demographic changes affect the experience of the elderly. New political approaches are needed, and health systems must embrace a holistic approach, incorporating access to appropriate analgesia when determining care for ageing populations and those approaching the end of life. More evidence is needed to demonstrate the need and cost-effectiveness of investment in elderly and palliative care, whilst also framing arguments in terms of human rights and social justice.

KEY POINTS

- Ageing and dying are complex biological processes that are significantly affected by social, psychological, cultural and economic factors.
- The world's population is ageing significantly, and this is one of the most pressing global challenges.
- Cultural and religious perspectives on ageing and dying must be considered in the provision of quality care for the older or dying person.
- Palliative care provides a holistic approach to caring for the dying patient; however, it is unavailable in many parts of the world.

Further reading

Commission on Dignity in Care for Older People: *Delivering dignity: securing dignity in care for older people in hospitals and care homes*, 2012. Available from: <http://www.ageuk.org.uk/Global/Delivering%20Dignity%20Report.pdf?dtrk=true>.

United Nations: *Political declaration and Madrid International Plan of Action on Ageing*, New York, 2002. United Nations. Available from: <http://www.un.org/en/events/pastevents/pdfs/Madrid_plan.pdf>.

UN Single Convention of Narcotic Drugs, 1961. Available from: <https://www.unodc.org/unodc/en/treaties/single-convention.html>.

World Health Assembly 2014 Palliative Care Resolution. 67th World Health Assembly, May, 2014. Strengthening of palliative care as a component of comprehensive care throughout the life course. WHA Resolution 67.19. Available from: <http://apps.who.int/gb/ebwha/pdf_files/WHA67/A67_R19-en.pdf>.

World Health Organization: *World report on ageing and health*, Geneva, 2015. World Health Organization.

6.5 Mental Health

Kimberly Williams (Canada)

Introduction

Mental illness impacts on all areas of health. Major depressive disorder is the second leading cause of disability worldwide, affecting the health of the world's population to a greater degree than diabetes and coronary artery disease. Mental health is integral to ensuring good physical health.

What is mental health?

'Health is a state of complete physical, mental and social well-being and not merely the absence of disease or infirmity.'

WHO

An understanding of the concepts of mental health, mental illness and the specialty of psychiatry is important to appreciate the nature of global mental health. These are different but closely related concepts.

- Mental health is the *psychological state of a person*. This state is impacted by many factors, including relationships, biology and psychological resilience. Individual mental health can be either good or poor at any given moment. Good mental health can improve a person's functioning, whilst poor mental health can, but does not necessarily lead to dysfunction. It is possible to have poor mental health without having a mental illness.
- Mental illness is a *mental or behavioural pattern* or difference that causes suffering or impaired ability to function in ordinary life. This includes a combination of how someone thinks, perceives the experiences they have and feels and interacts with their environment. To receive a diagnosis of a mental illness, an individual must have experienced dysfunction in his or her life at some point in time caused by poor mental health.
- *Psychiatry is a medical specialty* devoted to the study, diagnosis, treatment and prevention of mental disorders. It is the study of both the biological sciences and the social sciences, and takes into consideration the subjective experiences of patients as well as their objective physiology. Psychiatry focuses on the treatment of dysfunctional manifestations of mental illness.

Mental and physical health interact in many ways. Evidence suggests that patients with depressive disorders are at increased risk of developing heart disease. Depression increases mortality and morbidity in patients with heart failure, regardless of the cause. Interventions that improve mental health can improve physical health.

Global mental health

Global mental health applies the principles of global health within the domain of mental health, and is not limited to cultural or international psychiatry. It seeks to improve the lives of people and their families affected by mental illness.

Depression in Malawi

Depression is a neglected disease in settings with a high prevalence of infectious disease; treatment options are very limited. This case study illustrates how mental illness can be forgotten as a possible diagnosis.
    A 20-year-old man, accompanied by his sister, walked into the ward in a hospital in Malawi. His sister said that he was not speaking any more, was coughing, felt weak and occasionally fell over.
    The junior doctor noted that the man was very quiet but did not identify any neurological or other physical abnormalities. His senior colleague, on reviewing the patient, spoke to him in his native language (Chichewa). Gradually, the man started speaking to him. The senior colleague diagnosed that the patient had depression. Mental health problems are often missed in Malawi because of the overwhelming prevalence of infectious diseases and malnutrition. The pharmacy had only three pills of amitriptyline available, and these were given to the patient. The lack of appropriate medication in this case compromised his recovery, a situation which is common in low-income countries because of a lack of resources.

Ragna Boerma (Netherlands)

It was once thought that mental disorders were a 'figment of a Western imagination and that the imposition of such concepts on traditional and holistic models of understanding amounted to little more than an exercise in neocolonialism' (Prince et al., 2007) but these ideas have since been contradicted. There is now strong evidence to confirm that mental illness impacts all cultures. It is caused by a multitude of factors – genetic, environmental, social, cultural, biological and psychological.

The presentation of mental illness differs between cultures. Mental illness can be experienced, expressed and understood in many different ways. All psychological distress is culturally bound; therefore clinicians must understand the multitude of ways in which mental illness may present.

Mind the gap

'The difference in the quality of medical care received by people with mental illness is one of the reasons why they live shorter lives than people without mental illness. Even in the best resourced countries in the world this life expectancy gap is as much as 20 years. In the developing countries of the world this gap is even larger.'

Vikram Patel

Access to effective treatment for patients with mental health issues is extremely variable. Despite the availability of high-quality diagnostics and treatments in some countries, many people with mental illness experience degrading treatment such as unauthorised and unmonitored detention, shackling and chaining.

The Global Burden of Disease study (2010) found that mental illness was in five of the top 10 contributors to the number of years in a person's life lived with disability. Among young adults, only HIV infection and AIDS had a bigger impact on leave from work for sickness and disability than depression. The study confirmed that in the previous 20 years the disability-adjusted life years attributable to mental, neurological and substance use disorders accounted for nearly one-quarter of all the years lived with disability globally. Mental, neurological and substance abuse disorders also contribute to mortality indirectly. For example, conditions such as cirrhosis caused by the misuse of alcohol rank among the leading causes of disease burden.

There is a large disparity in the resources allocated to treat mental illness between LIC, LMIC and High Income Countries. More than 75% of individuals identified with serious anxiety, mood, impulse control or substance abuse disorders in LMIC receive no care at all. In certain areas such as sub-Saharan Africa, more than 90% of those with schizophrenia and other forms of psychosis are untreated. The impact of these illnesses on society has only recently been appreciated. The World Bank and WHO analysis of the global burden of disease (2007) resulted in increased global attention on the social and economic impact that mental illness has on society. However, this focus has yet to translate into improved outcomes for people with mental disorders in LMIC.

Significant differences in health persist not only between, but also within nations. In some high-income regions, for instance in Western Europe, nearly half of those who have depression lack access to effective treatment as well as access to important support services. Those with mental illness often lack basic necessities such as food, clothing, shelter and security. To reduce health disparities, access to care must be addressed in the context of the underlying social, economic and political determinants of poor health outcomes.

Stigma

Views about mental illness differ considerably. Studies from West Africa found that an overwhelming majority of people believe that those with mental illness are dangerous and not suitable for normal social contact. Families in Asia hide mental illness as it may reduce the ability of other members of the family to marry and ensure economic stability. The way mental illness is described creates stigma.

Stigma has a large impact on people's health. It can be defined as 'a sign of disgrace or discredit, which sets a person apart from others' (Crabb et al., 2012), and often results in shame, blame and secrecy for those who experience it. Stigma means that those with mental illness are less likely to seek treatment. This may also affect their subsequent participation in society. To improve the likelihood of treatment success, stigma must be reduced.

Both biological and psychosocial factors have an impact on the severity of illness. Patients may experience inappropriate blame when the influence of their innate genetic factors is poorly appreciated. Individuals in sub-Saharan Africa most commonly attribute mental illness to alcohol and illicit drug use or possession by a spirit. These misperceptions greatly impact the lives of those with mental illness. A better understanding and social acceptance of the root causes of mental illness are necessary to reduce the stigma that surrounds it.

Mental illness is caused by many factors. These include genetics, brain defects or injury, infection, substance abuse, prenatal trauma, chemical imbalances and psychological conditioning. Stigma towards those with mental illness is an important global health and human rights issue. It can be reduced through the appropriate education of physicians, allied health workers, government policymakers and society in general. Knowledge of the causes of mental illness improves the prognosis of those who have it.

Within medical schools and amongst medical students, stigma around mental illness still exists. The 'hidden curriculum' often infers that psychiatry is a less valuable area of medicine, when in reality, mental illness is pervasive and causes one of the largest impacts on both the health and the economics of a society.

The way forward

'Determinants of mental health and mental disorders include not only individual attributes such as the ability to manage one's thoughts, emotions, behaviours and interactions with others, but also social, cultural, economic, political and environmental factors such as national policies, social protection, living standards, working conditions, and community social supports.'

WHO Mental Health Action Plan 2013–2020

Treating mental illness in resource-limited settings is challenging. However, efficacious medicines and psychological treatments for a range of mental disorders can be delivered effectively by *nonspecialist* health care workers, reducing the cost burden of treatments.

There are two ways in which services can be scaled up:

- *Effective integration of mental health care into primary care.* This requires few extra resources beyond those already available for other basic health care services such as chronic diseases, maternal and child health, and HIV and AIDS care.
- *Extending treatment to those who are the most vulnerable, including the deinstitutionalised.* Continuity of care is also important; clinicians should be able to follow up patients from the acute phase of their illness across their whole life course.

Reason for hope: schizophrenia in Tanzania

The prospect of abatement of mental illness sometimes seems unlikely, but this case study illustrates that effective management of even severe psychiatric disorders in resource-poor settings can be very effective.

Julius was born in Dar es Salaam. His parents hoped that he would become a teacher as he had a passion for biology and the outdoors. In his late teens, he took a job working on a local farm. He enjoyed his work, but would go through bouts of feeling quite sad, for reasons he did not understand. In his early 20s, he began to hear voices. Some of these were supportive, but others were very frightening. At first, he tried to ignore them, but then he started to wonder if this was a gift from God because he somehow had to suffer for the betterment of others.

Julius was assessed by a mental health nurse as his parents were aware that an uncle had been treated for schizophrenia. Julius was given medication for schizophrenia and, in the next few months, his symptoms abated and he returned to work.

For the next 10 years, Julius contained taking his medication, without any major symptoms. In his mid-30s the voices began to return, this time much worse than before. He stopped going to work, and required admission to a psychiatric ward, where his antipsychotic medication was changed. Within a few months he had returned home and to work. Julius is now 67-years-old, and although he has never married or had children, he has been a successful agricultural cultivator, often growing enough goods to support not only himself but also many of his extended family members.

Kimberly Williams (Canada)

Treatment efforts that have both vertical and horizontal programming have been shown to be effective models of care. The HIV/AIDS experience is a good example of how this model works. ARV therapy roll-out forced basic health infrastructure changes. Basic laboratory facilities needed to be provided, more health care workers were hired and task sharing was promoted through education of community members about the disease and its management.

The broad benefits of programmes that focused on HIV/AIDS prevention and care are good examples of how investment in mental health care could strengthen primary health care. Building capacity for treating mental illness may also, as was seen with HIV/AIDS, strengthen health systems. As HIV/AIDS treatment advocates have shown, treatment of complex disease in resource-poor settings can be effective.

There are numerous examples of current and innovative interventions to improve mental health globally, such as:

screening for neurodevelopmental and psychiatric disorders during vaccine campaigns

addressing depression through community radio

using a smartphone electroencephalogram to diagnose seizure disorders

extending psychological first aid via mobile clinics in postconflict settings

However, there are a number of potentially important areas for further development (**Box 6.5.1**).

BOX 6.5.1 ■ Potential further developments in mental health care

- Creation of programmes to combat the human resources shortage, including a lack of both specialist and community-based workers, which are adaptable to various communities, countries and cultures
- Development of an educational curriculum that can be utilised by a diverse set of professional groups
- Adaptation of diagnostic systems used in high-income countries to become less rigid and more applicable to LMIC
- Upscaling of research to ensure global mental health services are improved
- Intersectoral collaboration between physicians, mental health workers, policy makers and the community at large
- System-wide approaches which use evidence-based interventions
- Increased sensitivity to environmental influences
- Integration of prevention and treatment across the life-course
- Coordination of activities, policies and organisational structures at the local, national and global level

---

LMIC, *Lower middle-income countries.*
Reproduced with permission from Collins PY, Insel TR, Chockalingam A, et al: Grand challenges in global mental health: integration in research, policy, and practice, PLoS Med 10(4):e1001434, 2013.

Conclusion

Mental health has increasingly been recognised as an important contributor to physical health. Much remains to be done in addressing not only how mental health is perceived but also how it is addressed globally. Lack of access to treatment and stigma are ongoing global health challenges. It is important that trainees and health professionals advocate improvement of the lives of those with mental illness and ensure access to treatment. 'There is no health without mental health' (Prince et al., 2007).

KEY POINTS

- Mental health refers to an individual's psychological state.
- Mental illness is a mental or behavioural pattern or difference that causes suffering or impaired ability to function.
- Mental illness can present in many ways.
- Individuals with mental illness face global gaps in access to diagnosis, management and treatment.
- Individuals with mental illness often face stigma in accessing care.

Further reading

Collins PY, Insel TR, Chockalingam A, et al: Grand challenges in global mental health: integration in research, policy, and practice, *PLoS Med* 10(4):e1001434, 2013.
Crabb J, Stewart RC, Kokota D, et al: Attitudes towards mental illness in Malawi: a cross-sectional survey. *BMC Public Health* 12:541, 2012.
Kastrup MC, Ramos AB: Global mental health, *Dan Med Bull* 54(1):42–43, 2007.
Prince M, Patel V, Saxena S: No health without mental health, *Lancet* 370:859–877, 2007.
World Health Organization: *Mental health action plan 2013-2020*, Geneva, 2013, World Health Organization.

The Walking Egg

Established in 2010, the Walking Egg exists to address fertility as an important part of reproductive health in developing countries.

This project adopts 'a multidisciplinary approach to realise affordable and accessible infertility programmes', working in collaboration with the European Society of Human Reproduction and Embryology and the World Health Organization.

The approach is multifaceted. It calls 'for research on social, cultural, ethical, religious and judicial aspects of infertility in poor-resource countries', with plans to start a global network of research in this domain.

The project also focuses on advocacy, pointing out that 'global access to fertility care can only be implemented and sustained if it is supported by local policy makers and the international community'. The Walking Egg recognises the importance of 'training and capacity building'. It eventually hopes to 'establish low-cost fertility services in developing countries'.

This multipronged approach is one that has the potential to be robust and effective, and is a model that could be transferred to other areas of global health.

is often limited. These factors culminate in a multitude of risks for these young women. Every year, 3 million women aged 15–19 years undergo unsafe abortions. Babies born to adolescent mothers face a 50% higher risk of stillbirth or death within the first few weeks versus those born to mothers aged 20–29 years. Newborns born to adolescent mothers are also more likely to have low birth weight, with the risk of long-term adverse health effects.

Adolescent pregnancies also place a large economic and social burden on girls and young women, their babies, families and communities. This particularly disrupts girls' education, thus affecting future employment prospects and, in many cases, helping to promote poverty.

Maternal mortality, the millennium development goals and the post-2015 development agenda

The risk of maternal death in the developed world is 1 in 3700, whereas in resource-poor countries it is 1 in 38 (WHO, 2014). Given this strong association with level of development, the United Nations declared maternal health its fifth MDG, and aimed to:

- reduce by three-quarters, between 1990 and 2015, the maternal mortality ratio
- achieve, by 2015, universal access to reproductive health

Strategies to achieve these goals have included health system targets (e.g., increasing the number and training of skilled birth attendants) and incentivising delivery in health facilities. Other strategies focused on improving women's education as uneducated women are at 2.7 times higher risk of maternal death than their educated counterparts. In 2011 huge gaps remained in contraceptive access for one in eight women worldwide who were married or in a union. In Africa, this ratio was as high as one in four (WHO, 2014, 2017).

The SDGs have seen a shift away from a narrower focus on health to a broader agenda for development. However, maternal health remains a feature within goal 3 ('ensure healthy lives and promote well-being for all'). Within this goal, there are two specific targets directly addressing maternal health:

- by 2030, reduce the global maternal mortality ratio to less than 70 per 100,000 live births;
- by 2030, ensure universal access to sexual and reproductive health care services, including for family planning, information and education, and the integration of reproductive health into national strategies and programmes.

Conclusion

Maternal health is a vital component of global health as it strongly affects the health of both children and families. Maternal morbidity and mortality remain high, and the greatest burden is carried by the poorest in the poorest countries. This problem is compounded by gender inequalities, which often manifest themselves as stigma, decreased access to health care and lack of education. Improvements in maternal health require interventions which target the most affected and deal with multifactorial challenges. Access to family planning resources and the ability to choose when to have children are key to reducing risk to both the mother and the child. The health of families and communities is improved through addressing the particular needs of women.

KEY POINTS

- Maternal health encompasses the health of women during pregnancy, childbirth, and the postpartum period.
- Healthy mothers with healthy pregnancies are more likely to have healthy children.
- Barriers to care leading to morbidity and death in maternal health include lack of access to appropriate care facilities and birth attendants, delays in reaching those facilities and availability of care once at a facility.
- Less than half of deliveries in the developing world occurred with a skilled birth attendant in 2016 (WHO).
- An estimated 225 million women worldwide who want to avoid a pregnancy are not using adequate contraceptive methods.
- Access to reproductive and antenatal care is limited for many HIV-positive women, increasing the risk of a pregnancy. Pregnant women with HIV receive inadequate treatment that if received, would greatly reduce the risk of passing HIV to their child.

Further reading

Bustreo F, Say L, Koblinsky M, et al: Ending preventable maternal deaths: the time is now, *Lancet Glob Health* 1(4):e176–e177, 2013.

Langer A, Horton R, Chalamilla G: A manifesto for maternal health post-2015, *Lancet* 381:601–602, 2013.

Loaiza E, Blake S: *How universal is access to reproductive health: a review of the evidence*, New York, 2010, United Nations Population Fund. Available from: <https://www.unfpa.org/sites/default/files/pub-pdf/universal_rh.pdf>.

World Health Organization: *Ensuring human rights in the provision of contraceptive information and services: guidance and recommendations*, Geneva, 2014, World Health Organization.

6.7 Child Health

Jelte Kelchtermans (Belgium) ▓ Avin Taher (Iraq)

> *'The desire for our children's well-being has always been the most universally cherished aspiration of mankind.'*
>
> **Kofi Annan, former UN Secretary General**

Introduction

In 2015 an estimated 5.9 million children younger than 5 years died; more than half of these deaths were attributable to preventable or treatable conditions (WHO). This represents a tragic failure of the global community to protect some of its most vulnerable members but it is also a sign of hope as it signifies a 53% decline in global under-5 mortality since 1990. The SDG agenda aims to end the preventable deaths of newborns and children younger than 5 years and to reduce under-5 mortality rate to less than 25 cases per 1000 live births. Of the 79 countries that currently have an under-5 mortality rate of more than 25 per 1000 live births, 47 will not meet this SDG goal by 2030 if they continue with their current trends (Global Health Observatory). Key definitions are given in **Table 6.7.1**.

Current status of child health

There is enormous global variation in child mortality levels. The global causes of child death are shown in **Fig. 6.7.1**.

Almost half of deaths of children younger than 5 years in 2012 occurred in the African region. There is global discrepancy in child deaths, which is partly accounted for by preventable and treatable conditions. For example, 45% of all child deaths are linked to malnutrition. Neonatal deaths accounted for roughly 44% of deaths of all children younger than 5 years between 2000 and 2012; more than 80% of these deaths were attributable to prematurity, infections and intrapartum-related problems, including asphyxia. In the postneonatal period, pneumonia (13%), diarrhoea (9%), malaria (7%) and NCDs (7%) are the most frequent causes of child death. There have, however, been major improvements in child health; the average under-5 mortality rate dropped from 93 deaths per 1000 live births in 1990 to 41 per 1000 live births in 2016 (WHO, 2016). The overall decline in cause-specific child mortality is illustrated in **Fig. 6.7.2**.

Several issue-specific plans are under way to ensure continuing investment in child health after 2015. The Global Strategy (2016–2030) for Women's, Children's and Adolescents' Health focuses on support for country-led health plans, ensuring access to essential services, strengthening of health systems and improved monitoring and evaluation of results. It specifically calls on health care workers to collaborate to provide universal access to health care, identify areas with room for improvement, advocate better training and hold authorities responsible for the effects of their actions.

TABLE 6.7.1 ■ Key definitions

Under-5 mortality rate	Probability of dying between birth and exactly 5 years of age, expressed per 1000 live births
Child mortality	This is generally also accepted to refer to under-5 mortality
Infant mortality rate	Probability of dying between birth and exactly 1 year of age, expressed per 1000 live births
Neonatal mortality rate	Probability of dying between birth and 28 days of age, expressed per 1000 live births
Perinatal mortality	The number of stillbirths and deaths in the first 7 days of life (also referred to as *early neonatal mortality*)

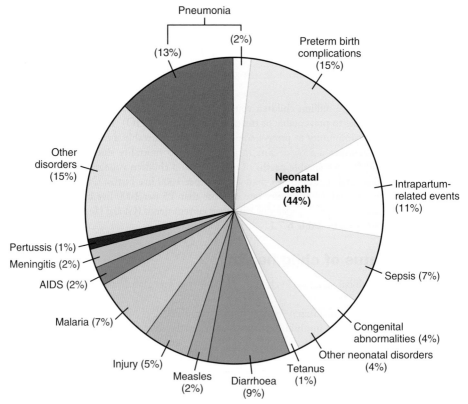

Figure 6.7.1   Causes of child deaths. *(Redrawn from Liu L, Oza S, Hogan D, et al: Global, regional, and national causes of child mortality in 2000–13, with projections to inform post-2015 priorities: an updated systematic analysis. Lancet 385:430–440, 2015.)*

Malnutrition

Malnutrition remains one of the greatest threats to child health. The UNICEF, WHO and World Bank Child Malnutrition Database shows the diversity and extent of this problem. In 2016, 160 million (23%) of all children younger than 5 years worldwide were 'stunted' (more than two standard deviations below median weight for height in a standard reference population). This represents an impressive decrease from 197 million in 2000, but remains unacceptably high.

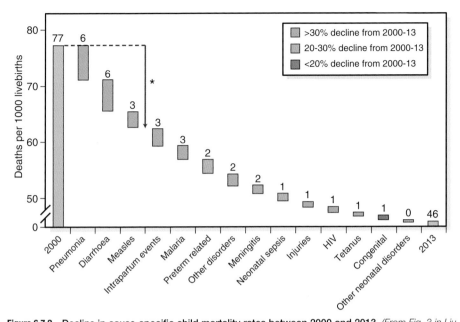

Figure 6.7.2 Decline in cause-specific child mortality rates between 2000 and 2013. *(From Fig. 3 in Liu L, Oza S, Hogan D, et al: Global, regional, and national causes of child mortality in 2000–13, with projections to inform post-2015 priorities: an updated systematic analysis. Lancet 385:430–440, 2015.)*

Paediatric mortality in Pakistan and Madagascar

This report describes a medical elective placement comparing experience in paediatric research in Karachi, Pakistan, and clinical care in Majunga, Madagascar. These locations differ hugely in terms of culture and geography, yet have similar health care challenges.

The infant mortality rate in Pakistan is 69 deaths per 1000 births (UNICEF, 2014). Most of these deaths occur in the poorest 20% of the country, primarily in rural areas. The prevalence of malnutrition in children younger than 5 years is around 30%—one of the highest levels globally (WHO, 2014). Madagascar, a former French colony, which gained independence in 1960, has an infant mortality rate of 41 deaths per 1000 live births. It is one of the poorest countries in the world (IMF, 2011), and health indicators have worsened since 2009. A coup against the president then led to the withdrawal of US$400 million of funding from international donors.

In both countries, a strong correlation was observed between the poverty of the patients and the severity of their presenting conditions. Children were often discharged early from hospital care because the parents had exhausted their funds.

Malnutrition amongst children in both countries contributed to the development of severe life-threatening disease as it reduced the children's ability to resist infection. Late presentation of patients to tertiary centres contributed to higher infant mortality rates. Personal and shared community experience of children dying in hospital reinforced a lack of trust in medical professionals. Provision of health care in rural areas was lacking when compared with the urban environment. However, community involvement of lay workers helped to reduce infant mortality.

Aaminah Verity (UK)

In 2012, approximately 99 million children younger than 5 years were underweight. In 2017 an estimated 50 million children younger than 5 years had wasting or severe wasting.

In contrast, 44 million children younger than 5 years (7%) were overweight. From 2000 to 2012 the prevalence of overweight children increased in all WHO regions, with the highest overall prevalence in southern Africa (18%), central Asia (12%) and South America (7%). In

2012 the World Health Assembly, as part of the 2010 Scaling Up Nutrition movement, set six global nutrition targets in the Comprehensive Implementation Plan on Maternal, Infant and Young Child Nutrition. These aim to:

- reduce stunting in children younger than 5 years
- reduce anaemia in women of reproductive age
- reduce the incidence of low-birthweight deliveries
- reduce the number of overweight children
- increase the number of children exclusively breastfed
- reduce the amount of childhood wasting

NGOs, in cooperation with local communities, national governments and international bodies, are the principal advocates through implementation of projects to promote evidence-based interventions. For example, kangaroo mother care, or early skin-to-skin contact between the mother and her baby, combined with continued breastfeeding, parental support and early discharge from hospital was associated with a 40% reduction of mortality in preterm neonates in a Cochrane review of 16 randomised trials.

Energy drinks: food for thought?

The popularity of energy drinks has increased worldwide. However, little is known about the potential dangers of the consumption of energy drinks amongst children.
These include:
1. childhood obesity, a worldwide growing health issue;
2. concerns about the presence of exotic herbals such as guarana and yohimbine whose effects on health are unknown;
3. concerns about the possible psychological side effects associated with the consumption of energy drinks;
4. the risk of addiction to energy drinks—20% of adolescents consuming caffeine on a regular basis experience withdrawal symptoms after stopping their consumption of energy drinks;
5. cardiovascular complications following the consumption of energy drinks.

Additionally, these drinks provide calorie intake with no nutritional benefit.

Many children are unaware of the potential dangers of energy drinks. More research should be conducted on the consumption of energy drinks amongst children and their potential harm.

Pravesh Gadjradj (Netherlands)

Perinatal and neonatal health

Children are extraordinarily vulnerable during the perinatal and neonatal period. Approximately two-thirds of infant deaths each year occur during the first 4 weeks of life. Two-thirds of those deaths occur during the first week of life. Unfortunately, the neonatal mortality rate has been falling at a slower rate than the overall under-5 mortality rate. To address this trend, the WHO and UNICEF developed the Every Newborn Action Plan (ENAP), which has the ambitious goal of ending preventable newborn deaths and stillbirths by 2035. The aim of ENAP is to reduce the neonatal mortality and stillbirth rate to below 10 per 1000. The action plan is organised around five strategic objectives:

- strengthening and investing in care for newborns and mothers
- improving the quality of maternal and infant care
- ensuring more equitable access to perinatal care
- improving newborn data and programme tracking
- involving parents, families and communities in the process of improving neonatal health

Child health in China

China has made exceptional progress by reducing its under-5 mortality rate from 61 per 1000 in 1991 to 12 per 1000 in 2013.
This was made possible by several ambitious projects and a thorough cooperation with organisations and institutions outside the traditional health sector. One programme aiming to eliminate neonatal tetanus was launched in 2000. It depended on health education, infrastructure changes and social mobilisation. By training health workers, creating referral networks and lowering the hospital delivery cost, it succeeded in eliminating neonatal tetanus in China by 2012. A second example is the Children Nutrition Improvement Pilot Project in Poverty-Stricken Areas. This programme required partnership between the Chinese government and the All-China Women's Federation. It made free nutritional supplements available and organised training courses and various other activities, helping greatly in reducing the overall under-5 mortality rate.

Jelte Kelchtermans (Belgium), Avin Taher (Iraq)

Nongovernmental organisations (NGOs) and health professionals can help by creating and executing advocacy plans for ENAP and its strategic objectives.

Infectious diseases

Pneumonia is the single most important cause of death in children younger than 5 years in all regions of the world. In 2015 it caused 920,136 child deaths, and 16% of all deaths in children younger than 5 years. The global strategy to prevent deaths from pneumonia has used three main approaches:

- *protection*—focusing on ensuring adequate nutrition and improving the environments in which children live
- *prevention*—focusing on vaccinating children against the main causative microorganisms of pneumonia in children and preventing HIV transmission
- *treatment*—focusing on increasing access to appropriate care and essential medicines

Globally, there are an estimated 1.7 billion cases of diarrhoeal disease every year (2013). Each year it kills 760,000 children younger than 5 years. With diarrhoea, the global community has focused on treatment and prevention. Access to low-osmolarity oral rehydration salts and zinc tablets is essential for effective treatment. Progress towards prevention can be made in the availability of safe drinking water, sanitation and hygiene as well as improvements in underlying health and nutritional status, including vitamin A supplementation. A vaccine is now available to protect against rotavirus, which causes an estimated 40% of hospital admissions due to diarrhoea amongst children younger than 5 years worldwide. The integrated Global Action Plan for Pneumonia and Diarrhoea aims to end preventable childhood deaths due to pneumonia and diarrhoea by 2025.

Malaria infection during pregnancy is associated with low birthweight

Of the estimated 660,000 malaria-related deaths in 2010, approximately 86% involved children younger than 5 years, thus making it one of the most deadly diseases in children. It is also an important contributing factor to anaemia and subsequent growth retardation in childhood.

Effective medical therapies exist for many of the conditions that cause death in children younger than 5 years. Access to essential medicines is a widely recognised problem in global health. The World Health Assembly adopted a resolution in 2007 calling for improvement in children's access to medications. The WHO's Model List of Essential Medicines for Children was developed to improve access to effective therapy for children with infectious diseases. However, many challenges still remain, and the WHO has called on governments to prioritise this issue and support continued research and development. The pharmaceutical industry and research communities have also been asked to address several fundamental knowledge and therapeutic gaps.

Child maltreatment and injuries

'There can be no keener revelation of a society's soul than the way in which it treats its children.'

Nelson Mandela

A taboo topic in many communities, child maltreatment is a dangerous and alarmingly common threat to child health. The WHO has defined child maltreatment to include several different concepts, including physical abuse, sexual abuse, neglect, emotional abuse and exploitation. The international statistics on child abuse are listed in **Box 6.7.1**.

Child labour is another form of child maltreatment. According to an International Labour Organization 2012 report from 2012, 168 million children work, and approximately 85 million of these work in hazardous environments. Whilst these numbers are still shocking, they represent a partial success story as the numbers of child workers have declined by two-thirds compared with the figures in 2000.

With child maltreatment, disruptions in biological and psychosocial development put children at increased risk of behavioural, physical and mental health problems throughout their lives. Furthermore, children who work are often deprived of their childhood; these children may drop out of school, and are frequently exposed to health-threatening environments.

The WHO has identified risk factors in children, caregivers, relationships and communities that permit understanding of the causes of child maltreatment whilst providing options for prevention of this abuse as well as support for affected individuals. The recommendations emphasise the importance of intervention early in a child's life whenever possible. In 2014 the World Health Assembly adopted a resolution on 'strengthening the role of the health system in addressing violence, in particular against women and girls, and against children'. Specifically targeting child labour, the International Labour Organization has launched the Red Card to Child Labour campaign, and, in cooperation with the European Commission, the International Programme on the Elimination of Child Labour project Tackling Child Labour Through Education. This strives to decrease child employment through providing alternative educational programmes, which are specifically aimed at reducing poverty.

Injuries are an important cause of death and morbidity amongst children (see Fig. 6.7.1). An estimated 630,000 children under the age of 15 years were killed by an injury (WHO, 2011). Childhood injuries are the leading causes of morbidity and death in rich as well as poorer countries. In the United States in 2008, more than 12,000 children and adolescents died of unintentional

---

BOX 6.7.1 ■ International statistics on child abuse

- Forty million children are subjected to abuse each year.
- Suicide is the third leading cause of death among adolescents worldwide.
- Thirty percent of severely disabled children in special homes in the Ukraine die before 18 years of age.
- Approximately 20% of women and 5%–10% of men report being sexually abused as children, whilst 25%–50% of all children report being physically abused.
- Three million young girls are subjected to genital mutilation every year.

Data from Ark of Hope for Children: <http://www.arkofhopeforchildren.org>

injuries, and more than 9.2 million were treated for nonfatal injuries (Centers for Disease Control and Prevention, 2015).

Child refugees

Strong and sustainable gains in child health are possible only when the social determinants of health, including environmental determinants, are addressed. In 2011 more than 12 million children were forcibly displaced. This had major implications for their physical safety, mental health and access to essential resources, including education. The United Nations High Commissioner for Refugees is mandated to protect these children and ensure that their right, as established by the United Nations Convention of the Rights of the Child, are protected. The United Nations High Commissioner for Refugees has therefore created the Framework for the Protection of Children. Priorities for addressing this difficult issue include creating a safe environment in which children can live, learn and play; empowering children by involving them in decision-making processes; ensuring children's access to their legal documentation such as birth certificates; and creating targeted support for children with specific needs, such as those at increased risk of abuse.

The Carolina Abecedarian project

The Carolina Abecedarian Project was a carefully controlled scientific study of the potential benefits of early childhood education for poor children. Four cohorts, born between 1972 and 1977, who were living in or near North Carolina, United States, were studied. Of these 111 children, 57 were randomly assigned as infants to the early educational intervention group and 54 were randomly assigned as infants to the control group.

The project consisted of two stages of treatment. The first stage, early childhood, involved periods of cognitive and social stimulation interspersed with caregiving and supervised play throughout a full 8-hour day (from birth to age 5 years). This stage also included a nutritional and health care component. Treated children had two meals and a snack at the childcare facility. They were offered primary paediatric care, with periodic check-ups and daily screening. The second stage, school age, focused on improving early mathematics and reading skills (from age 6 years to age 8 years).

Up to 30 years later the outcomes were analysed.

The treated group were:

- four times more likely to have graduated from a 4-year college education (23% vs. 6%);
- more likely to have been employed consistently during the previous 2 years (74% vs. 53%);
- five times less likely to have used public assistance in the previous 7 years (4% vs. 20 %);
- delayed in becoming parents by an average of almost 2 years.

These findings suggest that education is an important determinant of child health, emphasising the importance of the social determinants of health in global health, and the necessity for early intervention to improve outcomes.

Altagracia Mares de Leon (Mexico)

Conclusion

Perinatal and neonatal death present an ongoing challenge for child health, particularly in areas of sub-Saharan Africa. Malnutrition is the largest contributor to unnecessary morbidity and death amongst children. Despite the availability of cost-effective prevention and treatment interventions, infectious diseases, including pneumonia, diarrhoeal diseases and malaria, significantly contribute to child mortality. Child maltreatment and injuries as well as child labour practices also pose a threat to child health. Continued improvements in child health require a coordinated multisector approach.

KEY POINTS

- Each year, more than 5.9 million children younger than 5 years die worldwide; more than half of these deaths are due to preventable or treatable conditions.
- Neonatal death accounts for more than 40% of deaths in children younger than 5 years.
- Malnutrition is the largest contributor to unnecessary morbidity and death amongst children.
- Infectious diseases, including pneumonia, diarrhoeal diseases and malaria, significantly contribute to child mortality globally.
- Child maltreatment is a threat to child health, and includes physical abuse, sexual abuse, neglect, emotional abuse and exploitation.

Further reading

Global strategy for women's, children's and adolescents' health (2016-2030), <www.everywomaneverychild.org>.

Lancet's 2013 Maternal and Child Nutrition series <http://www.thelancet.com/series/maternal-and-child-nutrition>.

United Nations Children's Fund: *Ending preventable child deaths from pneumonia and diarrhoea by 2025. The Integrated Global Action Plan for Pneumonia and Diarrhoea (GAPPD)*, Geneva, 2013, World Health Organization. Available from: <http://www.unicef.org/media/files/Final_GAPPD_main_Report-_EN-8_April_2013.pdf>.

United Nations: *Convention on the Rights of the Child*, 1996–2017. <http://www.ohchr.org/en/professionalinterest/pages/crc.aspx>.

United Nations High Commissioner for Refugees: *A framework for the protection of children*, Geneva, 2012, United Nations High Commissioner for Refugees. Available from: <http://www.unhcr.org/50f6cf0b9.html>.

World Health Organization: *Violence and injury prevention—child injuries*, 2011. Geneva, WHO. Available from: <http://www.who.int/violence_injury_prevention/child/injury/en/>.

World Health Organization: *Every newborn: an action plan to end preventable deaths*, Geneva, 2014, World Health Organization. Available from: <http://www.everynewborn.org/Documents/Full-action-plan-EN.pdf>.

World Health Organization: *Global Health Observatory (GHO) data: under-five mortality*, 2016. Geneva, WHO. Available from: <http://www.who.int/gho/child_health/mortality/mortality_under_five_text/en/>.

6.8 Global Dental Health

Elizabeth Kay (UK) ▪ Martha Paisi (UK)

Introduction

The WHO defines oral health as 'a state of being free from mouth and facial pain, oral and throat cancer, oral infection and sores, periodontal (gum) disease, tooth decay, tooth loss, and other diseases and disorders that limit an individual's capacity in biting, chewing, smiling, speaking, and psychosocial wellbeing' (2012). Dental health is thus a crucial part of an individual's overall health and well-being. Oral diseases have a significant negative impact on the quality of life of individuals, their family and society as a whole.

The burden of oral diseases

Oral diseases are 'major public health problems' with significant cost implications as they are the fourth most expensive health problem in the world. The Global Burden of Disease 2010 study which provided estimates of the impact of 291 diseases and injuries between 1990 and 2010 indicated that oral conditions affected 3.9 billion people worldwide. Estimates in this study showed that amongst all conditions evaluated, tooth decay in the permanent dentition had the highest prevalence (35% of all age groups). Severe periodontitis and untreated decay in the primary teeth were ranked the sixth and 10th most prevalent diseases respectively, affecting 11% and 9% of the population worldwide. Both severe periodontitis and caries were included amongst the 100 most common causes of disability. It was also estimated that oral conditions combined amounted to 224 years of health loss on average per 100,000 population.

Tooth decay

Despite being preventable, tooth decay is considered a major public health problem, and has been previously characterised as 'a silent epidemic'. It affects 60%–90% of school-age children. Improvements in the caries profile of populations worldwide have been evident in the last 30 years. These have been attributed primarily to the increased and effective use of fluorides through toothbrushing or water fluoridisation, schools-based programmes and better management of the condition. However, the burden of tooth decay remains high in some countries, and progress in reducing this burden has stagnated or even regressed in some cases, often compromising the well-being of very young children.

Tooth decay is more prevalent in females than males and is age dependent. Evidence from the Ten-State Nutrition Survey (1968–70), which analysed data on more than 10,000 participants aged 5 to 20 years, showed that decay starts after the teeth erupt, increases to late adolescence and then stabilises during early adulthood. The greater impact of tooth decay amongst females may be explained by their longer exposure to a cariogenic environment as teeth tend to erupt in females earlier than in males. Other reasons for sex differences include dietary preferences, snacking during food preparation and cultural, hormonal and genetic factors.

Periodontitis

Severe periodontitis is estimated to affect 10%–15% of the adult population. Gingival bleeding is the first and most prevalent sign of periodontal (gum) disease. The Centres for Disease Control and Prevention (2015) has estimated that 47.2% of adults in the United States aged 30 years or older have some periodontal disease (Eke et al., 2012). Periodontitis is responsible for 30% of tooth loss amongst people aged 65 to 74 years. It is the most common chronic inflammatory disease affecting individuals. In the United Kingdom, estimates show that almost half of the adult population is affected, whilst the percentage is higher (60%) for those aged 65 years or older.

The National Health and Nutrition Examination Survey (National Institute of Dental and Craniofacial Research, 2014) suggests that periodontal disease in adults decreased between 1970 and 2004. In upper middle-income countries, the prevalence of tooth loss is higher (35%) than in LMIC (10%). Although mild gingivitis can affect both children and adults, the presence of *severe* periodontal disease is uncommon in young people and is more profound in older age groups. It is also more common in men than women.

Inequalities in oral health

The improved overall dental health of populations, particularly in industrialised countries, has not been matched by similar improvements in all areas of the world.

The WHO has predicted that the incidence of dental caries is expected to increase in Africa because of the limited availability of fluoride and changes in living conditions which are accompanied by an increase in sugar intake. In developed countries, evidence from longitudinal and cross-sectional studies indicates that individuals of lower socioeconomic status have a higher burden of this condition in terms of prevalence and severity. In addition, children from lower socioeconomic status groups have been shown to have greater treatment needs when compared with their affluent peers. For example, in the United Kingdom, there are significant regional and socioeconomic inequalities in both the prevalence and the severity of tooth decay in children. Children from lower-income families are more likely to have oral disease. Amongst children between the ages of 5 and 15 years, the difference in the prevalence of severe or extensive tooth decay is approximately twofold higher in those who are eligible for free school meals. The latest National Dental Epidemiology Programme for England also showed that oral health was worse in the more deprived areas. Disadvantaged individuals may be more vulnerable to tooth decay through lack of knowledge, placement of low value on oral health, high perceived barriers to oral health behaviour and low perceived susceptibility to oral diseases.

There are also significant inequalities in the prevalence of periodontitis and tooth loss. Periodontitis particularly affects individuals from minority groups and from lower socioeconomic backgrounds. Thus African Americans are two times more likely to have periodontal disease compared with white Americans. Although overall periodontal health appears to be improving, particularly in industrialised countries, differences in the prevalence of this condition exist both between and within countries. Poor periodontal health is commoner amongst poor people, and these differences relate to socioeconomic conditions, dental health systems, behavioural risk factors and general health status. It seems that current approaches to controlling oral disease may have actually benefited those in the least need and increased inequalities in oral health.

Causes and common determinants of oral diseases

The causes of oral diseases are multifactorial, and include individual characteristics and traits as well as environmental and societal factors. The risk factors for oral disease are similar to those for many other NCDs. In the case of tooth decay, although tooth morphology, saliva composition and presence of bacteria are important in the development of disease, lifestyle factors such as fluoride use and frequency of sugar consumption determine the development of the condition. Sugar is considered to be a necessary factor in the initiation and progression of tooth decay, and it has been suggested that there would be no need for preventative measures such as fluoride if sugar consumption were adequately tackled. With periodontitis, the presence of certain bacteria is essential for the development of disease. The severity of this condition is determined in large part by lifestyle factors such as tobacco use, unhealthy dietary habits, excessive alcohol use and stress. It is clear that the social determinants of health have a major impact on the oral health of the population.

Consequences of poor oral health

Oral diseases can have a significant adverse impact both on the individual and on society. Their estimated cost accounts for 5%–10% of all health care resources. The global economic impact of oral diseases in 2010 was estimated to be US$442 billion, whilst in the European Union it has been estimated that if current trends continue, the annual cost for dental care could increase from current figures of €79 billion up to €93 billion in 2020.

Tooth decay has immediate and long-term consequences. Individual quality of life is adversely affected because of pain, whilst infections can lead to altered dietary habits and the potential need for extraction of the affected tooth. Extraction of a tooth early in life can cause early eruption of teeth, and may alter the alignment of permanent teeth, raising the need for orthodontic treatment. In addition, damaged teeth need long-term follow-up and treatment. This may result in loss of time from work or absence from school. The presence of decay and early tooth extraction have been shown to affect individual self-esteem, whilst early childhood caries may affect children's growth.

Early carious lesions have also been shown to increase the risk of developing caries in later life. In addition to the impact on individual health and quality of life, tooth decay has a significant economic impact. In the United Kingdom, tooth extractions for children aged 18 years or younger between 2012 and 2013 cost the National Health Service £30 million (UK Department of Health, 2013).

The consequences of periodontal disease are similar to those of tooth decay, but periodontitis has also been shown to be associated with systemic diseases such as heart disease and diabetes. The economic burden of periodontitis is substantial both for the individual and for society. Although data on the treatment of the whole spectrum of this disease are scarce, this may be due to the inappropriateness of current approaches used to manage the condition. In Malaysia, it was estimated that the cost of treating all cases of periodontitis was RM32.5 billion, which is higher than the economic burden of some chronic diseases in that country.

Common risk factor approach

Most NCDs, including oral diseases, are affected by similar social determinants. This fact provides evidence for the application of a common risk factor approach to target and prevent specific health conditions. The common risk factor approach constitutes one of the most important concepts in the prevention of oral diseases, and its application has been widely promoted. The approach is based on the concept that the targeting of a small number of risk factors which are common to many diseases will result in a major impact on several diseases whilst using fewer resources. As this approach targets the broader determinants of health and aims to address the health of the general population and those at high risk, it should also, potentially, be a major tool for reducing health inequalities.

Approaches to promoting dental health

Many approaches in promoting good dental health have traditionally focused on modifying the underlying behavioural risk factors through education. This is based on the assumption that improvement in knowledge related to oral health will actually lead to changes in people's behaviours. Using a number of approaches, these interventions have occurred primarily in clinical and school settings as well as in other places, such as residential homes. A major drawback of this approach is that it does not take into account the broader determinants of health and how these must be targeted in the wider context of promoting dental health.

Dental health is determined by individual choice as well as by societal factors. Oral health promotion has evolved in attempting to address the underlying determinants of dental health from a holistic approach. The WHO Ottawa Charter for Health Promotion (WHO, 1986) recognised the need to address several factors beyond the individual to improve health. It can be considered as a cornerstone of an effective approach in promoting dental health and lists the following as the prerequisite for health:

- peace
- shelter
- education
- food
- income
- a stable ecosystem
- sustainable resources
- social justice
- equity

Conclusion

A healthy lifestyle and behaviours are paramount for the establishment and maintenance of good oral health. Individual behaviours beneficial to oral health include a reduction in the frequency of sugar consumption, good oral hygiene and limited alcohol and cigarette consumption. Sustainable improvement in oral health requires political will to address the broader determinants of oral diseases.

KEY POINTS

- Oral health is an essential part of overall health and well-being.
- Oral diseases can have a profound impact on the individual and society.
- Maintenance and promotion of dental health should take into account the broader determinants of health.
- The common risk factor approach appears to be a promising means to reduce health inequalities.

Further reading

Batchelor P: Is periodontal disease a public health problem?, *Br Dent J* 217:405–409, 2014.

Benjamin RM: Oral health: the silent epidemic, *Public Health Rep* 125(2):158–159, 2010.

Eke PI, Dye BA, Wei L, et al: Prevalence of periodontitis in adults in the United States: 2009 and 2010, *J Dent Res* 91(10):914–920, 2012.

Listl S, Galloway J, Mossey PA, Marcenes W: Global economic impact of dental diseases, *J Dent Res* 94(10):1355–1361, 2015.

Marcenes W, Kassebaum NJ, Bernabe E, et al: Global burden of oral conditions in 1990-2010: a systematic analysis, *J Dent Res* 92(7):592–597, 2013.

Petersen PE, Ogawa H: The global burden of periodontal disease: towards integration with chronic disease prevention and control, *Periodontology* 60:15–39, 2012.

World Health Organization: *The Ottawa Charter for Health Promotion*, 1986. <http://www.who.int/healthpromotion/conferences/previous/ottawa/en/>.

6.9 Violence and Injury

Christopher Fourie (South Africa)   Michael Van Niekerk (South Africa)

Introduction

Injury is a major cause of global deaths, and accounted for 9.2% of the world's deaths in 2014. It represented 18.6% of the global burden of disease in 2004. Injury is defined by the WHO as the result of 'acute exposure to physical agents such as mechanical energy, heat, electricity, chemicals, and ionizing radiation interacting with the body in amounts or at rates that exceed the threshold of human tolerance.' In cases such as drowning and frostbite, injury is caused by a sudden lack of critical agents such as heat or oxygen. Injuries encompass all trauma, covering both intentional and unintentional injury. Apart from the profound effects of trauma and injury on the individual, injury can also immeasurably affect families and communities.

Although some injuries are listed as accidental, this does not mean that injuries are unavoidable or unpredictable. Recognising that injuries are preventable events allows organisations to develop programmes and implement policies to prevent injury and improve outcomes when they do occur.

Classification and epidemiology

According to the 10th revision of the International Statistical Classification of Diseases and Related Health Problems (WHO), injuries can be divided into two groups:

1. *Unintentional*, historically known as *accidents*;
2. *Intentional*, also known as *violence*.

Approximately two-thirds of all injuries globally are unintentional (**Fig. 6.9.1**). The WHO further highlights eight major causes of injury, grouped by prevalence in populations globally and the ability for global health policy to reduce morbidity and mortality. Most public health experts and organisations use this classification scheme in discussion of global injury surveillance and prevention.

The nature and scope of injuries differs considerably by region, age, sex, type of injury and, especially, socioeconomic status. Men are more commonly involved in violent injury, whereas toddlers have a greater propensity for road traffic injuries and drowning. The identification of populations vulnerable to specific types of injuries allows the development of targeted prevention plans for those populations at risk.

The greatest burden of disease attributable to injury is in LIC and conflict zones. The WHO estimates that more than 90% of deaths attributable to injury occur in LIC or middle-income countries. Even within countries, there is a strong correlation between deaths from injury and the rate of nonfatal injury and poverty.

This uneven distribution of injuries among the less advantaged is related to a number of factors:

- living, working and travelling in less safe conditions
- decreased focus on prevention efforts from local policymakers
- decreased access to emergency trauma care and rehabilitation services
- greater financial burden related to injury in both direct and indirect costs

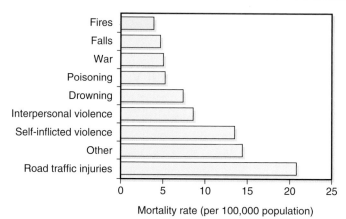

Figure 6.9.1   The global mortality rate per 100,000 population for types of injury.

There are also interesting *regional variations* between types of injury. For example, the burden of disease due to violence is relatively higher in Africa and the Americas, whilst war causes a relatively greater burden in the eastern Mediterranean region. Self-harm represents a relatively greater burden in Europe and Southeast Asia.

There are significant discrepancies between different *age groups*. Injuries are the leading killer of individuals aged 15–29 years worldwide, and rank in the top five (road traffic injuries in particular) from ages 5 to 49 years.

In terms of *sex*, almost twice as many men die as a result of injuries compared with women, with the exception of intimate partner violence and sexual violence, which affects 35% of women. An estimated 20% of girls are sexually abused at some point in their childhood compared with 10% of boys. Thus for men, the three leading causes of death from injuries are road traffic injuries, suicide and homicide, whereas for women, the top three are road traffic injuries, falls and suicide. **Fig. 6.9.2** illustrates the relative mortality for different causes between men and women. Male mortality exceeds female mortality in every category.

The impact of injury

Injury can have a profound impact on individuals, families and communities. Consequences include the physical injury with resulting disability, mental and emotional effects, financial burdens resulting from lost work or future opportunities, and the direct costs of medical care. All of these can be enduring, and lead to lifelong changes in the lives of those affected. Injuries may also lead to behavioural changes, especially following violence and abuse. These can contribute to practices such as drug and alcohol abuse and unsafe sexual practices resulting in sexually transmitted infections with their resultant health implications. Sedentary lifestyles resulting from injury-related disability can further contribute to the development of NCDs and their sequelae. For those in poverty, these events can be amplified (**Fig. 6.9.3**).

Measures of the burden of disease such as disability adjusted life years do not accurately reflect the individual impact of injury as this varies according to occupation and financial resources.

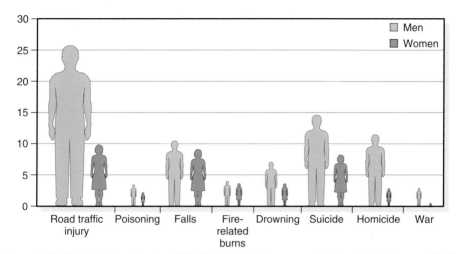

Figure 6.9.2   Global death rates (per 100,000 population) by cause of injury divided by sex (2012). *(Redrawn from World Health Organization: Injuries and violence the facts 2014, Geneva, 2014, World Health Organization. Available from <http://apps.who.int/iris/bitstream/10665/149798/1/9789241508018_eng.pdf? ua=1&ua=1&ua=1>)*

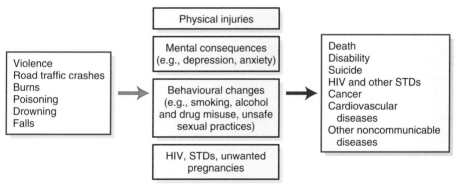

Figure 6.9.3   The consequence of violence and injury (2010). *(Redrawn from World Health Organization: Injuries and violence the facts, Geneva, 2010, World Health Organization. Available from <http://whqlibdoc. who.int/publications/2010/9789241599375_eng.pdf>)*

Community and economic impact

The true cost of injury to communities and to the economy is very difficult to estimate because of the large number of variables. Economic impacts on families can be immense, and most significantly affect the poor, who have fewer financial and social resources.

Direct costs of injury include medical care costs such as ambulance transport, hospital stays, medications, office visits, laboratory testing, physical therapy, medication, prostheses and other medical devices. Nonmedical costs include legal costs, security services in the case of violent injury and modifications to the home that may be required to cope with an injury (e.g., the provision of wheelchair ramps).

Indirect costs include lost resources and opportunities, such as the loss of working time, productivity and earnings, and reduced productivity of a caregiver in the family. Property values in violent neighbourhoods are often depressed, and community investment in these areas is often limited. Violence also affects communities by creating a culture of fear, with significant emotional and psychological impact for affected people.

In the WHO 2009 global status report on road safety, less than half of the participating countries conducted studies on the cost of road traffic deaths and injuries. In those that did, the study methodology was inconsistent, and generally underestimated the costs to countries and communities. Despite these difficulties, it is estimated that road traffic accidents cost most countries 1%–2% of their GDP, with the global cost estimated at US$518 billion.

Specific causes and prevention

Road traffic accidents

'The SDG target of a 50% reduction in road traffic deaths and injuries by 2020 offers a powerful focus around which governments and the international community can galvanize action – the challenge now is to seize the opportunity to do so, and to turn the current plateau in road deaths into a measurable decline.'

Margaret Chan, former WHO Director General

In 2013 1.25 million people were killed in road traffic accidents. These accidents are the ninth leading cause of death, and half of those killed are 'vulnerable road users' (defined as any user without a 'protective shell', such as pedestrians, motorcyclists and bicyclists). This burden is highest in LIC and LMIC (90% of all deaths) (WHO, 2017). The factors contributing to road traffic accidents include the increasing number of road users, poorly maintained vehicles lacking in safety features (e.g., seat belts and airbags) poorly maintained and poorly lit roads, and inadequate enforcement of traffic safety laws.

In 2010 the UN General Assembly declared 2011–20 the 'Decade of Action for Road Safety' with the aim of improving the safety of roads in more than 110 participating countries. **Table 6.9.1.** summarises the report's primary areas of action. This commitment was reaffirmed in line with SDG 3, Target 3.6, at a meeting of the WHA in 2016.

Falls

Falls are the most common injury-related death in adults aged older than 70 years and less commonly affect younger individuals. The risk factors for these injuries include occupations at elevated heights, overcrowded housing, alcohol or substance use, adverse effects of medication, poor mobility, poor cognition and impaired vision.

Falls can be prevented by the screening of living environments for fall risks, regular review of medications in the elderly, management of low blood pressure and correction of visual impairment. Community exercise programmes for the elderly may increase strength and improve balance and thus reduce the risk of falling. Treatment of conditions such as osteoporosis will reduce the morbidity associated with falls when they do occur.

Burns

'My life was different because after this no one wanted to play with me and don't want to talk with me because I look different from others.'

Tonmoy, facial burns survivor, Bangladesh

TABLE 6.9.1 ■ Key interventions to improve road safety

Area of action	Why it is a problem	Key interventions
Speed	Every 1 km per hour increase in speed correlates to a 3% increased risk of crashing Contributes to 30% of road traffic accidents	Enforcing speed limits Traffic calming measures (e.g., speed bumps) Education and public information
Alcohol	A significant increase occurs at blood alcohol concentrations greater than 0.04 g/dL	Enforcing blood alcohol concentration limits, random breath testing, tough and swift penalties for offenders, breath test devices as ignition interlocks Mass media campaigns
Seat belts and child restraints	Seat belts reduce serious injury by 40%–65%, making them the most effective road safety intervention Child restraints reduce infant deaths by 70% when installed correctly	Use enforcement and encouragement: fines/tickets, audible seat belt reminders Publicity campaigns
Helmets	Head trauma is the leading cause of death in drivers of motorcycles and bicycles Motorcycle helmets reduce deaths by 40%	Enforcing use of helmets Enforcing standards for motorcycle helmet production
Distractions	Mobile phones are currently the greatest distraction because of talking and texting	Legislation and public campaigns discouraging the use of distractions whilst driving
Visibility	Motorised vehicles using daytime running lights have a crash rate 10%–15% lower than those that do not	Daytime running lights Reflectors (vehicles) and reflective clothing (people) Street lighting

Footnote: 2010, the United Nations General Assembly declared 2011–2020 the Decade of Action for Road Safety. www.who.int/roadsafety/decade_of_action/plan/global_plan_decade.pdf.

Fires and burns are highly preventable public health issues, as evidenced by the effectiveness of public health interventions in high-income countries. Burns most severely affect those with the lowest socioeconomic status. In poorer settings, there is also decreased access to proper medical care for severely burnt patients. Home remedies such as papaya seed paste dressings, banana leaf dressings or honey have been investigated and have been found to be effective low-cost methods of wound care.

The risk factors for burns include occupational exposure to fire, poverty, overcrowding, the use of open fires for light and cooking, unsupervised children, and alcohol abuse and smoking (where individuals fall asleep with lit cigarettes). These factors lend themselves to a set of effective interventions, including development of safe stoves and lamps, particularly in low-income settings. Other interventions include installation of smoke alarms in homes, exploration of resource allocation towards severe burns centres and investment in low-cost wound care.

Drowning

Drowning is the third leading cause of unintentional injury death worldwide, and accounts for 7% of injury-related deaths. There are an estimated 360,000 annual drowning deaths worldwide

(WHO 2015). More than 90% of deaths occur in LMIC. Young people are those most at risk, with more than half of cases occurring in individuals younger than 25 years.

The Saving of Children's Lives from Drowning project

In Bangladesh, drowning causes 42% of deaths in children aged 1–4 years. For this reason the Saving of Children' Lives from Drowning project was designed.

The Saving of Children' Lives from Drowning project aims to take a multipronged approach to tackling this significant public health problem in Bangladesh, where most incidents of children drowning occur in natural water (as opposed to swimming pools, for example). The first principal intervention is the distribution of playpens to ensure children playing at home when not under direct supervision are kept safe from straying to dangerous water. Secondly, the project incorporates crèche programmes, where children are supervised in a communal environment for the highest risk period of the day for drowning (usually mornings).

The plan for the project includes education and awareness raising for families and communities regarding drowning. The project is strongly founded in research, and a comprehensive plan for evaluating and, hopefully, demonstrating its success has been laid out.

It is anticipated that this project will have other secondary benefits, such as employment opportunities for local individuals through staffing of crèches and production of playpens. The provision of crèches for young children should also benefit their education.

Key interventions include controlling access to water hazards, increased supervision of children around water, training in drowning rescue and resuscitation, enforcing safety regulations on boating, shipping and ferries, and robust flood and disaster management plans.

Intentional injuries (violence)

The WHO defines violence as 'the intentional use of physical force or power, threatened or actual, against oneself, another person, or against a group or community, that either results in or has a high likelihood of resulting in injury, death, psychological harm, maldevelopment, or deprivation.' Violence, in all of its forms, leads to the deaths of 1.3 million people annually. It is more difficult to track nonfatal violence, particularly sexual violence, as it often goes unreported.

Self-directed violence includes self-mutilation as well as suicide and attempted suicide. Suicide (SDG indicator 3.4.2) is the second leading cause of death in individuals aged 15–29 years. Despite this, the rate of suicides is highest in individuals aged 70 years or older. The risk factors are multifactorial, and include difficulty in accessing health care, the stigma of mental health issues, substance abuse, easy availability of means to commit suicide, sensationalised reporting of suicides and a history of suicide attempts. Self-mutilation is associated with a twofold morbidity: the direct effects of the self-harming behaviour and the associated preceding psychological turmoil. Key interventions include restriction of access to common means of suicide, ensuring access to appropriate mental health care (particularly for those with a history of suicide attempts) and responsible suicide reporting in the media.

> *'More needs to be done, particularly to increase investment in intimate partner violence prevention, to support women experiencing intimate partner violence (most women killed by a partner have been in long-term abusive relationships), and to control gun ownership for people with a history of violence.'*
> **Heidi Stöckl, UK**

Interpersonal violence is a broad category including violence between family members, strangers, friends and acquaintances, youth and gang violence, elder and child abuse and neglect, and intimate partner and sexual violence. Homicide is the third leading cause of death in males aged 15–44 years. Reducing access to weapons and alcohol and promoting gender equality, along with effective victim support programmes, are important in tackling this problem.

Collective violence is defined as instrumental violence inflicted by larger groups such as nation states, militia groups, and terrorist organisations to achieve political, economic or social objectives.

Conclusion

Injury is a significant and overlooked cause of morbidity and death in all age groups, especially in young people. A number of programmes worldwide demonstrate that appropriate interventions can help to prevent many of these injuries. This has particular relevance with regard to both health care and economic needs, for poorer individuals and societies. Information about possible strategies for injury prevention needs to be more widely available.

KEY POINTS

- Violence and injury are major causes of preventable global morbidity and death.
- Injuries can be classified as *intentional* or *unintentional*.
- Injuries disproportionately affect those in low- and middle-income countries, where there are the least resources to effectively treat them.
- The true effects of injury are difficult to quantify, and encompass direct physical effects, psychological effects and the resultant economic costs.
- Injuries and violence can be prevented by appropriate interventions.

Further reading

Jamison DT, Breman JG, Measham AR, et al: *Disease control priorities in developing countries*, ed 2, Washington, 2006, World Bank. Available from: http://www.ncbi.nlm.nih.gov/books/NBK11728/.

World Health Organization: *Drowning—Fact Sheet 347*, Geneva, WHO, 2015 data, updated May 2017. Available from: <http://www.who.int/mediacentre/factsheets/fs347/en/>.

World Health Organization: *Developing policies to prevent injuries and violence—guidelines for policy-makers and planners*, Geneva, 2016, Wold Health Organization. Available from: <http://www.who.int/violence_injury_prevention/publications/39919_oms_br_2.pdf>.

World Health Organization: *Violence and injury prevention*, 2017. <http://www.who.int/violence_injury_prevention/en/>.

The Environment

Junior Editor: Alexandre Lefebvre (Canada)

Introduction

'Young people should care about climate change because of all society, we will be on our planet longest. I want to be part of the long legacy of people trying to protect our environment.'

Sid Janota, student climate change activist

Approximately 25% of the global disease burden is due to modifiable environmental factors (WHO). The environment should therefore be a top priority for the health sector. The management of environmental issues requires close collaboration between national ministries, transnational companies and governments, as well as between intergovernmental organisations, in pursuit of strong global governance for health. The United Nations Framework Convention on Climate Change (UNFCCC) and the Sustainable Development Goals (SDGs) are major governance processes involving both the health sector and the nonhealth sector.

The 2015 Nepal earthquakes

This national disaster displaced more than 3 million people overnight. Hospitals were immediately overloaded, and several (in Ramechhap, Nuwakot and Sindhupalchowk) were damaged. Disaster management teams helped to mitigate this catastrophe. In the immediate aftermath of the earthquake, the emphasis was on finding survivors and those who required urgent medical help. This was hampered by bad weather and the fear of aftershocks.

Food was scarce, and food insecurity will persist for many years. Water and sanitation became a major issue, and outbreaks of diarrhoea affected many people, especially children. This scenario compromised the longer-term health requirements and, as resources were scarce, it was easy for friction and conflict to arise. Transport infrastructure was destroyed, and rural communities were isolated. Many of the survivors are still living in overcrowded areas, which significantly increases the risk of infectious diseases such as cholera.

Such disasters provide an opportunity for governments to ensure that this level of displacement never happens again. Climate change increases the likelihood of natural disasters. Nepal has little capacity to tackle or manage global issues such as climate change in the absence of a global collaborative approach.

7.1 Climate Change and Energy

Nick Watts (Australia)

'Climate Change is the biggest global health threat of the 21st century. Effects of climate change on health will affect most populations in the next decades and put the lives and wellbeing of billions of people at increased risk.'

The Lancet and UCL Commission, Managing the Health Effects of Climate Change (2009)

Introduction

The links between ecosystem services (clean air, food and nutrition, fresh water for drinking and sanitation, and shelter) and human well-being are well known. Climate change is linked to health and the work of health professionals in five key ways:

- *Impacts:* It has a negative impact on human health, disrupting social and environmental systems, whilst threatening to undermine recent major advances in global health.
- *Adaptation:* Health systems can adapt to some of these impacts through a range of specific strategies directed at the building of community and system resilience.
- *Mitigation:* The health system has a role to play in reducing its own emissions. Low-carbon health systems are often associated with reduced costs and improved patient care.
- *Health impact assessments:* Many of the interventions needed to respond to climate change (both mitigation and adaptation) have their own positive side effects. Replacing a coal-fired power plant with a wind farm leads to cleaner air, reducing local rates of cardiovascular and respiratory disease. Health impact assessments are a useful tool in planning for and unlocking these positive externalities.
- *Advocacy:* Climate change has long been recognised as an environmental crisis but little has been done to address this challenge. Health professionals are ideally placed to articulate a positive response to climate change in pursuit of human health and well-being. They are well able to reframe the public discourse on climate change whilst calling for stronger political leadership to protect health.

With strong engagement from the health profession and with a better understanding of the health co-benefits of mitigation and adaptation, 'tackling climate change could become the greatest global health opportunity of the 21st century' (Lancet Commission, 2015).

Impacts of climate change

Climate change affects human health and well-being both directly and indirectly. Three complex systems—the climate system, human social systems and the natural biophysical system—interact to determine the impact of climate change (**Fig. 7.1.1**). Geography and a reduced capacity for adaptation mean that these impacts disproportionately affect populations in low-income countries (LIC) and lower middle-income countries (LMIC), often the countries and people least responsible

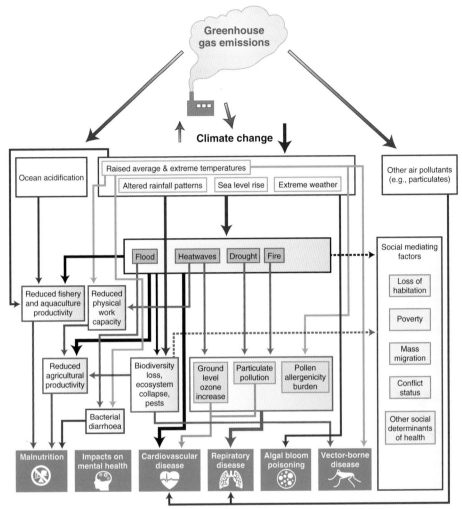

Figure 7.1.1   The health impacts of climate change. Overview of the links between greenhouse gas emissions, climate change and health. *(Redrawn from Watts N, Adger WN, Agnolucci P, et al: Health and climate change: policy responses to protect public health. Lancet 386:1861–1914, 2015.)*

for causing climate change. Many of these effects are being felt *today*, and their severity is set to increase dramatically in the coming century.

Extreme weather events

As a key ecosystem service, essential for both drinking water and sanitation, any change to the availability of clean and fresh water has important implications for public health. Through altered patterns of rainfall and increased temperatures, climate change threatens the availability of drinking water, leading to a rise in flooding in some areas, and droughts in others. The Intergovernmental Panel on Climate Change (IPCC) has reported that the number of people living in cities affected by chronic water scarcity is set to rise by almost 1 billion by 2050. In currently dry regions, such as the eastern Horn of Africa, there is an acknowledged likely increase in the severity and frequency of droughts, threatening current sanitation efforts. Increased susceptibility to flooding brings higher rates of diarrhoeal disease and injury, as well as substantial economic loss and damage to property. Areas such as the Maldives and large sections of Bangladesh which are very low lying are likely to suffer significant flooding from marginal increases in sea level.

The frequency and severity of extreme weather events are predicted to increase if climate change continues at the present rates. The effects of worsening storms, extremes of temperature, floods and droughts may be mitigated when populations are able to adapt appropriately. However, poorer individuals often lack the financial means needed to avoid harm as well as access to storm-ready housing or social safety nets. Extremes of temperature often disproportionately affect the elderly and people with chronic illnesses.

Infectious disease

Through changes in temperature and rainfall, climate change has already begun altering the pattern and distribution of a number of vector-borne diseases. 'Climate-sensitive' diseases (such as malaria and dengue fever) are those sensitive to changes in their local climate. Increased temperatures are more suitable for reproduction, and greater rainfall creates new breeding reservoirs for vectors. This is particularly problematic when the local health system is unprepared for the disease as health professionals require retraining and new surveillance systems must be put in place. At a more systemic level, the IPCC notes that mid-range warming scenarios 'will result within this century in abrupt and irreversible regional-scale change in the composition, structure and function of terrestrial and freshwater ecosystems, especially in the Amazon and the Arctic, leading to substantial additional climate change.' Such dramatic changes to these ecosystems threatens to limit the availability of food from fisheries and negatively impact local cultures and indigenous peoples.

Food and nutrition

Variation in the rainfall and temperature patterns of local climates (with associated increases in the frequency of floods or droughts) impacts on food security. The IPCC has identified a number of regions where the effects of climate change on food availability are already apparent. It notes that the extent to which this alters nutrition depends greatly on local social systems. These include the ability to pay for higher-priced food, or to respond quickly to an impending famine with foreign imports. Any decline in food availability increases susceptibility to infectious diseases, as well as the rates of stunting, anaemia and cognitive impairment in children. A global temperature rise of just 1°C may drastically reduce yields of major crops (rice, maize, wheat) and result in a rapid increase in global food prices, further exacerbating food security problems.

The downstream effects

Detrimental impacts for human health arise as a result of environmental change. Of particular concern, the downstream effects of climate change on social systems exacerbate poverty and social inequality. Many of the subsequent health impacts have the greatest effects on poorer populations. Coastal populations and small island states are at particular risk of mass displacement caused by rising sea levels and worsening storms. Resource scarcity and forced mass migration are known to create the conditions necessary for violent conflict. The IPCC has noted that climate variability is often a large factor in promoting conflict, and that climate change will 'increasingly shape both conditions of security and national security policies.'

Major institutions in global health now recognise that the achievement of their mainstream development goals is likely to be impossible in the absence of action to address climate change.

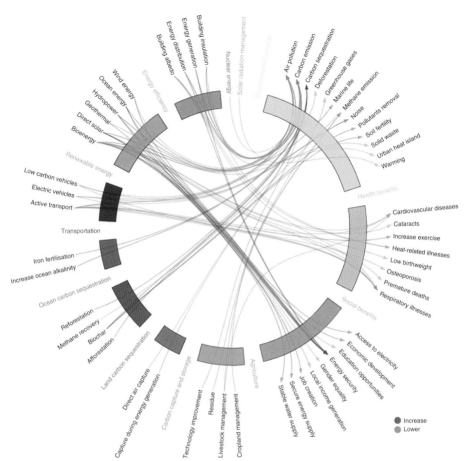

Figure 7.1.2 Frequently cited co-benefits of major mitigation techniques. *Red arrows* between a mitigation technology and an effect indicate that the technology will increase the effect; *green arrows* indicate the opposite trend. *(Redrawn from Watts N, Adger WN, Agnolucci P, et al: Health and climate change: policy responses to protect public health. Lancet 386:1861–1914, 2015.)*

Co-benefits of climate change mitigation

Avoidance of many current risks to health requires that global average temperatures are kept from rising more than 2°C. This means that total CO_2 emissions caused by human activity must be kept below 2900 billion tonnes (29 Gt CO_2). The reduced health care costs associated with the achievement of this carbon-reduction goal exceed the costs of the initial investment. The health co-benefits of climate mitigation are illustrated in **Fig. 7.1.2**.

Food and agriculture

In high-income countries, a shift to healthier diets rich in seasonal fruit and vegetables, combined with a reduction in red meat consumption, reduces rates of obesity, heart disease and colorectal cancer. Interventions aimed at encouraging these healthier diets have the added benefit of reducing carbon emissions from the agricultural system. In LIC, poor indoor air quality (often the result of poor household ventilation and unclean cooking stoves) is one of the largest environmental health risks faced by women and children. Policy interventions that follow the World Health

Organization (WHO) *Indoor Air Quality Guidelines for Household Fuel Combustion* by encouraging clean fuels and advanced-combustion cookstoves can both reduce the burden of disease on women and children and reduce emissions of black carbon (a short-lived climate pollutant).

My new stove

Mothers' Union of Rwatsinga Church is a grassroots community group in western Uganda, and one of many projects seeking to introduce clean cooking stoves throughout sub-Saharan Africa. Proviah feels that her stove has transformed life for her and her family.

'Before my new stove, I had many challenges. I used wood and dung from our goat to keep a fire alight for cooking in the centre of my house. The youngest of my three children was badly burnt three months ago on my open fire. The house was always black on the inside and it was hard to breathe when you entered. My husband has bad lungs and my family were always coughing—the community health worker said this is because of the fire.

The stove has changed my life. The Mothers' Union of Rwatsinga Church adapted the design of the stoves so that we could use fuel available in the local community. They then made stoves available to the poorest people and funded this activity through the cost savings resulting from reduced overall fuel requirements. I am so happy with my stove as I know it is safe for my children and it stays hot for so long. I spend much less time getting fuel, which means I have more time to do my other tasks and be with my children.'

Aston Baker Bagarukayo and Hope Bagarukayo (Uganda)

Electricity generation and clean air

Whilst fossil fuels have been historically important in providing energy to rapidly developing countries, the advent of cheap renewable energy now means that cleaner and healthier alternatives are available. Coal and diesel are major sources of CO_2 and damaging particulates ($PM_{2.5}$). They are often classified as carcinogens. Coal-fired power plants damage the cardiovascular and respiratory health of local communities by releasing these particulates into the atmosphere. Switching to cleaner sources of energy (i.e., wind power, solar power or hydropower) avoids these adverse health effects. They are readily available as microgrids for communities without reliable access to centralised electricity grids, and such low-carbon energy solutions are especially valuable for health care facilities in the remote rural areas of LIC.

Transport

The transport sector was responsible for 27% of global emissions (6.7 Gt CO_2) in 2010, and this proportion is expected to rise dramatically by 2050. Policies which encourage shifts away from cars towards walking and cycling provide a number of health benefits, whilst urban planning with good pedestrian access is associated with improvements in mental health and road safety. The detrimental health effects of local air pollution from motor vehicles contributes to the increasing rates of asthma, ischaemic heart disease and chronic obstructive lung disease. A shift to low-carbon fuel sources, coupled with healthy lifestyle changes, results in improved population health.

Health response to climate change

In many high-income countries, the health system may be an important contributor to national carbon emissions. Decreased carbon emissions can be attained through the application of currently available technologies. Alternative models of care which are less resource intensive include a strong emphasis on the availability of primary care, which decreases the reliance of the health system on hospitals and other tertiary centres.

Student advocacy in health sector fossil fuel divestment

The UK Fossil Free Health campaign encourages health organisations to divest themselves from their associations with fossil fuel organisations. Students have played a vital role throughout, and the campaign has had major successes.

Health organisations internationally acknowledge the need for radical climate change mitigation, on account of the health risks of inaction coupled with the co-benefits of lower-carbon energy for food and transport. Fossil fuel combustion drives climate change, and is also a major contributor to air pollution, responsible for one in eight premature deaths worldwide. There is a common perception that industry has spent huge sums of money attempting to subvert the scientific consensus on climate change, and in lobbying governments to reject or weaken environmental legislation. When confronted with a health threat of a similar magnitude, and an industry opposed to protective legislation, health organisations divested themselves from tobacco. This was crucial, as it stigmatised health-damaging business practices such that restrictive legislation became politically feasible. The fossil fuel divestment campaign seeks to bring similar pressure to bear to accelerate the transition to a lower-carbon energy system.

CAMPAIGN SUCCESSES

In 2014 the British Medical Association (BMA) was the first health organisation to vote in favour of divestment from fossil fuels. At the 2014 WHO Summit on Health and Climate, an international health sector coalition drew on this example to call divestment, and reinvestment in sustainable energy, a public health imperative. *Unhealthy Investments*, a report on fossil fuels, health and divestment copublished by a coalition of UK health charities, was reported extensively in the press.

STUDENT ACTION

The fossil fuel divestment movement began with student activism, and students have been integral to health sector successes. The UK Fossil Free Health campaign began as a collaboration between student group Healthy Planet UK and the health nongovernmental organisation Medact. Student advocacy at the BMA meeting in 2014 turned a niche financial issue into a key organising action for doctors concerned about climate change.

Alistair Wardrope (UK)

'People can feel helpless in the face of such a huge and overwhelming issue, but there is plenty that they can do – both as individuals and part of their organisations. These range from walking or cycling instead of using a car and taking care not to leave electrical appliances on standby, right up to carrying out a carbon audit, making sure environmental impact assessments become a routine part of all activities and developing a robust action plan. We in the health service are in a unique position to use the [health service's] immense influence and purchasing power to lead by example. If we do not act now, the consequences are unthinkable.'

Griffiths J and Stewart L, Sustaining a Healthy Future (FPH Guide)

The international policy response to climate change is housed within the negotiations of the UNFCCC. The UNFCCC has provided the forum for the world's governments to discuss and formulate a policy response to climate change. In 2016 the global response to the threats posed by climate change was strengthened when the 2015 Paris Agreement, signed by 197 parties, entered into force. This commits nations to undertake ambitious efforts to combat climate change and to adapt to its effects.

In the past 2 decades, the international health community has become increasingly involved in climate change policy formation, research and advocacy. The WHO has led the health policy response to climate change, working on a range of issues including the preparation of climate-ready health systems, the coordination of political engagement from a range of countries and actors, and close collaboration with the UNFCCC. However, this work is mostly limited to one department in the WHO, and there is an urgent need for greater financial and political support. The World Bank Group has recently implemented an impressive reform agenda to respond to this problem.

A thriving global research community supported by prominent universities and public health institutes is attempting to clarify the links between human health and global environmental change. This research has previously been focused on attempts to understand the impacts as well as the health co-benefits of climate change mitigation. Future work will seek to refine our understanding of the interactions between a wider range of sectors, including transport, agriculture and energy.

The Switch Off campaign

'The student Switch Off campaign is a nation-wide campaign which aims to encourage university students to reduce their carbon footprint, motivating students through inter-university competition. It advocates for simple changes such as not overfilling kettles, putting lids on saucepans and turning off lights or electrical appliances rather than leaving them on stand-by (hence the campaign's name).'

Lucinda Jones, UK

Conclusion

Urgent action to adapt to and mitigate the consequences of climate change is required. The health co-benefits of mitigation against climate change should prompt the health sector to take a leadership role. Whilst climate change is a global problem with global solutions, many of these will not be realised in the absence of local political support.

KEY POINTS

- Climate change impacts all sectors of activity as well as the environment.
- Social inequalities are a downstream impact of climate change as the poorest and most vulnerable populations are the most affected.
- Health co-benefits arising from mitigation against climate change are understated and undervalued.
- Advocacy, led by the WHO, for a climate and health perspective is gaining momentum and political traction.
- Health professionals play a crucial role in building local political support.

Further reading

Costello A, Abbas M, Allen A, et al: Managing the health effects of climate change: Lancet and University College London Institute for Global Health Commission, *Lancet* 373:1693–1733, 2009.

Friel S, Dangour AD, Garnett T, et al: Public health benefits of strategies to reduce greenhouse-gas emissions: food and agriculture, *Lancet* 374:2016–2025, 2009.

Intergovernmental Panel on Climate Change: Summary for policymakers. In Field CB, Barros VR, Dokken DJ, et al, editors: *Climate change 2014: impacts, adaptation, and vulnerability. Part A: global and sectoral aspects. Contribution of Working Group II to the Fifth Assessment Report of the Intergovernmental Panel on Climate Change*, Cambridge, 2014, Cambridge University Press, pp 1–32.

NHS Sustainable Development Unit: *Sustainable, resilient, healthy people & places: a sustainable development strategy for the NHS, public health and social care system*, Cambridge, 2014, NHS England and Public Health England.

Watts N, Adger N, Agnolucci P, et al: Health and climate change: policy responses to protect human health, *Lancet* 386:1861–1914, 2015.

7.2 Natural Disasters

Yassen Tcholakov (Canada)

Introduction

Disasters and the humanitarian response to disasters is a rapidly evolving field in global health. Unlike many areas, it has a very limited evidence-base because of the complexity of the issues it addresses. This environment fosters the innovation, quick thinking and passion that are crucial for successful outcomes.

Some initial definitions

Disasters are adverse events that overwhelm the response capacity (i.e., the resources available to a community to achieve its goals). An *emergency* is a serious set of events which can be resolved by use of the community's own response structures. Disasters can occur on a subnational, national or international level. According to the United Nations International Strategy for Disaster Reduction definition, disasters cause serious disruption to the functioning of a community or society as they involve widespread human, material, economic or environmental losses and impacts.

Disasters occur because of a preexistent *vulnerability* (i.e., the propensity to incur harm to certain populations, infrastructures or social structures). Vulnerability is not a characteristic of an event: it can differ from group to group and change over time. The opposite of vulnerability to a disaster (in this context) is *resilience*.

Hazards are events that have the potential to cause harm. A simple way of classifying hazards is to distinguish between *natural hazards* (such as earthquakes, storms and droughts) and *man-made hazards* (such as infrastructure failure, industrial incidents, civil conflict, war and terrorism). The *risk of a hazard* occurring is defined as the product of its likelihood of occurrence and the consequences expected. The relationship between hazards, vulnerabilities and disasters is shown in **Fig. 7.2.1**.

Disaster management

There are two ways in which health and disasters are linked. Firstly, most disasters have a significant impact on the health of the affected population. This can occur through direct injuries caused by the primary event or as a result of the subsequent failure of infrastructure, resulting in disease and psychological trauma.

The immediate aftermath of a disaster focuses on acute injuries, food and housing; many of the health impacts may not be revealed for months or years. These include mental health problems, an increase in gender violence and loss of ability to pay for health care. Refugee camps, a common requirement following a disaster, are cramped and lack access to shelter, food and water. This facilitates the spread of infectious diseases. Damage to both health facilities and transport infrastructure further compromises the availability of relief to those affected by a disaster. Other health-related challenges are posed by exposure to hazardous products such as toxins, radiation or biological hazards.

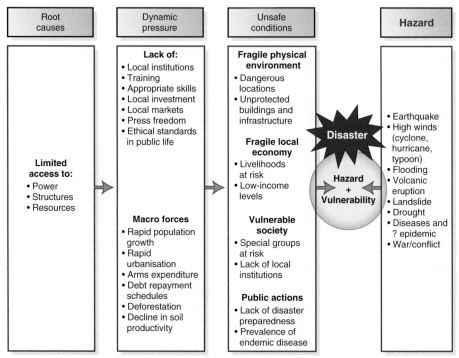

Figure 7.2.1   The causes of a disaster. *(Redrawn from Logistics Operational Guide: Intervention types, 2015. <http://log.logcluster.org/preparedness/intervention-types/index.html>.)*

Disaster management follows a four-phased approach, and health needs must be considered at each step of the process:

1. *Mitigation.* Mitigation is the process of reducing the risk of a hazard. This can be done both by reducing the likelihood of the hazard happening and by taking measures to diminish its consequences. Mitigation can scale down the hazard from a disaster level to that of an emergency. It may also prevent some hazards.

2. *Preparedness.* Preparedness refers to the process of planning how best to manage a potential hazard before it occurs. Once a hazard is evident, a speedy response with clear lines of communication is necessary to avoid confusion and error.

3. *Response.* Response involves the actions following a hazard that has occurred and whose goal is to limit loss and suffering.

4. *Recovery.* Recovery is the process of returning to the prehazard baseline following a disaster. Recovery can take from months to years. It can also serve as an opportunity for communities to strengthen their resilience in the hope of avoiding further disasters or, at least, limiting their consequences (**Fig. 7.2.2**).

Actors in disaster response

The response to disasters involves many individuals and organisations. These include national governments, nongovernmental organisations (NGOs) and international organisations (**Box 7.2.1**).

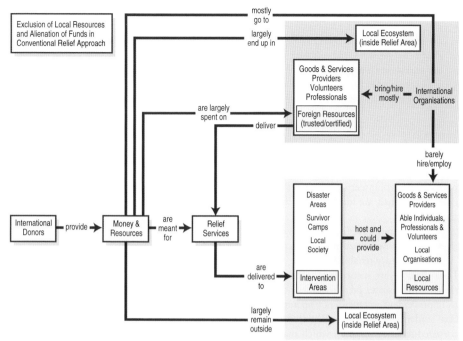

Figure 7.2.3 Exclusion of local resources and alienation of funds in conventional relief approach. *(Modified from Miranda Levy C: Entrepreneurial response: disaster relief with dignity, inclusion, generation and distribution of wealth. National University of Singapore, 2010. <https://www.changemakers.com/economicopportunity/entries/relief-20-enterprise>.)*

> *I come from Ethiopia. I had always wanted to engage in community development work, towards the betterment of the lives of children and women, but I also felt I was not equipped enough for the task. Therefore I decided to study "Community Well-being in Disaster and Development" at Northumbria University, UK. Here I met Martin Zuch, who also did the same course. He helped me to establish Give Hope Ethiopia, which is now helping hundreds of orphaned and vulnerable children recover from famine by training thousands of young people (with a focus on female high-school and tertiary-level students), and helping women to access finance and engage in income-generating activities to help them make their own money and restore their possessions and way of life.*
>
> **Tilahun Bekele Tesfaye, Director of Give Hope Ethiopia, Ethiopia**

Effective coordination is necessary in the processes which deliver longer-term recovery. Negative outcomes may ensue when these processes are hastily developed. For example, adequate urban planning, the building of resilient infrastructure and the building of resilient homes, are all time-consuming tasks that should be planned with care. The recovery phase also demands attention to specific areas, such as education provision, in pursuit of longer-term societal needs.

During the recovery period, chronic health conditions are a particular burden on the health system. Mental health issues are often poorly recognised and are also underfunded, whilst the provision of comprehensive mental health services is rarely a focus for international aid organisations. The incidence of severe mental illness doubles in the months following a mass disaster. For example, in the aftermath of Typhoon Haiyan in 2013, only two aid organisations, International Medical Corps and CBM (an international Christian disability and development organisation), were planning and providing specialist mental health services.

'I was supported by CBM to visit the Philippines and assess the need for international support in providing specialist mental health services to survivors in the Typhoon-affected areas. I found that the existing hard-pressed mental health services were, with few exceptions, highly centralised. This meant that for many, the only hope of treatment involved a long journey. The plan I recommended uses outside aid funds and a short burst of international training and project development expertise to create a model that would embed sessions of a local psychiatrist into clusters of the more remote municipalities affected by Typhoon Haiyan.'

Nick Rose, psychiatrist, UK

The role of health care professionals

Health care professionals should be equipped and ready for a local disaster, and many health care professionals volunteer to assist in the response to national and international disasters. Health care professionals are ideally placed to volunteer in national or regional disaster response efforts such as:

- provision of care (including psychosocial support)
- resource mobilisation (such as fundraising activities)
- community rehabilitation

Local health care institutions, especially in areas known to be prone to disasters, should offer training for disaster preparedness and health emergency management. Clinicians can contribute to improvement in emergency operation plans and to the training of local staff, including health care students. They are well placed to promote health equity by identifying the key areas of preparedness and response which may result in better outcomes for vulnerable groups.

'The recent increased threat of terrorism, coupled with the ever-present dangers posed by natural disasters and public health emergencies, clearly support the need to incorporate bioterrorism preparedness and emergency response material into the curricula of every health professional. A main barrier to health care preparedness in this country is a lack of coordination across the spectrum of public health and health care communities and disciplines. Ensuring a unified and coordinated approach to preparedness requires that benchmarks and standards be consistent across health care disciplines and public health, with the most basic level being education of health profession students.'

Markenson D, DiMaggio C and Redlener I, University of California

Conclusion

Disaster management and the subsequent humanitarian response is a rapidly evolving and complex multidisciplinary field. As climate change and conflict increase the likelihood of disasters, health care professionals and individuals with an interest in public and global health need to be familiar with the essential components of effective disaster management so that they can help to minimise adverse societal outcomes.

KEY POINTS

- Natural disasters have multiple systemic impacts which can affect health.
- There are four phases to disaster management: mitigation, preparedness, response and recovery.
- The health sector is intimately involved in all steps of disaster management and humanitarian response.
- Health care professionals face numerous challenges in emergency situations, including exposure to infectious disease, violence and long-term mental stress.

Further reading

Intergovernmental Panel on Climate Change: *Special report: managing the risks of extreme events and disasters to advance climate change adaptation*, Cambridge, 2012. Cambridge University Press.

United Nations Office for Disaster Risk Reduction: *Sendai framework for disaster risk reduction 2015-2030*, New York, 2015. United Nations. Available from: <http://www.unisdr.org/we/inform/publications/43291>.

World Health Organization: *Emergency response framework*, Geneva, 2013. World Health Organization.

7.3 Conflict and Health

Nazia Malik (UK)

'War is a direct threat to life. For millions of people world-wide, surviving war is the predominant objective in their daily existence.'
WHO Conflict and Health Working Paper Preventing Violent Conflict—The Search for Political Will, Strategies and Effective Tools, *Krusenberg, 19–20 June 2000.*

Introduction

Approximately 300 million people are currently affected in some way by armed conflict. This has a profound impact on the physical and mental health of both military combatants and civilians. The direct and indirect impact of violence is a leading cause of death and morbidity worldwide, and exceeds that of any other major disease. In recent years (**Fig. 7.3.1**), the magnitude and frequency of armed conflict have increased, leading to major crises in public health. Unfortunately, the health consequences of war are often overshadowed by underlying geopolitical issues and so fail to command public attention.

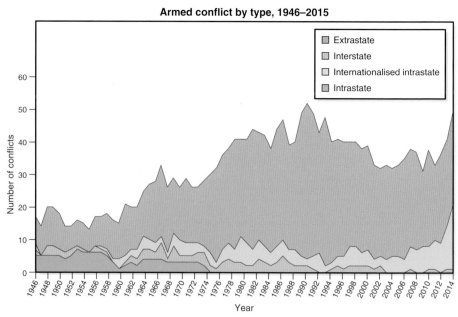

Figure 7.3.1 Global conflicts 1946–2014 showing a steady increase in conflict during this period. *(Re-drawn from Melander E, Pettersson T, Themnér L.: Organized violence, 1989-2015, J Peace Res 53(5):727–742, 2016.)*

TABLE 7.3.1 ▓ **Key terms used in discussing conflict**

Term	Description
Conflict	A state of serious disagreement based on conflicting 'needs, values or interests'
War	A form of armed conflict which occurs between two or more opposing sides. It is often rooted in politics where discord between opposing factions often involves protracted periods of violence with considerable casualties
Civil war	Armed conflict *within* a nation against governments or occupying forces
Terrorism	Politically motivated violence or the threat of violence, usually against civilians, with the intent to instil fear
Refugee	Individuals who cross borders into neighbouring countries to escape violence or the threat of armed conflict
Internally displaced persons	Individuals who are forced to flee their home but remain within the borders of their country and must adapt to this forced displacement
Combatants	Military personnel, child soldiers, prisoners of war and military peacekeepers
War stress	Any form of stressful exposure or experience that may have a psychological impact on an individual. Examples of war stresses include witnessing a war-related death or violence (bombardment, mutilation, firing of tanks and heavy artillery); having one's life threatened; torture; displacement; being forced to serve as a child soldier; being physically or sexually assaulted

Violence and instability created by conflict also carry significant longer-term consequences for health. For example, the collapse of health services and displacement of populations has an ongoing impact on health in affected areas. The survivors of war are left with physical and psychological scars which profoundly affect their quality of life, especially when individuals are left with chronic disabilities.

The key terms relevant to discussions regarding war, conflict and terrorism are defined in **Table 7.3.1**.

How does conflict affect health?

The immediate and ongoing health needs created by conflict are similar to those created by natural disasters. The effects of both disasters and conflicts on populations include death, disability and displacement. Despite their similarities, the 'political complexities' of conflict intensify the health and protection needs of civilian populations. Armed conflict affects the health of military personnel directly involved in combat as well as that of noncombatants, including refugees and internally displaced people.

Mortality

An estimated 191 million people were killed as a direct or indirect consequence of war during the 20th century. An increasing number of violent war-related deaths occur amongst innocent bystanders who may have been caught in crossfire or specifically targeted during conflict. These include health care workers specifically targeted by military forces (**Fig. 7.3.2**).

The causes of death attributable to conflict are outlined in **Fig. 7.3.3**. Another example of death as a result of conflict is demonstrated by the civil conflict in Darfur, where 5.9 to 9.3 deaths per 10,000 people occurred per day, and 68% to 93% were attributed solely to the violent nature of the conflict.

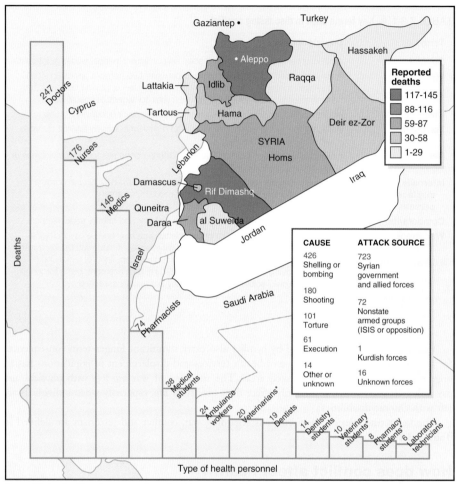

Figure 7.3.2 Profile of a war crime: health workers killed in the Syrian conflict, 2011–16. *(Redrawn from Fouad FM, Sparrow A, Tarakji A, et al: (2017) Health workers and the weaponisation of health care in Syria: a preliminary inquiry for The Lancet–American University of Beirut Commission on Syria, Lancet 390(10111):2516–2526, 2017.)*

The lives of civilian populations are threatened by the indirect consequences of war, such as malnutrition, infectious disease and diminished public health services. These may cause more death and disability than the direct injuries caused by conflict. Increases in the mortality rates of infants and children younger than 5 years reflect specifically how these factors affect the health of children.

Morbidity

War is also directly responsible for a growing number of serious physical and psychological disorders. One important public health concern is the rising threat of communicable diseases such as polio. The WHO has reported that polio eradication faces major challenges in all

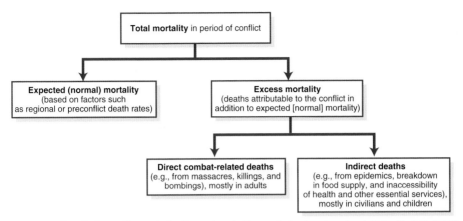

Figure 7.3.3 **Deaths in conflict periods.** *(Reproduced with permission from Leaning J, Guha-Sapir D. (2013) Natural disasters, armed conflict, and public health. N Engl J Med 369(19):1839, 2013.)*

countries affected by armed conflict. During the Iraq War, for example, one-fifth of children failed to receive neonatal polio immunisation, and similar failures of vaccination programmes against malaria and tuberculosis have occurred in countries affected by conflict. Conflict destabilises society and hampers international efforts against communicable disease, particularly in sub-Saharan Africa.

Frontline violence, roadside bombings and drone attacks leave many innocent bystanders with injuries requiring urgent medical and surgical attention. In conflict zones, the rates of amputations vastly exceed preconflict rates, and surgical admissions outweigh the capacity of hospitals.

The indirect impact of conflict on health

Armed conflict has a subtle indirect impact on health care in two ways: it diverts limited resources away from health services and damages the infrastructure supporting these services. Before an armed conflict, governments may redirect valuable health resources to favour military expenditure. This diverts funding from urgent public health work, and the discrepancy between investment in health and military spending may be extreme. For example, in 1991, Iraq cut its health budget by 90% in preparation for the impending Gulf War. This lack of resources resulted in avoidable deaths.

The health infrastructure is often a target of war. In addition to damage to health facilities, homes and roads are destroyed and access to safe food, water and shelter is suddenly limited. This accounts for much of the indirect morbidity and mortality in civilian populations. The insecurity associated with displacement means that individuals are particularly vulnerable to death and disability as an indirect consequence of war. Following the Iraq Gulf War and the subsequent 12 years of economic sanctions, most of the estimated 350,000 preventable child deaths were due to malnutrition, contaminated water and inaccessible health care. Additionally, the recovery of vital health care infrastructure was hampered by the prewar diversion of resources.

Conflict and the effect on health care workers

Conflict results in a decrease in the availability of health care professionals, which may be exacerbated by the direct targeting of health care workers by the warring parties. Violations of human rights are frequently ignored as the care of those acutely injured is prioritised.

TABLE 7.3.2 ■ Jordanian national health indicators 2013–14

Indicator	2013 without Syrians (6.4 million)	2014 with Syrians (8 million)
Physicians per 10,000 population	28.6	23.4
Dentists per 10,000 population	10.4	8.5
Nurses (all categories) per 10,000 population	44.8	36.6
Pharmacists per 10,000 population	17.8	14.5
Hospital beds per 10,000 population	18	15.1
Hospital beds per 10,000 population in Mafraq	8	6
Coverage by health care services (%)	98	90 (estimated)

Data from Musa T Ajlouini. The impact of Syrian refugees on the Jordanian health sector: 2014 (Slide 29).

Syrian refugees and Jordan's health sector

The Syrian civil war has become one of the worst humanitarian crises of the 21st century. More than nine million people have been internally displaced or have fled across borders to neighbouring states. Jordan currently hosts 1.38 million Syrians (20% of its population). A minority of these displaced individuals have relocated to purpose-built refugee camps such as the Zaatari camp. This camp houses more than 120,000 Syrian refugees, and is currently the second largest refugee camp in the world. The remaining 83% of displaced individuals have taken up housing in urban centres, placing an unprecedented pressure on these communities for education and health care services (**Table 7.3.2**). This has dangerously overstretched resources, and has affected the stability of the country. Health care facilities are short of workers and medicines, and long-eradicated diseases such as poliomyelitis have recurred.

As a medical student, my clinical experience has involved the care of refugees from war. I have therefore focused on communicable diseases that were previously scarce among the local population. A huge rise in demand for surgical procedures has resulted from amputations, burns and acute surgical conditions. The conflict has placed a heavy burden on the Syrian people and the host communities in which they reside. Jordan needs more help from the international community and donor governments, as the country can no longer bear the financial and social impacts alone. Support should be focused on longer-term partnerships until the displaced are able to return to their homes.

Yazan Mousa (Jordan)

The psychological impact of conflict

Soldiers and civilians are exposed to traumatising war stress, and the psychological scars of conflict are often the hardest to treat. Women and children are at the greatest risk of ongoing mental health issues following exposure to war. Violence also has indirect consequences on mental health long after a war is over. Such violence, during and after armed conflict, is frequently targeted at women in the form of domestic and sexual violence, resulting in depression, anxiety and suicidal thoughts. Rape is also used as a weapon of war. During the conflict in Bosnia and Herzegovina, military personnel mercilessly raped more than 10,000 women. In Palestine, where most living generations have known only conflict, children grow up with a dangerously prolonged exposure to violence, and this undermines civil society.

Posttraumatic stress disorder (PTSD) is an anxiety disorder which develops as a consequence of a severely stressful or distressing incident. PTSD commonly occurs following conflict, and affects civilians as well as military personnel. Psychosomatic disorders also commonly occur after a war, and may be difficult to evaluate on account of their nonspecific symptoms. The WHO recognises that mental health services are an integral component of public health programmes in the postconflict recovery phase in developing countries. Such programmes should be designed in accordance with community needs, taking into account cultural frameworks for mental health.

Conflict and mental health in Liberia: 'The crazy people's friend'

Almost half of the adult population experienced posttraumatic stress disorder (PTSD) following a brutal civil war in Liberia, a country with only one resident psychiatrist. One study found that 44% of the adult population suffered from PTSD and 40% experienced major depressive disorder.

Between 1989 and 2003 a civil war in Liberia left more than 250,000 people dead. Almost one million Liberians fled to neighbouring countries, whilst those remaining lacked basic health amenities. Individuals with mental health disorders were stigmatised, and only 1% of the population had access to mental health services.

In 2012 *The Guardian* published the story of 33-year-old Dakemue Kollie, the sole survivor of his family following the civil war. With the support and training of Doctors of the World, he would travel upwards of 200 km a day on his motorbike treating and counselling mental health patients in rural villages. He was known as *the crazy people's friend*, and was inspired to change minds and promote mental health in his native land.

Rockie Kang (Canada)

Twenty-first century threats

The threats of conflict are changing as weaponry and defence systems have become more sophisticated and destructive. Some states now possess armaments sometimes referred to as *dirty bombs*. These include biological, chemical, nuclear or radiological weapons as powerful as the atomic bomb used in 1945 against Japan. Many countries have accumulated massive stockpiles of nuclear warheads as part of their defence portfolio (**Fig. 7.3.4**).

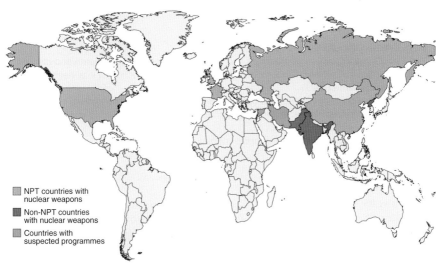

NPT countries with nuclear weapons

Non-NPT countries with nuclear weapons

Countries with suspected programmes

Figure 7.3.4 **The international nuclear family.** Map showing countries with confirmed and suspected nuclear weapons programmes. *NPT,* Nonproliferation Treaty. *(Redrawn from The Economist: Gunning for Trident, 2010. <http://www.economist.com/node/17151137>.)*

Massive attacks using sophisticated bombs are a major threat to global peace, especially on account of constant threats by politically motivated terrorist organisations. Landmines deployed in previous conflicts remain a constant health threat in areas where they have not been systematically cleared. Signatories to the Ottawa Treaty (1997) agreed that they will not produce, stockpile or trade in antipersonnel mines, but 35 countries, including the United States, Russia and China, are not signatories to this treaty.

Challenges in post-conflict recovery

Postconflict recovery, in the context of health, is compromised on account of any failure to comprehend the full extent of damage and the extensive rebuilding of hospitals and services required to meet the unprecedented health needs of the remaining population. The collapse of vital registration systems and high population mobility inevitably conceal the true extent of damage. The absence of timely information means that the aid response is often inadequate and, during this postconflict phase, when health care capacity is at its lowest, health needs are at their highest.

The influx of external agencies which commonly form a significant part of emergency relief initiatives may compromise and further destabilise the provision of health care when multiple parallel systems of health care are established. The abrupt departure of these relief services leaves patients without follow-up care, and is an ongoing burden on the recovering health system. The resolution of administrative and transitional issues is key to addressing the health needs of civilian populations moving on to a postconflict society.

Conclusion

Conflict affects the morbidity, mortality and general well-being of military combatants and civilian noncombatants both physically and psychologically. The health impact of war is commonly ignored or inadequately addressed. Health professionals should aim to prevent or minimise the indirect as well as the direct impacts of armed conflict on health.

KEY POINTS

- Wars threaten the stability of society.
- War has a huge impact on combatants and noncombatants. It causes death and disability as a direct result of violence and, indirectly, owing to the destruction of vital health-supporting infrastructure.
- The psychological consequences of conflict are extensive and long-standing.
- Public health services are neglected during conflict as funding is diverted towards military initiatives.
- Terrorist activities and dirty bombs represent new societal threats.

Further reading

Sidel VW, Levy BS: War, terrorism, and public health, *J Law Med Ethics* 31(4):516–523, 2003.
Sidel VW, Levy BS: *War and public health*, New York, 2007, Oxford University Press.
World Health Organization: *Mental health and emergencies: mental and social aspects of health of populations exposed to extreme stressors*, Geneva, 2003, World Health Organization. Available from: <http://www.who.int/mental_health/emergencies/MSDMER03_01/en/>.

7.4 Food and Agriculture

Guendalina Anzolin (Italy)   Samantha Pegoraro (Italy)

Introduction

Food production, nutrition and health are closely linked. Health professionals and health-focused NGOs have a responsibility to promote policies which increase the availability and access to food.

Defining food

Undernourishment, commonly interpreted as hunger, is defined by the Food and Agriculture Organization (FAO) as a condition in which the 'dietary energy consumption is continuously below a minimum dietary energy requirement for maintaining a healthy life and carrying out a light physical activity.' Undernourishment can hugely affect a patient's general health and reduces their resilience to illness. Undernourishment occurs as a result of an individual's lack of accessibility to food, whilst *food insecurity* refers to a community or a region's lack of accessibility to food. The FAO (1996) defined food security as 'when all people at all times have access to sufficient, safe, nutritious food to maintain a healthy and active life.' Food security is based both on the availability and accessibility of food and on *food stability*, the ability for communities to obtain adequate food over time. This concept implies that government policies are required to protect the population from market and food availability fluctuations. Major risks to food security include population growth, fossil fuel dependence, land use change and climate change.

The term *food sovereignty* refers to a population's 'right to healthy and culturally appropriate food produced through ecologically sound and sustainable methods, and their right to define their own food and agriculture systems' (Declaration of Nyéléni, 2007). The term emerged from the La Via Campesina movement, which is an organisation of farmers, peasants and landless workers' movements with more than 200 million combined members in 73 countries. It promotes the adoption of democratic agricultural policies and aims to benefit consumers and small-scale producers to ensure local access to food and greater social justice. This movement developed as a response to the growing concept of food security which focused only on food accessibility and gave little importance to how and where food is produced. Food sovereignty proponents want to halt the progression of trade liberalisation where food is involved.

Food sovereignty is a matter of freedom of choice. Proponents of food sovereignty uphold the right of people and communities to define their food and agricultural policies, in contrast to a market-driven production. Measures to implement food sovereignty can occur at personal, local community, and national and international levels (**Fig. 7.4.1**).

Lack of food availability is commonly associated with famine-affected areas, and results in undernourishment and illness. However, according to the Indian economist and philosopher Amartya Sen, famine is not solely the result of the lack of food availability. Food security and food sovereignty are strongly linked to the political, social and economic factors which influence the right and the entitlement to nourishment.

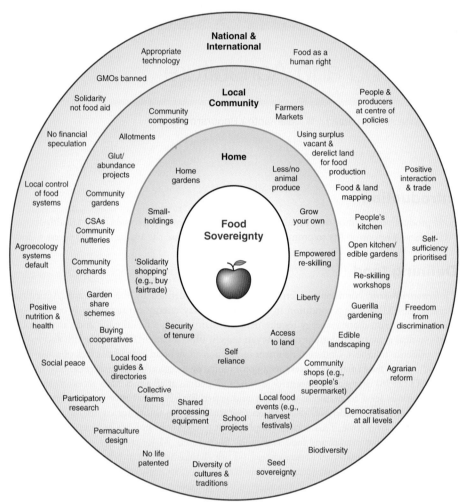

Figure 7.4.1 Designing for food sovereignty. *CSAs,* Community-supported agriculture farms. *GMOs,* genetically modified organisms. *(Redrawn from Gaia University: <http://portfolios.gaiauniversity.org/view/view.php?id=637>.)*

> 'I attempted to see famines as broad "economic" problems (concentrating on how people can buy food, or otherwise get entitled to it), rather than in terms of the grossly undifferentiated picture of aggregate food supply for the economy as a whole.'
>
> **Amartya Sen, India**

Food safety concerns all policies and regulations aimed at avoiding potential food-related pathologies. The 2011 *Escherichia coli* 0104:H4 outbreak in Germany was a food safety issue. This outbreak affected 3965 people and caused 54 deaths. It exemplified the importance of establishing effective food standards to protect the public from the risks of eating contaminated food. National and international organisations such as the US Environmental Protection Agency and the European Food Safety Authority together with governments, institutes and research centres have a responsibility to ensure food safety.

Eat the Rich—a student-led bottom-up experience: from food poverty to food sovereignty

Italian students in Bologna set up a canteen providing high-quality organic food as a reaction to the expensive and unhealthy food available in their local area. This enabled their local community to access healthy locally produced food for the cost of a donation.

Food poverty is a growing phenomenon. In Italy in 2013, a group of students, recent graduates and workers initiated an alternative way to eat high-quality food inexpensively. Eat the Rich is the first self-managed canteen in Bologna. The aim is to provide access to high-quality food for all and to become an alternative community mechanism that can be exported and reproduced across Italy.

The canteen is located in the city centre, and is open on Wednesdays for lunch. The price is by donation so as to be as inclusive as possible. Anyone can volunteer to help out to serve the 'social meal'. Local producers who are committed to produce high-quality organic food are also members of the project provide the ingredients. Eat the Rich is now trying to recreate similar experiences elsewhere in Italy with the hope of raising awareness about food poverty and bottom-up solutions. Furthermore, it strives to utilise its new network of farmers, students and community associations to advocate, at a political level, an equitable food system.

Samantha Pegoraro (Italy)

Malnutrition: beyond just a lack of food

Malnutrition is one of the main causes of child death in LIC and middle-income countries. It refers to the deprived state the body develops when it does not receive an adequate amount of proteins, vitamins, minerals and nutrients. It can also be defined as the insufficient, excessive or imbalanced consumption of food. A malnourished state may occur both in undernutrition and overnutrition situations.

Malnutrition kills more people every year than AIDS, malaria and tuberculosis combined. In 2012 there were 165 million stunted children under 5 years of age, worldwide (WHO/UNICEF/WB 2012). Of these, 56% lived in Asia and 36% in Africa. At the same time, 44 million children younger than 5 years were overweight, and 37% lived in resource-poor countries. Poor nutrition causes 45% of deaths in children younger than 5 years (2.6 million children each year).

NGOs and international institutions have prioritised the fight against malnutrition on account of the catastrophic effects it has both on affected children and on society. Tangible responses include the provision of ready-to-use therapeutic foods, which are energy dense and are enriched with specific minerals and vitamins. An example of this is Plumpy'Nut, a peanut-based paste. It provides high energy and can be given to a child whatever his or her degree of malnourishment.

'In my clinic, we see children every day who need more nutrition. Many have malaria, diarrhoea or a chronic disease that they do not have the strength to fight. So many lives have been saved through Plumpy'Nut; in just 6 weeks the child is unrecognisable, and clinic figures suggest ~9/10 severely malnourished children who are given Plumpy'Nut alongside condition-specific treatment recover. Children like the taste and find it easy to digest and it doesn't need special storage or to be mixed with water to swallow (clean water is hard to access in my local community). The only challenge is turning away those who are only 'moderately' malnourished and don't meet the funding criteria for Plumpy'Nut – parents are always very distressed.'

Anonymous community health worker, Niger

Political efforts to combat malnutrition include the Global Alliance for Improved Nutrition (GAIN), created in 2002 by the Special Session of the UN General Assembly on Children. GAIN has been the pioneer in creating a new partnership model which includes the active participation of the private sector in collaboration with governments, international agencies, academic institutions and civil society organisations. This alliance involves more than 600 companies in 30 countries and has created more than 50 multisectorial partnerships. GAIN's immediate primary objective is to feed nutritious food to 1.3 billion people by 2017.

In 2014 the WHO estimated that 1.9 billion adults (39% of the world's adult population) were overweight and 600 million were obese. Except for famine-stricken countries, overweight and obesity are globally responsible for more deaths than undernutrition. This is a massive health burden on the populations in these countries, and is thought to be one of the most serious 'epidemics' of modern times. Obesity is a major risk factor for both noncommunicable diseases (NCDs) and musculoskeletal disorders—a major cause of disability. LMIC are now facing a 'double burden' of disease. They face 'traditional' global health issues (i.e., infectious diseases and undernutrition), but NCDs are surging in prevalence as a result of dietary changes and physical inactivity. Health professionals can help to communicate the importance of healthy living to their populations.

Transnational food and beverage companies, such as Coca-Cola, Nestlé and PepsiCo, are now responding to the WHO *Global Strategy on Diet, Physical Activity and Health* by supporting healthy lifestyle programmes in resource-poor countries. The main objective of the strategy is to curb and prevent obesity as well as chronic diseases. The strategy states that food and beverage companies need to limit the amounts of saturated fats, *trans*-fatty acids, free sugar and salt in their products. There is, however, an obvious potential conflict of interest for companies as they also directly contribute to global malnutrition and the double burden of disease in resource-poor countries by selling sugary drinks and unhealthy foods.

The 2008 global food crisis

'We allow multinational food corporations and speculators to decide every day who is eating and living, and who is starving and dying.'

Jean Siegler, UN Special Rapporteur on the Right to Food (2012)

In 2008 the world experienced the worst food crisis since the 1970s. The price of commodities, such as wheat, maize and rice, suddenly doubled (**Fig. 7.4.2**), leading to a surge in the number of undernourished people and in food insecurity across regions. The crisis affected most of sub-Saharan African and South Asian countries.

This global food crisis was caused by a synergy between short-term and long-term factors. These factors included:

Short-term factors
- increased speculation in commodity futures markets
- drought-induced crop failure
- the surge in biofuel production

Long-term factors
- population growth
- lack of proper food security policies
- climate change
- trade liberalisation causing export-oriented agriculture focus, and a high dependency on imported foods and the international market

Commodity futures have traditionally been viewed by investors as stable assets, and thus were largely ignored by speculators. Commodity index speculation increased by 1900% between 2003 and 2008, from US$13 billion to US$260 billion. Higher investments increased commodity indexes, and this, in turn, increased consumer food prices. This situation has been described by Jean Ziegler, UN Special Rapporteur for the Right to Food, as a 'man-made' disaster and 'a massive mass murder'.

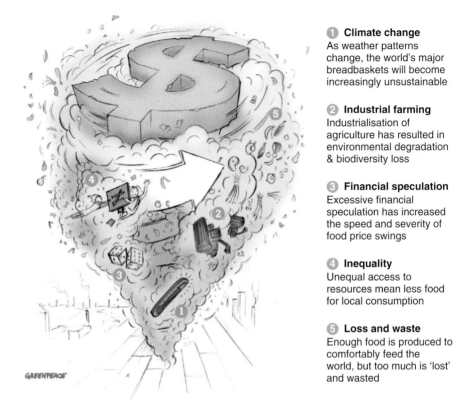

① Climate change
As weather patterns change, the world's major breadbaskets will become increasingly unsustainable

② Industrial farming
Industrialisation of agriculture has resulted in environmental degradation & biodiversity loss

③ Financial speculation
Excessive financial speculation has increased the speed and severity of food price swings

④ Inequality
Unequal access to resources mean less food for local consumption

⑤ Loss and waste
Enough food is produced to comfortably feed the world, but too much is 'lost' and wasted

Figure 7.4.2 **The causes of spiralling food prices.** *(Reproduced with permission from Greenpeace: Causes of the food crisis, 2016. <http://www.greenpeace.org/international/en/multimedia/photos/Causes-of-the-food-crisis/>.)*

At the same time, the need for cheaper energy meant that biofuel production was massively increased. The resulting diversion of more than 120 million tons of cereal from human consumption, enough to feed more than 350 million people for a year, may have resulted in the 75% increase in global food prices (World Bank, unpublished data). Other factors contributing to the increase in food prices included population growth, the reduction in agricultural subsidies and overfishing in many parts of the world.

Risks of population growth

The global population will likely reach 9.6 billion inhabitants by 2050 (**Fig. 7.4.3**). By 2028 both India and China, the two most populated countries in the world, are projected to have 1.45 billion residents each. This increase in population has important consequences for global food supply. Whilst current global food production is adequate for the entire world population, inequalities force 800 million people to be undernourished, whilst 600 million are obese. For example, Mexico is the country with the highest percentage of obesity (37.5% of adult women), and many programmes have been developed to palliate this epidemic. On the other hand, the country has implemented a national programme to fight undernutrition as 7.4 million Mexicans are living in extreme poverty and lack access to adequate nutrition.

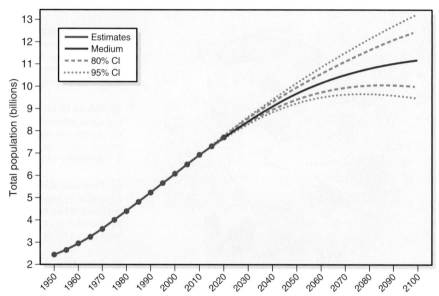

Figure 7.4.3 World population prospects. Population of the world: estimates, 1950–2015, medium-variant projection and 80% and 95% confidence intervals, 2015–2100. *CI*, Confidence interval. *(Redrawn from United Nations, Department of Economic and Social Affairs, Population Division: World population prospects: the 2015 revision, New York, 2015, United Nations.)*

The most populated countries are LMIC in which national living standards are improving rapidly. This development has resulted in a major increase in demand for quality food and meat. Meat consumption has more than doubled in the past 50 years, and this has significantly contributed to the increase in greenhouse gas emissions, adversely affecting climate change. A 30% reduction in meat consumption per capita would reduce the prevalence of heart diseases by approximately 16% in the city of São Paolo (Brazil) and by 15% in the United Kingdom. Some countries, such as China, are especially vulnerable to climate change from a food security perspective. China needs to feed 20% of the world population with just one-tenth of the worldwide arable land.

Population growth and food-quality: is China ready?

China is a country which has undergone rapid and dramatic population growth. It faces serious challenges regarding the sustainability of its national food security as a result of geography and previous land exploitation.

In 2002 China became a net exporter of food as a result of aggressive policies aimed at achieving food security. The country is now the world's largest importer of food. China needs to feed 20% of the global population, but only 10% of the country's land is arable. In April 2014 a government report stated that 20% of its arable land was polluted because of industrial and agricultural activities such as irrigation with polluted water and improper use of pesticides. This resulted from inadequate environmental laws, a lack of proper irrigation infrastructure and poor popular education on environmental sustainability.

Eight in 10 Chinese people connect the word *security* with food. There is a firm belief that there is no safe food in China, and there is an increasing demand for 'safe' imported foods.

Yiyou, a student in Shanghai, highlights the change in values of the Chinese youth: 'Most of the people, especially young generations, see food as the most urgent issue for China.' She is calm but visibly disappointed: 'there has been rapid economic progress in the past 15 years but no one knows the costs it passed on to future generations in terms of climate change and food security.' Yiyou, as many other youths in China, is concerned about the future of food in China. She firmly believes that youth movements are, and will be, a key actor in pressuring national governments to think of long-term food security strategies, as they are the people most directly affected by these detrimental short-term actions.

Guendalina Anzolin (Italy)

Food and agriculture: a governance matter

The food and agriculture landscape is considerably impacted by global policy. Policymakers have largely agreed that climate change is anthropogenic and that climate sustainability is a collective responsibility. Agenda 21 is an action programme adopted by many states (though not the United States) at the UN Conference on Environment and Development, held in Rio de Janeiro in 1992. It is a pillar of the sustainable development approach, and includes the statement that 'adjustments are needed in agricultural, environmental and macroeconomic policy, at both national and international levels, in developed as well as developing countries, to create the conditions for sustainable agriculture and rural development (SARD). The major objective of SARD is to increase food production in a sustainable way and enhance food security.'

The Future We Want, a document approved in 2012 at the Rio+20 conference, contains an implementation road map of Agenda 21, but remains nonbinding. At Rio+20, great attention was drawn to the SDGs, and voluntary commitments by countries were undertaken regarding agricultural policies. Moreover, the involvement of civil society organisations strengthened the involvement and impact of grassroots approaches in the decision-making processes.

> *'In general, a great challenge in the next decades is to force policymakers to allow a level playing field for agriculture and food trade. In many cases progress can be made only by breaking conflicts of interests and forcing all policymakers to give up part of the national or private interests. Many rural farmers can organize themselves to achieve political representation and make their voices heard. In developed countries, a new concept of food, with improved quality and decreasing quantities, is becoming more interesting to the public. More attention is likely to be paid to the ethical origin and the content of food. Awareness is growing with regard to food waste and food distribution too.'*
> **Enrico Labriola, former Food and Agriculture Organization and World Food Programme consultant (2014)**

Land grabbing: essential step or violation of human rights?

'Now no land, no farm, no food'

Local woman in West Nigeria

The term *land grabbing* indicates the buying or leasing of land in developing countries by governments, individuals or domestic and international companies. The issue has gained significant attention following the 2007–08 world food crisis as deregulation enabled easier large-scale land acquisitions. Arguments in favour of these massive land investments included a commitment to develop coveted areas which have been defined by organisations such as the World Bank as empty, marginal or degraded. Land grabbing is both a new form of capital accumulation and a method to accumulate foreign political power.

Political and corporate interests have often overruled the respect of human rights and priorities of local populations for financial profit or political gains. Land grabbing is a clear threat to some of the most important human rights: the right to own the land where people have lived for generations and the right to adequate food and water. For many resource-poor countries, subsistence farming is one of the only means of living, especially in rural areas. Land grabbing, for these communities, causes financial as well as food insecurity.

In Cambodia, dubbed the *land of the smiles*, 90% of the population does not own the land on which they work. In 2001 a new land law was passed with the objective of protecting poverty-stricken communities. It recognised that inhabitants no longer were required to hold official documentation of land ownership to officially claim ownership of a piece of land. Unfortunately, this law was never enacted, and in 2007 some former senior military officers made land claims that resulted in many villagers being displaced because of the lack of official documentation on ownership rights. It is estimated that around 400,000 Cambodians have been affected by land concessions since 2003.

Addressing the land-grabbing issue is a necessity to protect basic rights. It enables developing countries to ensure food security and protect themselves from foreign influence and resource mismanagement.

Local action to improve nutrition

Whilst many of the challenges relating to food security need to be tackled at national and international levels, many of the most effective programmes tackling food poverty act locally. For example, the Trussell Trust provides food banks offering emergency food supplies to those in need from local churches across the United Kingdom. It estimates that more than 900,000 individuals accessed its supplies in 2013–14, an increase which it attributes to low income and welfare problems.

A similar programme is run by churches in western Uganda, where more 80% of the local population are farmers. Every Sunday, all members of the church offer 10% of their produce to the church (a tithe). Some of this food is then sold back to members of the church by auction. This increases the variety of food available to the congregation, and any remaining food or profit is given to the most deprived members of the community.

Examples of successful initiatives undertaken by students to improve nutrition in their local populations include:

- establishment of healthy eating opportunities in their university canteen
- improvement in the nutritional status of meals provided in the local school
- promotion of a healthy eating and living campaign in the local community
- creation of a student vegetable garden
- establishment of local 'food cycling' of food reaching its 'sell-by date', or 'meals on wheels' schemes providing fresh food for those who are housebound or unable to cook and shop for themselves

Conclusion

Issues regarding food and agriculture are directly linked to population health. The establishment of food security is an important international challenge. Academic institutions, health professionals and civil society should be advocates for the right to food whilst promoting good nutritional practices. Land-grabbing practices compromise the well-being of disadvantaged communities, and there remains a need to change our current food and agricultural structures to a more sustainable model.

KEY POINTS

- Food production and health are closely interrelated societal challenges.
- Food security may be compromised by political considerations.
- Sustainable food production is especially challenging in the face of a rapidly increasing global population.
- Good governance in food and agriculture is essential for a healthy society.

Further reading

Food and Agriculture Organization of the United Nations, International Fund for Agricultural Development, World Food Programme: *The state of food insecurity in the world 2014. Strengthening the enabling environment for food security and nutrition*, Rome, 2014, Food and Agriculture Organization of the United Nations.

La Via Campesina: *Declaration of Nyéléni*, 2007. <https://viacampesina.org/en/declaration-of-nyi/>.

Smith P, Bustamante M, Ahammad H, et al: Agriculture, forestry and other land use (AFOLU). In Edenhofer O, Pichs-Madruga R, Sokona Y, et al, editors: *Climate change 2014: mitigation of climate change. Contribution of Working Group III to the Fifth Assessment Report of the Intergovernmental Panel on Climate Change*, Cambridge, 2014, Cambridge University Press.

World Health Organization, UNICEF, World Bank: *Levels and trends in child malnutrition*, WHO/UNICEF/WB, 2012.

World Health Organization: *Obesity and overweight. Fact sheet no311*, 2016. <http://www.who.int/mediacentre/factsheets/fs311/en/>.

7.5 Urbanisation and Transport

Angeli Guadalupe (Philippines)

Introduction

The first year during which more than half of the world's population lived in urban areas was 2007, and by 2050, it is projected that 66% of the global population will be living in cities. Up to 90% of the future population growth will occur in the cities of LMIC. One-third of city dwellers reside in slum conditions due to the high inflow of poor rural residents.

The definition of *urban areas* differs. In Australia, urban areas (or *urban centres*) are defined as population clusters of 1000 inhabitants or more with a density of at least 200 inhabitants per square kilometre. In contrast, the definition of urban areas in China is a city or town with a population density greater than 1500 inhabitants per square kilometre. The United Nations defines urban areas as settlements that are considered to be 'urban' by the national statistical agencies. Urbanisation is the process whereby a rural area has transitioned to a more urban society (**Fig. 7.5.1**).

Urbanisation has been promoted by improved access to educational and employment opportunities in cities. The increased availability of services and economic opportunities (**Table 7.5.1**) has accelerated migration from rural areas. It can be challenging to provide medical services in a rural setting, because the drivers which affect population migration also affect the availability of health care professionals. The lack of health facilities in rural areas also encourages migration to cities.

The challenge of recruiting health care professionals in rural India

The lack of health care facilities in rural environments discourages workers, including health professionals, from accepting positions there.

Indian cities are well provided with hospitals and clinics. There is a severe shortage of doctors in rural areas, where 76% of India's population resides. I work in a rural mission hospital in western India. It is 10 km from the nearest shop and 60 km from the railway station. It offers basic outpatient and inpatient facilities, and home-based HIV/AIDS and palliative care services. This facility is run by a single doctor and one staff nurse.

Common reasons for the reluctance to serve in rural areas include poor access to training and the latest technological medical advances and low salaries. Other disincentives include the lack of work opportunities for spouses and educational facilities for children. However, working in a rural area provides a sense of fulfilment and self-satisfaction through selfless service to the marginalised.

Health care professional (anon.)

Urbanisation as an environmental stressor

Air pollution is a major cause of morbidity and death because of the increased risk of cardiovascular and pulmonary diseases. In developing countries, roughly 130,000 premature deaths and 60 million cases of pulmonary disease occur every year because of urban air pollution.

Emissions of particulate matter and ozone pose the greatest risks to health. In Mexico City, it is estimated that 75% of the ambient air pollution is due to motor-vehicle exhaust. Tobacco

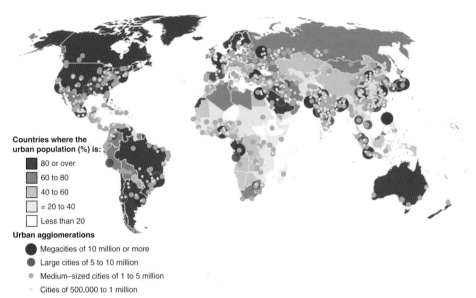

**Countries where the
urban population (%) is:**

- 80 or over
- 60 to 80
- 40 to 60
- = 20 to 40
- Less than 20

Urban agglomerations

- ● Megacities of 10 million or more
- ● Large cities of 5 to 10 million
- ● Medium–sized cities of 1 to 5 million
- Cities of 500,000 to 1 million

Figure 7.5.1 Percentage and locations of urban agglomerations with at least 500,000 inhabitants (2014). The designations used and the presentation of the material on this map do not imply the expression of any opinion whatsoever on the part of the Secretariat of the United Nations concerning the legal status of any country, territory, city or area of its authorities, or concerning the delimitation of its frontiers or boundaries. *(Redrawn from World urbanisation prospects, 2014 version. <esa.un.org>.)*

TABLE 7.5.1 ■ **Benefits and drivers of urbanisation**

Drivers of urbanisation	Benefits of urbanisation
Natural population increase (births, demographics and health transition)	Greater access to educational and employment opportunities
Internal migration (rural to urban)	Higher concentration of health care and complex health services
International urban migration	Greater leisure and recreational facilities
Changes in classification of urban areas	Access to more information and more advanced technologies

smoking and use of coal, kerosene and wood in cooking, especially in resource-poor nations, are the primary sources of indoor air pollution. Many countries, including the United Kingdom, have introduced indoor smoking bans in public places to minimise the adverse impact on population health.

Urban sprawl is defined as the development of individual housing in car-oriented neighbourhoods on the fringe of urban centres. This leads to increased use of private motor vehicles and a substantial increase in greenhouse gas emissions. Improved public transportation infrastructure and compact urban growth are heavily promoted to reduce both air pollution and carbon emissions.

Urbanisation is a major threat to the water cycle and water availability through damage to the local aquatic habitat and the associated accumulation of toxic pollutants. Seventy percent of industrial waste is dumped unfiltered in nearby water sources in resource-poor countries.

A major challenge in LIC and LMIC is water availability, which is compromised by the increased demand for drinking water in growing cities, especially during the dry season. UN

WATER predicts that 1.8 billion people will be living in an environment of absolute water scarcity by 2025. This will have a major effect on food production.

Vector-borne diseases

'Exponential urban growth is having a profound impact on global health. Because of international travel and migration, cities are becoming important hubs for the transmission of infectious diseases, as shown by recent pandemics. Physicians in urban environments need to be aware of the changes in infectious diseases associated with urbanisation. Furthermore, health should be a major consideration in town planning to ensure urbanisation works to reduce the burden of infectious diseases in the future.'

Alirol, Getaz, Stoll, Chappuis, Loutan (Lancet Infectious Diseases, 2011)

Urbanisation is an ongoing threat to population health from infectious disease because of the creation of high-density areas. New strains of viruses, especially influenza, proliferate in this environment and may be difficult to contain. Improved public health and food and safety regulations are needed to prevent disease transmission. An example of vector-borne disease migration secondary to urbanisation is leishmaniasis. This is transmitted via sand flies mostly confined to forests but now has become common in the cities of Latin America because of the development of urban areas in habitats which were previously the preserve of wildlife.

Impacts on the economy and health inequity

Urban areas should provide excellent economic opportunities and health care services to all, given the increased proximity to services. However, rapid unplanned urbanisation may be associated with increased levels of inequity and poverty. Mass rural to urban migration, as well as international migration, has led to the creation or the amplification of slums and precarious housing. In 1990 almost half the urban population in developing regions were living in slums. By 2005 the proportion had been reduced to 36%. However, a large majority of urban dwellers in sub-Saharan Africa (62%) were still living in slums. According to UN-Habitat, one-third of all urban dwellers in resource-poor countries were living in slums in 2012.

These settlements lack adequate water and sanitation systems, access to health services, and adequate security and permanency. This predisposes inhabitants to poorer economic and health outcomes. Slums are regarded as illegal settlements by local governments, which therefore fail to provide basic services. In these environments, infectious diseases spread rapidly, and the control of any outbreaks is challenging.

Women are at a particular disadvantage in the slums, and pregnancy rates remain high, with associated risks to maternal and child health. Urban areas allow better proximity to skilled birth attendance and access to emergency obstetric services; however, proximity does not translate into improved accessibility to maternal and child care. The mortality rate of children younger than 5 years is 40% higher in Nairobi's slums than in rural Kenya and, 15 times higher than in than in high-income areas of the city.

The United Nations proclaimed 2010 as the International Year of Youth, recognising the increased importance and benefits of youth involvement towards achieving the Millennium Development Goals (MDGs) and building resilient communities. Youth represent nearly half of the global population and more than 60% of all urban dwellers. This *youth bulge* needs to be addressed as nearly 42% of the global youth population lived on less than US$2 per day (2003 data) and today's youth face poor employment prospects. In 2016, global youth unemployment was 71 million (13.1% of all young people). This had increased by 0.2% since 2015 (ILO). High levels of unemployment, poverty and poor education amongst the youth population promote unacceptable marginalisation and civil unrest.

An insight into the drivers of urbanisation and the health challenges of slum living

Rapid urbanisation is occurring in the Philippines. Erino moved to Manila, where her family have poor health and nutrition.

A 24-year-old woman, Erino tries to support her five children and husband in the capital of the Philippines by selling candies, corn and cigarettes along the sidewalk (pavement) of Manila. She came to Manila from the countryside in 2006 to work at a linen factory. She said, 'I thought money is easy here in Manila. I really wanted to send my siblings to school. I don't want them to be like me who just finished grade 4.'

At the age of 17 years, she gave birth to her first son, and consequently lost her job. She then fell into a series of odd jobs—street sweeper, hotdog vendor, shoe repair woman. In 2010 she met a tricycle driver, who eventually became the father of her four younger children. They settled in a small house made of cardboard and plywood, located near a government hospital. 'We preferred to live here. My children are very sickly. Whenever they get cough and colds, the hospital is just a few steps away from us. Consultations and medicines are free here; unlike in the rural areas where there are no medicines or even doctors in the hospital.'

She and her husband earn an average of US$10.00 in a day, just enough to feed a family of seven one meal per day. When asked if she wanted to go back to the province, she was very clear that the answer was no. 'I think life is better here in Manila. When you're hungry, you can just ask alms from anyone who looks rich. In the province, you will be hungry all day long because everyone there has no food as well. I haven't seen or talked to my family for more than 5 years now. I just pray that they get to eat at least once every day.'

Erino's story demonstrates some of the challenges of urban living for those living in slum conditions. As a health care professional involved in her family's care, it is clear to me that many of the medical ailments her family are experiencing result directly from the conditions in which they are living. However, it also shows how strong the 'pull' factors can seem, particularly to those who may not understand the social determinants of health and may not recognise the impact that slum conditions can have on their well-being. 'Life here is not easy. But you have to endure it. After all, our future here is much better', concludes Erino.

Kim Patrick Tejano (Philippines)

'*Young people remain disengaged from the process of city planning and decision making. Decisions are routinely made without sufficient participation. We want to be heard and we want to be heard in powerful ways. We are active stakeholders who need to participate. Together we have a role in ensuring that our urban future together is a bright and prosperous one.*'

UN-Habitat Youth Advisory Board members, statement at sixth World Urban Forum 2012

Transport and urbanisation

Transport systems in cities have struggled to adapt to increased urbanisation. Roads are oversaturated with vehicles, and this has negative consequences for health and the environment. Arrangements for the provision of urban infrastructure, including public transport, are often inadequate. Investment in active transport (walking, cycling) provides significant population health benefits. However, as 27% of global road traffic deaths involve cyclists and pedestrians (WHO), more work is needed to reduce the risks to these individuals.

Noncommunicable diseases and urbanisation

Urbanisation has resulted in a concentration of risk factors which underpin the development of NCDs. These include easy access to fast food and exposure to environmental pollutants, as well as the risks which arise from deficiencies in transport infrastructure.

Urbanisation and nutrition transition in the Bedouin of southern Israel

Route 31 cuts through a vast desert landscape dotted with clusters of tin-roofed shacks on the approach to the Bedouin township of Laqiya, in the Negev, a desert in southern Israel. Camels and goats graze on one side of the highway, whilst on the other, the ubiquitous golden arches of a McDonald's fast food outlet rise up over the dunes. The McDonald's restaurant symbolises the Bedouin's lifestyle shift. Their traditional agrarian lifestyle has been gradually abandoned as the population urbanises, and their diet has been dominated by convenience and processed foods high in sugar and oil. This lifestyle shift has resulted in a change in their disease burden from infectious diseases towards noncommunicable lifestyle-related disease.

Noncommunicable diseases, which were very rare until the 1970s, are rapidly increasing in incidence. A study in 1985 found that urbanised Bedouin men were significantly more likely than traditional Bedouin men to be obese and overweight. Potential areas of intervention and prevention of noncommunicable diseases in the Bedouin community include improving access to and utilisation of primary care prevention services, improving the cultural competence of health care providers, preserving their traditional diet, increased education and empowerment of women, and community-based prevention initiatives.

Angeli Guadalupe (Philippines)

Current initiatives towards a healthy urban area

'Cities have the capability of providing something for everybody, only because, and only when, they are created by everybody.'

Jane Jacobs, The Death and Life of Great American Cities

The negative impacts of urbanisation are predominantly linked to its rapid and unplanned nature. At the Rio+20 UN Conference on Sustainable Development, sustainable cities were one of the seven priority issues discussed for inclusion in the SDGs. The concept of sustainable cities or green urbanism covers a range of ideas from transport to housing and public spaces (**Fig. 7.5.2**).

A WHO-led initiative to help local and national officials to promote the identification and reduction of health inequity within urban areas is the Urban Health Equity Assessment and Response Tool. It uses indicators such as infant mortality rate, access to safe water, completion of primary education and unemployment to assess the current situation of a city. This tool aims to enable policymakers to promote evidence-based interventions which reduce disparities in health. Other initiatives such as the Alliance of Healthy Cities, the WHO Kyoto Center for Urban Health and various UN-Habitat programmes promote the implementation of 'smart' and 'healthy' cities.

Sustainable development in Curitiba, Brazil

Curitiba, Brazil, has been an international model for sustainable development and healthy urban living as a result of strategic and integrated urban planning.

Curitiba is the capital of Parana state, a prime agricultural state in southern Brazil. In the 1960s a group led by Jamie Lerner, formally known as Institute of Urban Research and Planning, advocated a lower-cost, people-first approach. This involved environmental, social and economic programmes.

Lerner created an eco-efficient transport system to integrate Curitiba's people with their living and working environments. Major roads were built in a radial fashion, where lanes were

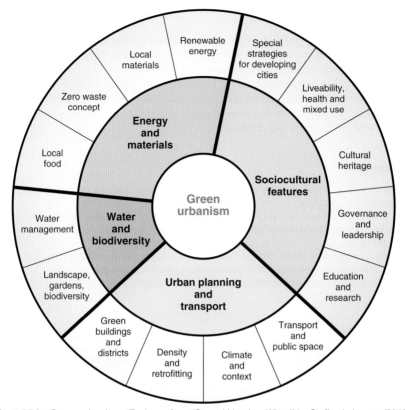

Figure 7.5.2   Green urbanism. *(Redrawn from 'Green Urbanism Wheel' by Steffen Lehmann (2010).*

designated for certain types of vehicles and the transit network provided express buses with lanes located in the centre. Express buses travel faster and have standardised ticket prices, regardless of the distance travelled. This fare pricing encouraged people to minimise the use of private cars, thereby reducing traffic and air pollution. It promoted social inclusion and equity especially for those low-income families who lived on the outskirts of the city. The integration of the transport system with land use management led to a healthy and wealthy Curitiba. The location of essential urban infrastructure maximised the use of express buses by making the public services more accessible.

Numerous other initiatives underpin Curitiba as an ecological capital. These include Green Swap, which encourages recycling, and the Green Space Initiative, which provides tax breaks to builders if green areas are included in their project. Green Swap also facilitates social inclusion; low-income families living in areas not serviced by the city's waste disposal infrastructure bring their bin bags to collection points in exchange for food and bus tickets.

The key elements that led to the environmental and economic sustainable developments in Curitiba include (1) the integrated nature of urban planning for solving practical problems, (2) the emphasis on efficient resource management, and (3) strong values of leadership and social justice. Other cities have much to learn from this innovative and impressive city.

Angeli Guadalupe (Philippines)

Conclusion

There are many complex interactions between urbanisation, transport and health. Rapid and unplanned urbanisation can lead to increases in both infectious diseases and NCDs, as well as increasing health inequity, particularly when urban slums develop.

International policy developments and summits offer hope for the development of sustainable cities which consider issues such as climate change, social justice and health throughout the urban planning process. Health professionals should advocate the inclusion and consideration of health in all aspects of urban design and development.

KEY POINTS

- Definitions of urbanisation differ and encompass demographical, geopolitical and socioeconomic aspects.
- The stresses of urbanisation on health are interrelated. These include air, water and land pollution, emerging and reemerging infectious diseases, and the promotion of obesogenic environments.
- The main stressors of urban transport systems include accidents, noise and air pollution.
- Major health challenges ensue from rapid and unplanned urbanisation.
- The creation of healthy and sustainable urban environments should be a key global priority.

Further reading

United Nations Population Fund: *State of world population 2015: shelter from the storm*, New York, 2015, United Nations.

United Nations, Department of Economic and Social Affairs, Population Division: *World urbanization prospects: the 2014 revision, highlights*, New York, 2014, United Nations.

World Health Organization: *Household air pollution and health. Fact sheet no292*, 2016. <http://www.who.int/mediacentre/factsheets/fs292/en/>.

7.6 Water, Sanitation and Hygiene

Isobel Braithwaite (UK)　　Maxwell Kaplan (Canada/USA)

Introduction

'Water is the driving force of nature.'

Leonardo da Vinci

As of 2010 approximately 768 million people, 11% of the world's population, lacked access to 'improved' water supplies. An improved water supply is defined by the WHO/UNICEF Joint Monitoring Programme for Water and Sanitation as 'one that, by nature of its construction or through active intervention, is protected from outside contamination, in particular from contamination with faecal matter.' The definition also stipulates access to at least 20 L of water per person per day, from a source within 1 km of the user's dwelling. Water quantity, which has implications for hand and personal hygiene, may be even more important than water quality.

Achieving 'improved' water and sanitation facilities

The drinking water target of the MDGs was met 5 years ahead of schedule as more than 2 billion people gained access to improved water sources between 1990 and 2010. However, 768 million people worldwide still lack access to water, of which 119 million are in China, 97 million are in India, and 66 million are in Nigeria. Most of these people live in rural areas; 19% of rural dwellers in sub-Saharan Africa and 39% of those in Oceania still rely on surface water for drinking and cooking. Progress on the sanitation MDG has been significantly slower than that targeting water; more than 2.5 billion people still lack access to an improved sanitation facility, and 1.1 billion still practise open defecation. More still are put at risk by unsafe hand-washing practices.

In 2012 an estimated 842,000 people, many of them children, died as a result of diarrhoea resulting from inadequate water, sanitation and hygiene. Much of the morbidity and many of the deaths associated with poor water and sanitation could be prevented through improved supplies, sanitation, hygiene and water resource management. The links between these mean that they are often considered as a 'composite' risk factor, affecting various water-related health outcomes in conjunction with one another (**Table 7.6.1**).

The WHO estimates that a combination of such interventions, scaled up globally, could prevent almost one-tenth of the total global burden of disease, and 5.5% of deaths amongst children younger than 5 years. Despite this, and the additional challenges posed by growing global population and a changing environment, water quality, sanitation and hygiene arguably have a lower public profile today than threats such as malaria or HIV. They have been called 'the forgotten foundations of health' (Bartram and Cairncross, 2010).

The health impacts of water-related diseases

There are several categories of water-related diseases, including faecal–oral, water-borne, water-washed, and water-based diseases (see **Table 7.6.1**). The pathways involved in their transmission can be varied and complex, as exemplified by the example of faecal–oral transmission (**Fig. 7.6.1**).

TABLE 7.6.1 ■ Categories of water-related diseases, and preventive strategies

Classification	Transmission	Examples	Preventive strategies
Water-borne (these can also be water washed)	Disease is transmitted by ingestion	Diarrhoeal diseases (e.g., cholera), enteric fevers (e.g., typhoid), hepatitis A	Improve quality of drinking water Prevent casual use of other unimproved sources Improve sanitation
Water washed (water scarce)	Transmission is reduced with an increase in water quantity and with improved hygiene (e.g., infections of the gastrointestinal tract, skin or eyes, and infections caused by lice or mites)	Diarrhoeal diseases (e.g., amoebic dysentery), trachoma, scabies	Increase water quantity Improve accessibility and reliability of domestic water supply Improve hygiene Improve sanitation
Water based	The pathogen spends part of its life cycle in an intermediate host which is water based. The pathogen is transmitted by ingestion or by skin penetration	Guinea worm, schistosomiasis, other helminth infections	Decrease need for contact with infected water Control vector host populations Improve quality of the water and sanitation (depending on the type)
Insect vector	Spread by insect vectors, particularly mosquitoes, which breed and/or bite near water	Malaria, dengue fever, onchocerciasis (river blindness), filariasis, trypanosomiasis	Improve surface-water management Destroy insects' breeding sites Decrease need to visit insects' breeding sites Mosquito netting Insecticides

Modified from Cairncross S, Feachem RG: Environmental health engineering in the tropics: an introductory text, Hoboken, 1983, John Wiley & Sons.

Additionally, chemical contamination of water supplies can lead to adverse health outcomes. For example, thousands of people in Bangladesh have developed arsenical skin lesions following the expansion of boreholes to extract groundwater. Water supplies may be contaminated by hydraulic fracturing, which uses substances known to be toxic or carcinogenic, along with many poorly studied chemicals. In the case of water-related vector-borne diseases such as malaria, non-WASH (Water Sanitation and Hygiene) -related interventions, such as bed-nets, are typically more effective than interventions relating to WASH.

The largest health impact of water- and sanitation-related diseases results from diarrhoea and associated malnutrition (**Fig. 7.6.2**). Thirty-five percent of all deaths amongst children younger than 5 years worldwide result from malnutrition. This malnutrition commonly results from chronic diarrhoea and parasitic infections, because they reduce the body's ability to absorb nutrients and energy from ingested food. Malnutrition is associated with significant reductions in children's growth, potentially compromising cognitive development. Children's height can be increased through sanitation programmes. Protein-energy malnutrition associated with diarrhoeal diseases and intestinal nematodes directly accounts for 2.9 million disability-adjusted life years (DALYs) lost per year. The disease burden from secondary consequences such as anaemia, stunting and immune deficiency, is far greater, accounting for 28 million DALYs lost.

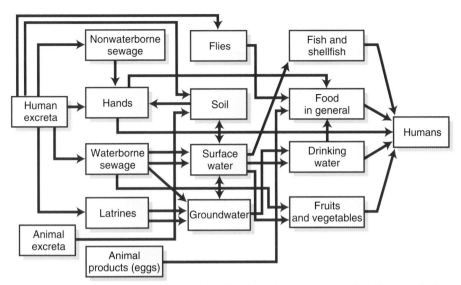

Figure 7.6.1 Faecal–oral contamination pathways leading to human exposure to pathogens. *(Redrawn from Prüss-Üstün A, Bos R, Gore F, Bartram J: Safer water, better health: costs, benefits and sustainability of interventions to protect and promote health, Geneva, 2008, World Health Organization.)*

The challenges of caring for children accessing contaminated water from the Matanza River

Industries in many parts of the world cause river pollution with heavy metals such as mercury, zinc, lead and chromium, affecting all who rely on the river as a source of water. This contamination results in a higher prevalence of disease and chronic illness.

One of the world's most polluted watersheds, the Matanza, is situated in Argentina. Despite 6 years of cleaning and sanitation, the water remains contaminated and of poor quality. Exposure to heavy metals from landfill sites and proximity to the Matanza affects the neurodevelopment of the local children, resulting in neurobehavioural disorders and learning problems. Many have been born premature and underweight. Amongst children younger than 6 years, 19.4% have anaemia and 25% present with problems in psychomotor development. Many children have been admitted to hospital with toxic lead levels. After the children have recovered, they need to avoid this water and have a special diet, but families often cannot afford that kind of food or an alternative water supply because of economic limitations. This is a clear example of the major impacts that a poor environment can have on our health.

Germán Ángel Emanuel Escobar (Argentina)

Assessing the adequacy of water services for health

According to IRCWASH (International Rescue Committee WASH), the most common indicators against which water services can be assessed include quality, quantity, distance, reliability and crowding (i.e., how many people share a point water source), although other factors such as cost, taste and population coverage are also important. Whilst contamination of drinking water by pathogens and chemicals above safe levels poses risks to human health, access to an adequate quantity of water may possibly be even more important as it allows people to perform key activities of daily life, such as hand and personal hygiene, washing clothes and cooking.

Target levels for water needs suggest that population health needs are appropriately met when individuals have access to 50 L/person per day. Lower levels (15–20 L/person per day) are used

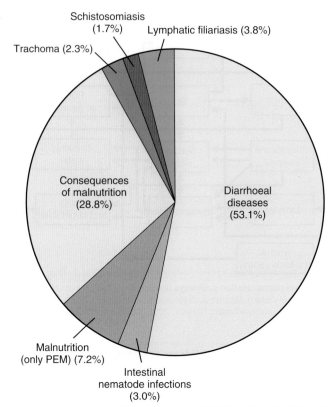

Figure 7.6.2 Percentage of water, sanitation and hygiene (WASH)-related disability-adjusted life years lost globally as a result of different diseases. *PEM,* Protein-energy malnutrition. *(Redrawn from Prüss-Üstün A, Bos R, Gore F, Bartram J: Safer water, better health: costs, benefits and sustainability of interventions to protect and promote health, Geneva, 2008, World Health Organization.)*

in some monitoring programmes (WHO/UNICEF), but these levels of access are still associated with significant health risks.

The arrangements for supply of water (**Fig. 7.6.3**) are important factors in improving water services, because the amount of water collected decreases as collection time increases, particularly after 30 minutes. The WHO estimates that 200 million work hours are spent collecting water every day worldwide. This burden has an important gender dimension; an estimated 76% of water for household use is collected by women and girls in resource-poor countries. Thus supplies nearer to people's homes can help to improve gender equity by freeing up women's and girls' time for other activities, including education and paid work.

> *'I am a community health worker living in Kamuli, Uganda. I was the first beneficiary of a tank donated by a collaboration of local and international NGOs. I was chosen because I teach others in my village about best practice of water hygiene and sanitation when they come to use my water tank. My village are delighted: prior to the building of tanks in our area, queues of 140 people would wait with buckets to access a borehole up to 4 miles from their house. I myself used to spend 5 hours daily collecting water 3 km from my home. The construction of this water tank has made my life easy; I have time to do my domestic chores.'*
>
> **Mrs Amuza, Uganda**

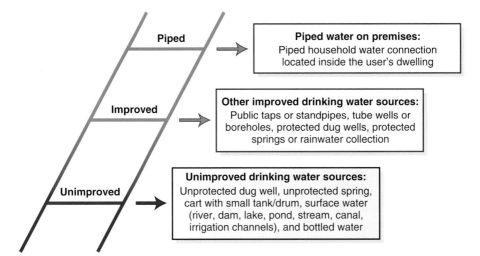

Figure 7.6.3   The water ladder. *(Redrawn from Kayser GL, Moriarty P, Fonseca C, Bartram J: Domestic water service delivery indicators and frameworks for monitoring, evaluation, policy and planning: a review, Int J Environ Res Public Health 10;4812–4835, 2013.)*

The current status of sanitation and hygiene practices

Improved sanitation requires access to a safe and functioning toilet or latrine which meets the WHO/UNICEF Joint Monitoring Programme for Water and Sanitation's minimum standards. It reduces the risk of drinking contaminated water. In 2013 approximately 2.5 billion people, mostly in rural areas, lacked access to improved sanitation, far exceeding the number lacking access to an improved water source.

Open defecation is still practised by 15% of the world's population, or 1.1 billion people, most of whom live in rural areas in LIC or middle-income countries. Inadequate sanitation can have many adverse health effects, ranging from faecal–oral transmission of pathogens or infection with eye diseases to interpersonal violence at isolated toilet sites.

The impacts of poor sanitation and open defaecation in India

Cultural taboo surrounding sanitation in India and the high prevalence of open defecation are thought to have significant impacts, including economic costs and high levels of gender violence and child mortality.

Poor sanitation and hygiene can have many impacts on long-term health and well-being, including stunting in children, lost work days and educational opportunities, and increased health care costs. According to a study by the World Bank's Water and Sanitation Programme, India's shortage of toilets costs its economy more than US$53 billion per year, or US$144 per person, most of which (72%) is accounted for by health impacts. Urban households in the poorest quintile bear the highest proportion of these costs (excluding premature death, for which data stratified by wealth are not available).

As of 2012, approximately 626 million people in India, or approximately 55% of the population, practised open defecation. Open defaecation creates risks for personal safety, particularly for women and girls as they wait until nightfall to walk to open fields, where they are vulnerable to harassment and violence. Survey data from part of Delhi indicates that 22.5% of women have suffered violent physical attacks while walking to defecate in the open, and more than 10% have suffered sexual assault.

Similar data from 2005 suggest that 67% of all Hindu households in India practise open defecation, whilst only 42% of Muslim households do so. Even though Muslims on average have a lower socioeconomic status and less access to clean water in India, survival of children younger than 5 years is 1.7% higher in Muslim families, with the most likely explanation being the differences in the rates of open defecation.

Isobel Braithwaite (UK)

The washing of hands with soap and water after defaecation and before preparation of food is an important way to mitigate health risks associated with unhygienic sanitation facilities or open defecation at communal sites. Hand hygiene is also key to the reduction of health care–associated infections, especially when surgery or invasive procedures are performed. Good personal hygiene has also been shown to help prevent 'water-washed' eye and skin diseases such as trachoma and scabies. However, hygiene promotion remains comparatively neglected, and hand washing is still not common practice in many countries.

Poor hygiene and sanitation practices can also lead to the re-emergence of diseases. For example, poor hygiene and community resistance to vaccination enabled wild poliovirus to resurface in the Democratic Republic of the Congo. UNICEF worked with religious leaders, NGOs and community groups, and designed training sessions for communities involved in social mobilisation to promote re-vaccination and better hygiene and sanitation.

'I got motivated to be a mobiliser because as a priest and a professor, people in this village really listen to me. I tell people why it is important to vaccinate their children. Then I explain to parents who are concerned about the high number of campaigns that as long as there will be polio cases, there will be vaccination campaigns.'

Jeremie Kusunga Mayinga, Democratic Republic of the Congo

Measures to improve water, sanitation and hygiene

Interventions to improve hygiene and access to safe drinking water and sanitation are often difficult to evaluate, and their documented health benefits differ substantially. However, the public health benefits of interventions in WASH are often substantial (**Table 7.6.2**).

One major systematic review has estimated that hand-washing interventions alone could save approximately 1.1 million lives each year worldwide. Interventions in water and sanitation have been less thoroughly studied, but further review identified average reductions in diarrhoea incidence of 36% following sanitation interventions and of 25% following household water treatment.

The role played by active involvement of local community leaders, and particularly of women, is important in the design and implementation of community-based interventions.

Many interventions to improve water quality and access to sanitation exist, and they are often very cost-effective. Arguably, such measures are becoming increasingly important given the challenges to the water and sanitation sectors posed by global climate change.

Health care professionals can play a key role in advancing interventions in many of these areas. Public health professionals should consider water supply and disposal as a fundamental building block in city planning, disaster management and health system-strengthening initiatives. Clinical health care professionals are ideally placed to lead health behaviour interventions such as encouraging hand washing.

TABLE 7.6.2 ■ **Reported reduction in diarrhoeal disease morbidity from improvements in one or more components of water and sanitation**

Intervention	Reduction in diarrhoeal disease (%)
Hygiene	33
Sanitation	22
Water supply	22
Water quality	17
Multiple	20

Data from Fewtrell, L, Kaufmann RB, Kay S, et al: Water, sanitation, and hygiene interventions to reduce diarrhoea in less developed countries: a systematic review and meta-analysis, Lancet Infect Dis 5(1):42–52, 2005.

Teaching hand washing in my local primary school

Does your country take part in the WHO's Global Hand Washing Day? I was shocked when I found out that Kurdistan does not, so took it upon myself to change this locally. I gathered together a group of students interested in public health and we held an educational day in Ishik Gulan primary school.

We showed 60 schoolchildren, aged 7–9 years, a PowerPoint presentation explaining hand hygiene terminology such as *germs*, *hygiene* and *soap* and then we explained why, when and how we wash our hands. After we had shown the children the 'correct' method of washing their hands, with volunteers we also taught them that sneezing into your elbow is important to prevent the spread of germs. The students were then divided into smaller groups to do various activities, including hand painting, reading books or watching videos related to hand hygiene (**Fig. 7.6.4**). We repeated these activities for 300 students, and the students then raised their hands and took five promises/oaths to continue washing their hands. This was a simple, fun intervention that students everywhere can do in their local schools.

Chra Abdulla (Kurdistan)

Climate change and water

'We must connect the dots between climate change, water scarcity, energy shortages, global health, food security and women's empowerment. Solutions to one problem must be solutions for all.'

Ban Ki-Moon, former UN Secretary General

Many of the environmental shifts that have been predicted as a result of our changing climate for the coming decades have implications for human health. Each degree of warming is projected to reduce renewable water resources by at least 20% for an additional 7% of the world's population, with particular effects on those living in regions prone to droughts and near the equator (**Fig. 7.6.5**).

The frequency of droughts is predicted to increase with climate change in regions that are currently dry, whilst the likelihood of exposure to floods is projected to increase in Asia, Africa, Central America and South America. Flooding can result in high levels of death through drowning and hypothermia, increased communicable disease transmission when water treatment is compromised and contamination of drinking water, crops and home sewage. Current projections suggest that that wet regions and seasons will become wetter, on average, whilst dry regions and seasons will become drier with climate change. Mean rainfall is likely to increase on a global scale but there will be large variations amongst regions. Additionally, changes in the pattern of rainfall, as well as changes in the intensity of storms, will result in increased transmission of communicable disease as a result of both contaminated water and inadequate supply. It is therefore essential that

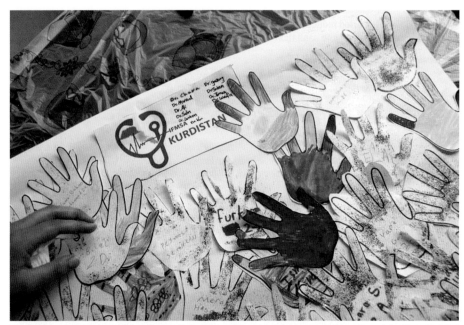

Figure 7.6.4 Students participating in Global Hand Washing Day in Kurdistan. *(Copyright Chra Abdulla.)*

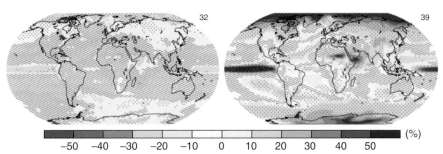

Figure 7.6.5 Change in average precipitation (1986–2005 to 2081–2100). How rainfall patterns are expected to change under alternative emission scenarios. Left: Low greenhouse gas emissions (RCP 2.6). Right: High greenhouse gas emissions (RCP8.5). *(Adapted from IPCC Fifth Assessment Report AR5, 2013.)*

policymakers, NGOs and others are aware of the need to create sanitation systems which are resilient to these climate-related shocks.

The outlook for freshwater availability

'When the well is dry, we learn the worth of water.'

Benjamin Franklin

Over the course of the current century, water scarcity will affect more areas of the world. Population growth, increasing domestic use, and increasing demand from agriculture, manufacturing and thermal energy generation further compromise access to water. By 2050 global water demand is predicted to increase by 50%. Worldwide, surface water withdrawals increased by approximately 1% per year from 1987 to 2000. At present, 20% of the world's aquifers are overexploited (i.e., removal rates are unsustainable), and the proportion is set to increase. To date, China has lost 27,000 rivers because of overexploitation, leading to an estimated 2.3% annual reduction in GDP, primarily due to adverse health effects. To combat reduced freshwater availability, many coastal countries have turned to desalination technologies, especially in the Middle East, and, more recently, in China. In some countries access to clean water is improved through the provision of water tanks and bore holes.

Building and protecting water springs to enable access to safe water in my local community

Isaac is a 27-year-old who set up a programme to build and protect springs in south-western Uganda. He is working with a multidisciplinary team of builders, community health workers and motivated members of the community to create a water, sanitation and hygiene movement: Africa Grow Forward.

I run a project which aims to ensure that the indigenous African communities in my local area have access to clean water. We are fortunate to have numerous natural underground water sources nearby; however, many local communities travel more than 3 km to the local river for water. The springs that are currently available are not protected, and therefore may be contaminated (**Fig. 7.6.6A**). Each new spring supports at least 30 members of the local community, and they are expected to last at least 50 years. Alongside building springs, we are educating local communities about health and sanitation practices (**Fig. 7.6.6B**). A key part of the project has entailed protection of existing water sources. I gathered together experts in my local area to put together a budget, and applied for (and gained) a seed grant for the programme.

The challenges met in running this project include:
- Territorial arguments over water sources by local families and land owners.
- Underestimating the cost of construction. The price of building materials fluctuates significantly. We expected each spring to cost at most £415; however, the cost has been nearer £500.
- Challenges for poor communities to contribute financially towards the successful running of the project; however, this is a key component of ensuring ownership of the project.
- My inexperience. This was the first project of this kind that I have run, and it has been a steep learning curve.

Through this project, I have learnt many things, including:
- Even when a community desperately needs some resources or services, often wealthier members are not aware of this need and distance themselves from the poorer individuals in their local area. Several local wealthy land owners have refused the community access to their land to build a spring.
- It is challenging to determine an accurate budget in a fluctuating economy, something many overseas donors fail to appreciate.
- It can be challenging to work in the community in which you were born when delivering a message from an external organisation. However, international organisations that support local leaders are more likely to deliver successful programmes.

Isaac Rukundo (Uganda)

Many countries rely on freshwater sources that cross international borders. These may be compromised in the event of conflict, and tensions may arise. For example, China has constructed large-scale dams and engaged in water diversion projects to move water from the Mekong River to the dry north of the country. This compromises irrigation arrangements in five surrounding countries.

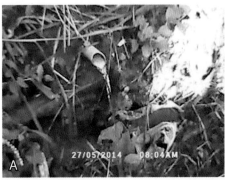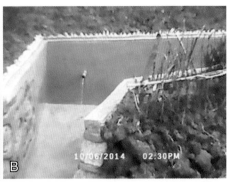

Figure 7.6.6 **Building and protecting water springs.** (A) Initial condition of the spring. (B) Condition of the water spring when nearing completion. *(Copyright Isaac Rukundo.)*

Conclusion

WASH are key to improving global health. Inadequate access or poor hygiene practices can cause major health morbidity and death especially in children. Despite substantial advances in the provision of clean drinking water, access to improved sanitation and adequate quantities of water remains limited in large parts of the world.

Interventions to improve WASH are known to be highly effective, with parallel benefits for education, poverty reduction and gender equality. Improvements in WASH have the huge potential to improve the lives of people around the world, and global health professionals should work to ensure that WASH receives an appropriate degree of attention.

KEY POINTS

- Despite significant progress towards the Millennium Development Goals, water, sanitation and hygiene (WASH), remain a major cause of early death and illness worldwide, particularly amongst children. Together they account for nearly one-tenth of the total global burden of disease.
- Many diseases are associated with poor water quality and lack of sanitation.
- Most diseases related to WASH are largely preventable.
- Improved access to water results in multiple social and health benefits.

Further reading

Bartram J, Cairncross S: Hygiene, sanitation, and water: forgotten foundations of health, *PLoS Med* 7(11):e10000367, 2010.

London School of Hygiene & Tropical Medicine: *Toilets for health*, 2012. <https://www.ircwash.org/resources/toilets-health-report-london-school-hygiene-and-tropical-medicine-collaboration-domestos>.

Prüss-Üstün A, Bos R, Gore F, Bartram J: *Safer water, better health: costs, benefits and sustainability of interventions to protect and promote health*, Geneva, 2008, World Health Organization.

WHO/UNICEF Joint Monitoring Programme for Water Supply and Sanitation (JMP). <http://www.unwater.org/publication_categories/whounicef-joint-monitoring-programme-for-water-supply-sanitation-hygiene-jmp/>.

Page numbers followed by '*f*' indicate figures, '*t*' indicate tables, and '*b*' indicate boxes.